Special Statutory Funding Program for Type 1 Diabetes Research

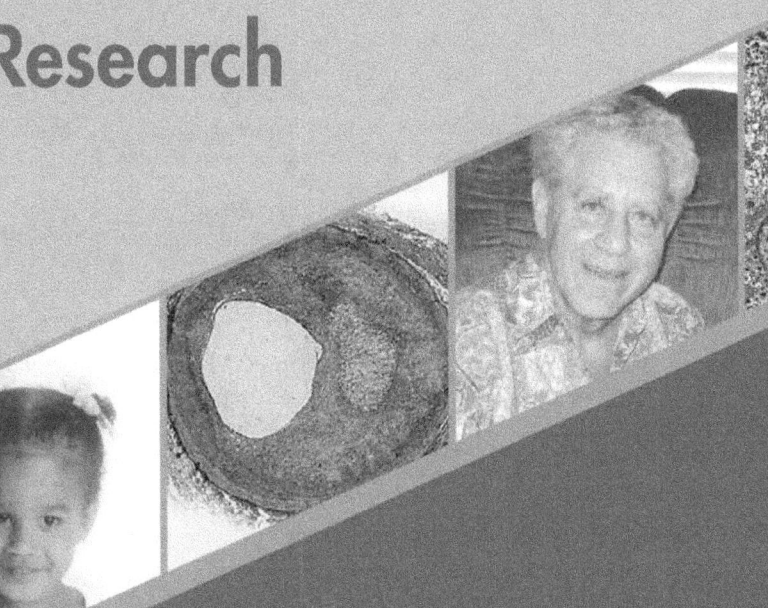

LEGISLATIVE HISTORY OF THE *SPECIAL STATUTORY FUNDING PROGRAM FOR TYPE 1 DIABETES RESEARCH*

A *Special Statutory Funding Program for Type 1 Diabetes Research* is mandated by Section 330B of the Public Health Service Act. The original enabling legislation was the Balanced Budget Act of 1997 (Public Law 105-33), which was later amended by the Fiscal Year 2001 Consolidated Appropriations Act (Public Law 106-554); the Public Health Service Act amendment relating to diabetes research (Public Law 107-360); the Medicare, Medicaid, and SCHIP Extension Act of 2007 (Public Law 110-173); the Medicare Improvement for Patients and Providers Act of 2008 (Public Law 110-275); and the Medicare and Medicaid Extenders Act of 2010 (Public Law 111-309). Section 330B states:

Sec. 330B.[254c-2] Special Diabetes Programs for Type 1 Diabetes

"(a) In General.—The Secretary, directly or through grants, shall provide for research into the prevention and cure of Type 1 diabetes."

"(b) Funding.—

(1) Transferred Funds.—Notwithstanding section 2104(a) of the Social Security Act, from the amounts appropriated in such section for each of the fiscal years 1998 through 2002, $30,000,000 is hereby transferred and made available in such fiscal years for grants under this section."

"(2) Appropriations.—For the purpose of making grants under this section, there is appropriated, out of any funds in the Treasury not otherwise appropriated –
(A) $70,000,000 for each of fiscal years 2001 and 2002 (which shall be combined with amounts transferred under paragraph (1) for each such fiscal years);
(B) $100,000,000 for fiscal year 2003; and
(C) $150,000,000 for fiscal years 2004 through 2013."

This *Program* also has Congressionally-mandated reporting requirements. Section 4923 of the Balanced Budget Act of 1997, as amended by Section 931 of the Fiscal Year 2001 Consolidated Appropriations Act, Section 1(c) of the Public Health Service Act Amendment for Diabetes, and Section 303 of the Medicare Improvement for Patients and Providers Act of 2008, states that "The Secretary of Health and Human Services shall conduct an evaluation of the diabetes grant programs established under the amendments made by this chapter."

Subsequently, the Secretary was required to submit to the appropriate committees of Congress –
(1) an interim evaluation report not later than January 1, 2000, to the Senate Health, Education, Labor and Pensions Committee and the House Committee on Commerce, Subcommittee on Health and Environment;

(2) a second interim evaluation report not later than January 1, 2007, to the Senate Health, Education, Labor and Pensions Committee; the House Energy and Commerce Committee; and the House Energy and Commerce Committee, Subcommittee on Health; and

(3) a third evaluation report not later than January 1, 2011, to the Senate Health, Education, Labor and Pensions Committee; the Senate Finance Committee; the House Energy and Commerce Committee; the House Energy and Commerce Committee, Subcommittee on Health; and the House Ways and Means Committee.

In parallel with the *Special Statutory Funding Program for Type 1 Diabetes Research*, Congress established the *Special Diabetes Program for Indians*, which is administered by the Indian Health Service.

Cover images—People participating in clinical research to combat type 1 diabetes and its complications (l-r): Nilia Olsen, Robert Watts, and Gina Ferrari. Scientific images (l-r): Artery occluded by lipid buildup (credit: NHLBI/NIH); human islet (credit: Steve Gschmeissner/Photo Researchers, Inc).

Special Statutory Funding Program for Type 1 Diabetes Research

CONTENTS

OVERVIEW OF THE

SPECIAL STATUTORY FUNDING PROGRAM FOR TYPE 1 DIABETES RESEARCH

This report is prepared in response to Section 330B of the Public Health Service Act, as amended by the Medicare Improvement for Patients and Providers Act of 2008 (Public Law [P.L.] 110-275), which calls for the preparation of an evaluation report to the Congress on the *Special Statutory Funding Program for Type 1 Diabetes Research (Special Diabetes Program* or *Program)* established under that Section.*

The last decade has seen extraordinary progress in our understanding and treatment of type 1 diabetes—*Nature*, April 2010.[1]

Type 1 diabetes—previously known as juvenile diabetes—is a devastating illness that often strikes in infancy, childhood, or young adulthood. The immune system mounts a misguided attack destroying the insulin-producing beta cells found in clusters called "islets" within the pancreas. Without the hormone insulin, the tissues of the body cannot absorb or use glucose (sugar), the major cellular fuel. If left untreated, this disease results in death from starvation despite high levels of glucose in the bloodstream. The discovery and purification of insulin by a team of medical researchers at the University of Toronto in 1921 quickly led to the realization that insulin was the key to restoring the body's ability to process glucose. This insight, which earned the investigators a Nobel Prize, provided a lifesaving treatment for type 1 diabetes in the form of daily insulin injections, and transformed type 1 diabetes from an acutely and uniformly fatal disease to a chronic one.

The treatment regimen for type 1 diabetes requires constant attention and is difficult to maintain even in the best of circumstances. On a daily basis, individuals with type 1 diabetes must check their blood glucose levels multiple times with invasive finger sticks, monitor their food intake and physical activity levels, and administer insulin through injections or a pump. Even the most vigilant patients are at risk for sudden, acute episodes of dangerously low or high blood glucose levels (hypoglycemia or hyperglycemia, respectively), either of which can be life-threatening in extreme cases. The constant burden of this disease greatly affects the quality of life of patients and their family members.

Persistent elevation of blood glucose levels, despite insulin therapy, slowly damages nearly all of the body's organs. Diabetes substantially increases the risk of blindness, kidney failure, chronic wounds and skin ulcers, nerve pain and other neurological problems, limb amputation, heart disease and clogged arteries, stroke, high blood pressure, periodontal disease, erectile dysfunction, bladder control problems, depression, and pregnancy-related complications. Because of these serious, long-term complications, type 1 diabetes is estimated to shorten the average life span by 15 years.[2]

Type 1 diabetes affects approximately 5 percent of the 18.8 million people in the United States diagnosed with diabetes.[3] In type 2 diabetes—which is the major form of diabetes and is closely associated with obesity—the body gradually loses or "resists" its ability to respond

---

* This report to Congress, submitted in December 2010, was supplemented with patient profiles and other ancillary material prior to printing. In order to prepare this evaluation to meet the statutory deadline, data collection on research progress was terminated in spring 2010.

[1] Reprinted by permission from Macmillan Publishers Ltd: Nature 464: 1293-1300, copyright 2010.

[2] Portuese E and Orchard T: Mortality in Insulin-Dependent Diabetes. In *Diabetes in America* (pp. 221-232). Bethesda, MD: National Diabetes Data Group, NIH, 1995.

[3] Centers for Disease Control and Prevention. National diabetes fact sheet: national estimates and general information on diabetes and prediabetes in the United States, 2011. Atlanta, GA: U.S. Department of Health and Human Services, Centers for Disease Control and Prevention, 2011. Accessed from www.cdc.gov/diabetes/pubs/factsheet11.htm

effectively to insulin, and the pancreatic beta cells cannot secrete a sufficient amount of additional insulin to overcome this insulin resistance. It is important to note that because both forms of diabetes involve malfunctions in the body's system for maintaining appropriate blood glucose levels, and because both also share many of the same complications, research directed toward type 1 diabetes also benefits people with type 2 diabetes.

Type 1 diabetes can be more serious and costly for patients because it tends to strike earlier in life. For example, while type 2 diabetes increases the risk of heart disease 2- to 4-fold,[4] heart disease risk is increased by up to 10-fold in people with type 1 diabetes compared to the general age-matched population.[5,6] Importantly, the longer a person has type 1 diabetes, the greater the risk of developing complications, and the more severe, difficult-to-treat, and costly they can become. Especially worrisome are data showing that type 1 diabetes is being diagnosed at younger ages, suggesting that something in the environment is triggering early onset of disease in children. Early onset of type 1 diabetes can set the stage for a lifetime of living with and medically managing the disease complications.

OVERVIEW OF THE SPECIAL STATUTORY FUNDING PROGRAM FOR TYPE 1 DIABETES RESEARCH

Special funding for type 1 diabetes research, in the total amount of $1.89 billion for Fiscal Year (FY) 1998 through FY 2013, was provided to the Secretary of the U.S. Department of Health and Human Services (HHS) through Section 330B of the Public Health Service Act. The

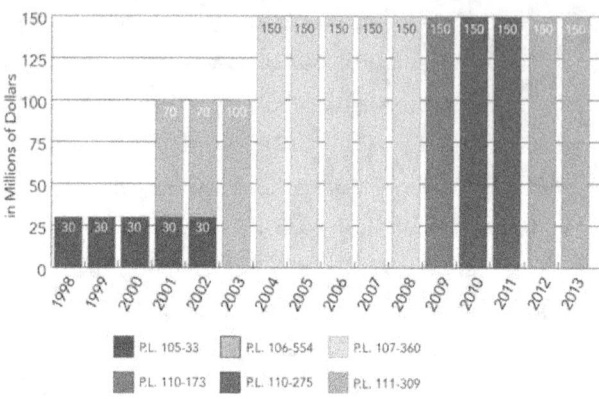

Figure 1: *Special Diabetes Program* Funding
Special Diabetes Program funding levels per year, Fiscal Year (FY) 1998-2011. The *Special Diabetes Program* was established by the Balanced Budget Act of 1997 (Public Law [P.L.] 105-33), and later extended by the FY 2001 Consolidated Appropriations Act (P.L. 106-554); the Public Health Service Act amendment relating to diabetes research (P.L. 107-360); the Medicare, Medicaid, and SCHIP Extension Act of 2007 (P.L. 110-173); the Medicare Improvement for Patients and Providers Act of 2008 (P.L. 110-275); and the Medicare and Medicaid Extenders Act of 2010 (P.L. 111-309).

Special Diabetes Program's original enabling legislation was the Balanced Budget Act of 1997 (P.L. 105-33), which was later amended by the FY 2001 Consolidated Appropriations Act (P.L. 106-554), the Public Health Service Act amendment relating to diabetes research (P.L. 107-360), the Medicare, Medicaid, and SCHIP Extension Act of 2007 (P.L. 110-173), the Medicare Improvement for Patients and Providers Act of 2008 (P.L. 110-275), and the Medicare and Medicaid Extenders Act of 2010 (P.L. 111-309) to extend the *Special Diabetes Program* in duration and funding levels (Figure 1).

This funding associated with the *Special Diabetes Program* augments regularly appropriated funds that the HHS receives for diabetes research through the House and Senate appropriations committees. The National

---

4   Laakso M: Cardiovascular disease in type 2 diabetes: challenge for treatment and prevention. J Intern Med 249: 225-235, 2001.
5   Krolewski AS, Kosinski EJ, Warram JH, et al: Magnitude and determinants of coronary artery disease in juvenile-onset, insulin-dependent diabetes mellitus. Am J Cardiol 59: 750-755, 1987.
6   Dorman JS, Laporte RE, Kuller LH, et al: The Pittsburgh insulin-dependent diabetes mellitus (IDDM) morbidity and mortality study: mortality results. Diabetes 33: 271-276, 1984.

Institute of Diabetes and Digestive and Kidney Diseases (NIDDK), through authority granted by the Secretary of HHS, has a leadership role in planning, implementing, and evaluating the allocation of these funds in a program that involves multiple Institutes and Centers of the National Institutes of Health (NIH), as well as the Centers for Disease Control and Prevention (CDC).

PURSUIT OF SIX MAJOR SCIENTIFIC GOALS

The *Special Statutory Funding Program for Type 1 Diabetes Research* and this evaluation report have been framed around six broad scientific Goals. The pursuit of research toward attaining each of these Goals is propelling progress toward the understanding, prevention, treatment, and cure of type 1 diabetes and its complications. While significant progress has been made toward each of these Goals, research challenges still remain in each of these areas.

SIX OVERARCHING GOALS OF TYPE 1 DIABETES RESEARCH

Goal I: Identify the Genetic and Environmental Causes of Type 1 Diabetes
Goal II: Prevent or Reverse Type 1 Diabetes
Goal III: Develop Cell Replacement Therapy
Goal IV: Prevent or Reduce Hypoglycemia in Type 1 Diabetes
Goal V: Prevent or Reduce the Complications of Type 1 Diabetes
Goal VI: Attract New Talent and Apply New Technologies to Research on Type 1 Diabetes

---

Goal I: Identify the Genetic and Environmental Causes of Type 1 Diabetes

To achieve the ultimate goal of preventing and curing type 1 diabetes, it is imperative to understand the causes of the disease. A complex interplay of genetic and environmental factors underlies the development of type 1 diabetes. Not all genes that play a role are known, although many have been uncovered in recent years. For genes that are known, research is needed to elucidate the biological roles that those genes play in health and disease. Scientists think that in some people, genetic susceptibility—which can cause a person to be predisposed to the disease—is "triggered" by an environmental agent leading the body's immune system to turn against itself. Potential environmental triggers may be infectious agents, dietary factors, environmental toxins, and psychological stress. To date, no single trigger has been conclusively identified. Identification and study of key genes, as well as environmental triggers, will not only help to more accurately predict who will develop the disease, but will also aid in the development of new prevention strategies and may suggest new avenues for treatment.

Goal II: Prevent or Reverse Type 1 Diabetes

Defining the molecular defects that provoke the immune system to attack and destroy the beta cells is key to predicting, diagnosing, treating, and ultimately preventing this autoimmune process. In addition, research to identify ways to halt or reverse beta cell destruction after disease onset could result in preservation or restoration of patients' insulin-producing capacity. Research has suggested that preserving patients' remaining beta cell function can have dramatic, long-term health benefits, and clinical trials are now testing the ability of agents to preserve beta cell function in people with newly diagnosed type 1 diabetes. Agents that are successful in preserving beta cell function in those newly diagnosed with type 1 diabetes can then be studied to determine whether they can prevent type 1 diabetes in those at high risk for the disease.

Goal III: Develop Cell Replacement Therapy

A real cure for type 1 diabetes could be achieved by replacing the insulin-producing beta cells that have been destroyed by the immune system, and scientists are aggressively pursuing this avenue of research. One possible approach to replace the insulin-producing beta cells is through a procedure known as islet transplantation. To date, only adult patients with severely unmanageable blood glucose levels, or who have had a kidney transplant and are already on immunosuppressive medications, have been eligible for islet transplantation due to the toxicity associated with the required immunosuppressive drugs. Research is ongoing to improve this experimental procedure so that it may be a viable option for more patients. Scientists are also pursuing other strategies to replace beta cells, such as inducing any remaining beta cells in the pancreas to generate additional beta cells, or directing other pancreatic cell types toward becoming beta cells. For these approaches to be clinically useful, it is imperative to protect the newly formed beta cells from the same immune system attack that initially destroyed the patients' own beta cells.

Goal IV: Prevent or Reduce Hypoglycemia in Type 1 Diabetes

Hypoglycemia (low blood sugar) is a distressing, acute complication of type 1 diabetes. It impairs brain and other bodily functions, including defenses against future hypoglycemia episodes, causing a vicious cycle of recurrent events. The immediate effects of hypoglycemia can include changes in cardiovascular and nervous system function, cognitive impairment, increased risk for unintentional injury, coma, and sometimes death. Furthermore, the potential for acute episodes of hypoglycemia is a severe limitation to the practice of intensive glucose control, which has been proven to prevent or delay onset of other diabetes complications. Newly developed continuous glucose monitoring devices can reduce the time that patients spend with low blood glucose values and sound alarms to prompt them to take steps to prevent life-threatening episodes of severe hypoglycemia. Linking glucose monitoring to insulin delivery—in essence, an artificial pancreas—could have a positive impact on patients' health and quality of life, and alleviate an enormous amount of patient burden.

Goal V: Prevent or Reduce the Complications of Type 1 Diabetes

Persistent elevation of blood glucose levels, despite insulin therapy, slowly damages the body's organs and can lead to life-threatening diabetes complications. Type 1 diabetes ravages nearly every part of the body: the heart, eyes, kidneys, nerves, lower limbs, mouth, and digestive and urologic systems. Insights into the underlying molecular mechanisms of these complications and new tools such as animal models and biomarkers to facilitate testing of therapeutic strategies are imperative for the development of new treatments. Until the prevention or cure of type 1 diabetes is possible, research toward preventing and treating the complications of the disease is critically important.

Goal VI: Attract New Talent and Apply New Technologies to Research on Type 1 Diabetes

Research on type 1 diabetes spans a broad range of scientific disciplines, including endocrinology and metabolism; immunology; genetics; epidemiology; clinical trials; neuroscience; behavioral science; bioengineering; cell, developmental, and vascular biology; and the physiology of the heart, eyes, kidneys, urologic tract, and nervous system. Continued research progress depends on attracting and training a workforce of scientists with diverse expertise. Furthermore, the scientific community has experienced an explosion of emerging technologies that allow scientists to conduct research more efficiently and to ask questions that were previously impossible to answer. New technologies have already led to major discoveries and continue to hold great promise for advancing the type 1 diabetes research field.

SUPPORT OF RESEARCH TOWARD ACHIEVING THE SIX SCIENTIFIC GOALS

In the first years (FY 1998-2000), the *Special Diabetes Program* primarily supported initiatives to solicit research from individual independent investigators on topics of urgent and unmet research challenge. When the *Special Diabetes Program* was augmented in FY 2001, the additional funds enabled the creation of unique, innovative, and collaborative research consortia and clinical trials networks. The majority of the funds since 2001 have supported these collaborative research efforts, with a goal of promoting progress in type 1 diabetes research that could not be achieved by a single laboratory. The *Special Diabetes Program* enabled the initiation of these large, high-impact research efforts at

an unprecedented scale. These efforts span a continuum from basic research to identify promising therapeutic targets and agents, to pre-clinical studies testing agents in animal models, to clinical trials in people with or at risk for type 1 diabetes. These consortia, as well as the research resources that they are generating, expand the scope and power of research efforts by making technological developments and tools available to the broad diabetes scientific community and beyond.

In addition to these major collaborative efforts, a large portion of the positive impact of the *Special Diabetes Program*-supported research comes from creative endeavors undertaken by excellent investigators working in small laboratories across the country, selected through a peer review, highly competitive process. The *Special Diabetes Program* has provided them with new key resources and solicited investigator-initiated research on topics of urgent and unmet need, such as development of artificial pancreas technology and beta cell imaging, and other issues of importance to the prevention and cure of type 1 diabetes and its complications, through announcements known as "Requests for Applications (RFAs)."

The *Special Diabetes Program* has also served to catalyze burgeoning fields of research by bringing together scientists from across disciplines to address specific research challenges. Furthermore, the *Special Diabetes Program* has invested in training programs to ensure a future generation of clinical diabetes researchers. Overall, the funds have been deployed in a scientifically focused, but flexible, budgeting process that allows a rapid response to emerging research topics of critical importance.

HIGHLIGHTS OF SCIENTIFIC ACCOMPLISHMENTS

While important findings have already come from research supported by the Special Diabetes Program, it is anticipated that even greater benefits to the health and quality of life of people with type 1 diabetes will accrue in the coming years as the findings from recent, long-term investments come to fruition. Thus, the advances already achieved likely represent the vanguard of the scientific discoveries enabled by the Special Statutory Funding Program for Type 1 Diabetes Research.

Greatly Improved Prognosis for Americans with Type 1 Diabetes: Because of research progress over the last 2 decades, including research supported by the *Special Diabetes Program*, people with the disease are living longer and healthier lives than ever before and experiencing lower rates of disease complications. A recent study of the clinical course of type 1 diabetes concluded that starting intensive control of blood glucose as soon as possible after diagnosis greatly improves the long-term prognosis for patients. The study also found that the outlook for people with longstanding type 1 diabetes has greatly improved over the past 20 years due to a better understanding of the importance of intensive glucose control, as well as advances in insulin formulations and delivery, glucose monitoring, and the treatment of cardiovascular disease risk factors. These findings come from analyses of the long-term health outcomes for people who participated in NIDDK's landmark Diabetes Control and Complications Trial (DCCT) and its ongoing, *Special Diabetes Program*-supported, follow-up study, the Epidemiology of Diabetes Interventions and Complications, which began in 1993. This study reinforced and extended the DCCT's initial findings that intensive blood glucose control dramatically reduces the risk of eye, kidney, and nerve damage due to diabetes. In particular, researchers found that, among DCCT participants who had received intensive glucose control during the trial, rates of vision loss and kidney failure had fallen to much lower levels than seen historically. Achieving and maintaining intensive glucose control is not easy for people with type 1 diabetes; the 21st century picture of clinical outcomes provided by this study can aid health care providers in discussing the tremendous health benefits of intensive control with their patients and reinforces the need for research to develop less burdensome approaches to help patients achieve these goals.

Newly Discovered Type 1 Diabetes Genes: Using new and emerging genetics technologies, scientists in the NIDDK-led and *Special Diabetes Program*-supported Type 1 Diabetes Genetics Consortium and their collaborators identified over 40 different genes or genetic regions that influence a person's risk of developing type 1 diabetes, bringing the total number of known regions to near 50—up from only three known genes a few years ago. Now, the challenge is to understand how those genes may influence disease development. Further research is ongoing to pinpoint the exact genes and understand their function in type 1 diabetes. Understanding the genetic underpinnings of type 1 diabetes can aid the ability to predict risk, as well as inform the development of new prevention and treatment strategies.

Adult Pancreas Cells Reprogrammed to Insulin-producing Beta Cells: Scientists in the NIDDK-led and *Special Diabetes Program*-supported Beta Cell Biology Consortium (BCBC) have made tremendous progress in understanding beta cell biology toward the goal of developing cell-based therapies for diabetes. For example, in order to promote the formation of new beta cells, BCBC scientists are determining when and how certain pancreatic progenitor cells become "committed" to developing into specific pancreatic cell types and discovering flexibility in these cells. In one study, scientists made an exciting discovery that a type of adult cell in the mouse pancreas, called exocrine cells, can be reprogrammed to become insulin-producing beta cells. Using a genetically engineered virus and a combination of just three transcription factors, the researchers were able to reprogram some of the exocrine cells into beta cells. The newly formed beta cells produced enough insulin to decrease high blood glucose levels in diabetic mice. If the same type of approach can be developed to work safely and effectively in humans, this discovery could have a dramatic impact on the ability to increase beta cell mass in people with diabetes.

In another study, scientists uncovered plasticity in another pancreatic cell type—the alpha cell. Using genetic techniques in mice, the researchers increased the levels of a protein called Pax4, which is known to be involved in promoting cells to develop into the pancreatic beta cell type. They found that mice with high levels of Pax4 had oversized clusters of beta cells, which resulted from alpha-beta precursor cells and established alpha cells being induced to form beta cells. In addition, in a mouse model of diabetes, high levels of Pax4 promoted generation of new beta cells and overcame the diabetic state. In another study, BCBC scientists observed spontaneous conversion in beta cell-depleted mice of alpha cells to insulin-producing cells. These discoveries—that adult pancreatic cells have the potential to convert to beta cells—generate a fuller picture of pancreatic development and may pave the way toward new cell-based therapies for diabetes.

Hemoglobin A1c (HbA1c) Standardization Improves Care for People with Diabetes: HbA1c is a component of blood that is a good surrogate measure of long-term blood glucose control and, as such, reflects risk of diabetic complications. Clinical guidelines for controlling blood glucose to reduce diabetes complications set targets for control of blood glucose as assessed by this key test based on results from two landmark clinical trials: the DCCT for type 1 diabetes and the United Kingdom Prospective Diabetes Study for type 2 diabetes. To enable translation of these targets for control of blood glucose into common medical practice, the CDC and NIDDK, with support from the *Special Diabetes Program*, launched the HbA1c Standardization Program in 1998. This program improved the standardization and reliability in measures of HbA1c so that clinical laboratory results can be used by health care providers and patients to accurately and meaningfully assess blood glucose control and risks for complications. The standardization effort has been a great success and has facilitated national campaigns to improve control of blood glucose. As a result, the percentage of Americans with diabetes who had excellent glucose control increased from 37 percent in 1999-2000 to 56 percent in 2003-2004.[7] The American Diabetes Association (ADA) built on the tremendous success of the HbA1c Standardization Program to set

---

[7] Hoerger TJ, Segel JE, Gregg EW, et al: Is glycemic control improving in U.S. adults? Diabetes Care 31: 81-86, 2008.

treatment goals for glucose control in all forms of diabetes based on the test and has recommended HbA1c as a more convenient approach to diagnose type 2 diabetes.

New Glucose Monitoring Tools for Controlling Blood Glucose Levels: Research supported by the *Special Diabetes Program* contributed to the development of U.S. Food and Drug Administration (FDA)-approved continuous glucose monitors, which reveal the dynamic changes in blood glucose levels. Alarms warn the patient if blood glucose becomes too high or too low, thereby reducing the need for invasive finger sticks to monitor blood glucose levels. This revolutionary technology can make it easier for patients to keep blood glucose at healthy levels and can enhance their ability to achieve the intensive control necessary to prevent or delay disease complications. In addition, this technology, when linked to insulin delivery (known as an "artificial pancreas"), has the potential to have a further positive impact on patients' health and quality of life, and alleviate an enormous amount of patient burden.

Novel Drugs for Treating Complications: The *Special Diabetes Program* has supported the development and clinical testing of new therapeutic agents for diabetic eye disease. For example, a recent comparative effectiveness research study, conducted by the National Eye Institute (NEI)-led Diabetic Retinopathy Clinical Research Network, found that a therapeutic called ranibizumab, in combination with laser therapy, was substantially better than laser therapy alone or laser therapy with a different drug, at treating diabetic macular edema, a swelling in the eye that often accompanies and aggravates diabetic retinopathy. Ranibizumab with laser therapy substantially improved vision among study patients, and could become the new standard of care for diabetic macular edema.

Advances in Islet Transplantation as a Therapeutic Approach for People with Type 1 Diabetes: The *Special Diabetes Program* supported the first islet transplantation trial in the United States using a procedure referred to as the "Edmonton protocol" that dramatically improved islet survival and rendered many patients insulin-free. Through the Immune Tolerance Network (ITN), which is led by the National Institute of Allergy and Infectious Diseases (NIAID), the *Special Diabetes Program* also supported the first international, multicenter trial of islet transplantation using the protocol. Additionally, research supported by the *Program* laid the foundation for an unprecedented islet transplant to an American airman, sparing him from a life-long insulin requirement after pancreatic damage from wounds suffered while serving in Afghanistan. Improved approaches to islet transplantation are important not only as an alternative to whole pancreas transplantation for treatment of type 1 diabetes but also to avoid diabetes through auto-transplantation after removal of the pancreas due to pancreatitis or injury. The *Special Diabetes Program* is supporting multifaceted research efforts to overcome barriers to making islet transplantation a viable therapy, such as the shortage of available islets and the toxicity associated with the life-long immunosuppressive medication.

Promise of Therapies that Target Specific Lymphocytes in Preventing and Reversing Type 1 Diabetes:
Previous clinical trials have suggested that preserving patients' remaining beta cell function can have dramatic, long-term health benefits. Researchers in NIDDK's Type 1 Diabetes TrialNet, which is supported by the *Special Diabetes Program*, reported that an immunosuppressive drug (rituximab), which destroys immune system cells called B lymphocytes, preserved the function of insulin-producing beta cells in people newly diagnosed with type 1 diabetes. Improved insulin production was maintained 1 year after the drug was administered, but the effect dissipated at 2 years. As drugs such as rituximab broadly deplete B lymphocytes, they can increase the risk of infection and therefore can have significant side effects. Nonetheless, the finding is very important because it will propel research to find drugs targeting the specific B lymphocytes involved in type 1 diabetes without the associated side effects of drugs like rituximab.

In another study, researchers in NIAID's ITN, also supported by the *Special Diabetes Program*, are building on an earlier study showing benefits of teplizumab, a humanized anti-CD3 monoclonal antibody that targets white blood cells known as "T cells" that are involved in the autoimmune attack on the beta cells. A pilot study of teplizumab showed that a single course of the antibody could delay progression of the disease over a 2-year period. The new trial is a larger follow-up study, in which two courses of the antibody are administered, 1 year apart, in an effort to extend its effects on beta cell preservation.

Testing Novel Type 1 Diabetes Prevention Strategies: Research supported by the *Special Diabetes Program* has enabled testing of new type 1 diabetes prevention strategies and demonstrated that it is possible to predict with great accuracy a person's risk of developing type 1 diabetes. Moreover, while an oral insulin type 1 diabetes prevention trial (now part of TrialNet) did not demonstrate protection in the entire study population, it suggested a possible effect in the subgroup with highest insulin antibody titers. This knowledge has set the stage for screening and enrolling patients into new type 1 diabetes prevention trials, including a new trial through TrialNet that is testing oral insulin in a subgroup of people with high levels of insulin autoantibodies.

Building on findings from successful trials in newly diagnosed patients, TrialNet has developed a new paradigm: therapeutics demonstrated to be effective in new-onset patients are then tested for their prevention potential. One such prevention trial was recently launched with teplizumab, a monoclonal antibody engineered to alter the balance between destructive and protective T cells. Based on promising results in preserving beta cell function in patients newly diagnosed with type 1 diabetes, teplizumab is now being studied in relatives of people with type 1 diabetes, who are at 80 percent risk of developing type 1 diabetes over the next 5 years. This effort builds not only on the earlier success with teplizumab but also on the proven accuracy of tests to predict type 1 diabetes risk.

How Research Supported by the *Special Diabetes Program* Contributes to the Pipeline for New Therapies: The *Special Diabetes Program* supports type 1 diabetes research along a pipeline that facilitates the identification and development of new therapies. Examples of studies that are feeding into this pipeline are described in the bottom panel.

Identifying Molecular Pathways of Disease Progression	Identifying Therapeutic Agents To Target Molecular Pathways	Pre-clinical Drug Development and Testing	Testing Promising Therapies in People with Type 1 Diabetes
Research to identify genes, environmental triggers, and underlying mechanisms of disease development help scientists find targets for therapy.	Knowledge about molecular pathways permits identification of drugs or other interventions to act on those pathways and intervene in the disease process.	Before agents can be tested in patients, there are many pre-clinical steps necessary to get agents ready for clinical trials, including testing in animal models.	After pre-clinical development, agents are ready to be tested in humans to see if they are effective.
In addition to progress from investigator-initiated basic research studying underlying disease mechanisms, the Type 1 Diabetes Genetics Consortium and its collaborators have identified over 40 genes or genetic regions associated with type 1 diabetes, and The Environmental Determinants of Diabetes in the Young study completed enrollment of over 8,000 newborns and is following them until they are age 15 to study environmental triggers.	Studies on the immune system have led to the identification of promising agents targeting the autoimmune destruction of beta cells. The Diabetic Retinopathy Clinical Research Network identified a new therapy for diabetic macular edema that targets aberrant new blood vessel formation in the eye, a finding that was built on basic research on the molecular factors that play a role in that process.	Type 1 Diabetes-Rapid Access to Intervention Development and the Type 1 Diabetes-Preclinical Testing Program promote translation of research from the bench to the bedside by providing resources for pre-clinical development and testing of agents. The Animal Models of Diabetic Complications Consortium is generating animal models that mimic human complications.	Clinical trials networks, such as Type 1 Diabetes TrialNet and the Immune Tolerance Network, are testing strategies for prevention and early treatment. As new agents are identified for potential prevention or treatment of type 1 diabetes, the standing infrastructure of these networks will be critical for testing promising agents in patients.

How Type 1 Diabetes Research Benefits People with Other Diseases: Research supported by the *Special Diabetes Program* is far-reaching, benefiting not only people with type 1 diabetes, but also people with type 2 diabetes and people with other autoimmune diseases. For example, research to understand insulin-producing beta cells, and to find ways to preserve and restore beta cell function, benefits all people with diabetes. In the same way, all people with diabetes gain from research directed at the disease complications that type 1 and type 2 diabetes share. Epidemiologic studies supported by the *Special Diabetes Program* are collecting data on both type 1 and type 2 diabetes in youth. Type 2 diabetes in youth is a growing epidemic—these data will aid the design and implementation of public health efforts to stop this alarming trend. The studies also found that children with rarer forms of diabetes are often misdiagnosed as having type 1 or type 2 diabetes and thus do not receive appropriate treatment. These results will benefit children with rarer forms of diabetes and improve their treatment. Emerging research also shows that factors in the immune system are not just important in type 1 diabetes, but are also involved in childhood type 2 diabetes and "hybrid" forms of diabetes that have characteristics of both type 1 and type 2 diabetes. Thus, research on the immune basis of diabetes broadly benefits children with diabetes.

Type 1 diabetes research also benefits people with other autoimmune diseases. Although many autoimmune diseases are rare, collectively they affect approximately 5 to 8 percent of the U.S. population.[8] Some of the type 1 diabetes genes identified through research supported by the *Special Diabetes Program* affect the immune system and are involved in other autoimmune diseases. Therefore, understanding the genetic underpinnings of type 1 diabetes could provide insights into the genetics and pathogenesis of other autoimmune diseases. As therapies effective in type 1 diabetes may involve modulation of the immune system, these treatments could also be effective for other autoimmune diseases.

Furthermore, clinical trials networks supported by the *Special Diabetes Program* are conducting "mechanistic" studies that examine how immune regulation is altered in type 1 diabetes. Understanding these defects may also shed light on other autoimmune diseases. Research could also uncover environmental triggers of celiac disease, a digestive disorder caused by autoimmunity directed at gluten proteins in wheat and other grains. Some genes confer susceptibility to both celiac disease and type 1 diabetes, and many people have both diseases. Studies supported by the *Special Diabetes Program* to identify environmental triggers of type 1 diabetes are also investigating celiac disease, which ultimately benefit patients suffering from both diseases.

PLANNING AND EVALUATION OF THE SPECIAL DIABETES PROGRAM

Planning Process: To ensure the most scientifically productive use of the *Special Diabetes Program* funds, NIDDK initiated a collaborative planning process that involves the participation of the relevant NIH Institutes and Centers, including the National Cancer Institute (NCI), National Center for Complementary and Alternative Medicine (NCCAM), National Center for Research Resources (NCRR), National Eye Institute (NEI), National Human Genome Research Institute (NHGRI), National Heart, Lung, and Blood Institute (NHLBI), National Institute on Aging (NIA), National Institute of Allergy and Infectious Diseases (NIAID), National Institute of Biomedical Imaging and Bioengineering (NIBIB), *Eunice Kennedy Shriver* National Institute of Child Health and Human Development (NICHD), National Institute of Dental and Craniofacial Research (NIDCR), National Institute of Environmental Health Sciences (NIEHS),

---

[8]   Accessed from http://www3.niaid.nih.gov/topics/autoimmune

National Institute of Mental Health (NIMH), National Institute on Minority Health and Health Disparities (NIMHD), National Institute of Neurological Disorders and Stroke (NINDS), National Institute of Nursing Research (NINR), National Library of Medicine (NLM), NIH Office of Research on Women's Health (ORWH), and other NIH Institutes and Centers that are represented on the statutory Diabetes Mellitus Interagency Coordinating Committee (DMICC);[9] and the CDC, Centers for Medicare & Medicaid Services (CMS), and other government agencies represented on the DMICC. The DMICC serves as an important venue for coordination and information sharing across the government, and DMICC members provide input on planning, implementation, and evaluation of the *Special Diabetes Program.*

The collaborative planning process also involves the two major diabetes voluntary organizations: Juvenile Diabetes Research Foundation International (JDRF) and American Diabetes Association (ADA).

Type 1 diabetes is an excellent model for a scientifically targeted and administratively integrated program because it is a systemic disease that is addressed by multiple NIH and HHS components. Type 1 diabetes involves the body's endocrine and metabolic functions (NIDDK) and immune system (NIAID); multi-organ complications affecting the heart and arteries (NHLBI), eyes (NEI), kidneys and digestive and urologic tracts (NIDDK), nervous system (NINDS, NIMH), and oral cavity (NIDCR); the special problems of a disease diagnosed primarily in children and adolescents (NICHD); critically important and complex genetic (NHGRI) and environmental (NIEHS) factors; the need for novel imaging technologies (NIBIB), specialized research

resources (NCRR), and data on disease incidence and prevalence in the United States (CDC); and services for pre-clinical testing of therapeutics (NCI). Thus, the *Special Diabetes Program* has catalyzed and synergized the efforts of a wide range of NIH and HHS components to combat type 1 diabetes and complications, making it a model trans-NIH and trans-HHS program.

Critical to the planning process is scientific input NIH has garnered from type 1 diabetes researchers and the broader research community. Sources of input include a variety of scientific workshops and conferences, as well as a series of planning and evaluation meetings to assess current research and future opportunities. At these planning and evaluation meetings, input was obtained from: distinguished scientists whom NIH convened in April 2000, to consider opportunities for allocations of *Special Diabetes Program* funds; a panel of scientific experts, who met in May 2002, to evaluate the use of the *Special Diabetes Program* funds and to assess opportunities for future research; a group of scientific and lay experts who met in January 2005, to perform a mid-course assessment of the large-scale research consortia and networks supported by the *Program* and identify future research opportunities; a panel of scientific experts who met in April 2008 to evaluate clinical research consortia supported by the *Special Diabetes Program* and indicate future research opportunities; and a group of scientific and lay experts who met in June 2009 to evaluate pre-clinical research consortia supported by the *Special Diabetes Program* and discuss future research opportunities. More information on the April 2008 and June 2009 meetings is found in the box.

---

[9]   For more information, please see: www.diabetescommittee.gov

Strategic planning, with broad external input, has also guided program planning. Two recent plans, *"Advances and Emerging Opportunities in Type 1 Diabetes Research: A Strategic Plan"* and *"Advances and Emerging Opportunities in Diabetes Research: A Strategic Planning Report of the DMICC,"* are guiding type 1 diabetes research directions, including research supported by the *Special Diabetes Program*.

EXTERNAL EVALUATION OF ONGOING CLINICAL AND PRE-CLINICAL RESEARCH CONSORTIA AND NETWORKS SUPPORTED BY THE *SPECIAL STATUTORY FUNDING PROGRAM FOR TYPE 1 DIABETES RESEARCH*

Major components of this evaluation of the *Special Diabetes Program* are two *ad hoc* planning and evaluation meetings at which NIDDK convened panels of scientific and lay experts to obtain external input on the progress and future directions of ongoing research consortia and networks. Scientific judgment of these external experts on clinical and pre-clinical consortia supported by the *Special Diabetes Program* was sought at meetings in April 2008 and June 2009, respectively.

At both meetings, panelists were asked to provide input on current efforts and future directions for each consortium or network, as well as on future research opportunities outside the context of ongoing research programs. In particular, because the *Special Diabetes Program* is limited in time, the panel members were asked to provide input on future directions if the *Special Diabetes Program* is extended in time.

To frame the discussion, the panel members were asked to address questions for each consortium being evaluated, such as:

- Does the consortium address a compelling scientific opportunity?
- How might scientific progress of each consortium be improved?
- Are processes in place to modify consortium plans in response to new scientific discoveries?
- Are there opportunities to better use resources generated by the consortium to advance type 1 diabetes research?
- Are there additional opportunities for coordination of consortia with each other and with other efforts?

At the April 2008 meeting, an external panel of scientists with expertise in clinical trials, autoimmune diseases, immunology, transplantation, epidemiology, and biostatistics performed a mid-course assessment of ongoing clinical research efforts supported by the *Special Diabetes Program* and discussed possible future directions for the programs. After reviewing the clinical consortia portfolio, the panel members provided input that cut across multiple research efforts. They commended NIH and CDC on the many accomplishments that have been achieved through the clinical consortia supported by the *Special Diabetes Program* in such a short period of time and noted that the research portfolio that has been established under NIDDK's leadership has been a very wise investment of funding.

At the June 2009 meeting, an external panel of scientific experts with expertise in beta cell biology, immunology, diabetes complications, and animal models, and a lay reviewer performed a mid-course assessment of ongoing pre-clinical research efforts supported by the *Special Diabetes Program* and discussed possible future directions for the programs. They were enthusiastic about the progress and accomplishments of the pre-clinical consortia supported by the *Special Diabetes Program*, and commended NIDDK and NIAID for their leadership of these consortia.

The input obtained at these evaluation meetings has been critically important for informing the government's program planning efforts for this time-limited appropriation. For example, at both meetings, panel members encouraged the government to enhance coordination across existing research consortia, to make the best use of existing resources and maximize research progress. One example of how coordination has been enhanced is through collaboration on a new clinical trial. Two research consortia—one with expertise in glucose monitoring technology and another with expertise in testing therapies for early treatment of type 1 diabetes—are collaborating on a clinical trial testing whether early and intensive blood glucose control at disease onset could preserve insulin production. In the trial, patients are placed on an inpatient closed-loop system and sent home with a sensor-augmented insulin pump. Thus, the combined expertise of the two consortia has been instrumental in enabling the conduct of this trial.

At the pre-clinical research meeting, the panel evaluated a consortium studying porcine to non-human primate models of xenotransplantation (solid organ, tissue, or cell transplantation between species). Panel members felt that the consortium's research was extremely valuable as an approach to relieve the shortage of solid organs for transplantation, but the research was less relevant to islet transplantation. Based on that feedback, the consortium is no longer supported by the *Special Diabetes Program*, but does continue to receive support from regularly appropriated funds for research on solid organ transplantation. Panel members at the clinical meeting felt that it was important to bolster research toward the development of an artificial pancreas. Based on this input, NIDDK developed new initiatives, with support from the *Special Diabetes Program*, to solicit research proposals from small businesses toward developing new technologies to inform development of an artificial pancreas. This example demonstrates how external evaluation led to a shift in use of the funds based on ongoing surveillance of scientific opportunities and how NIH has implemented input from the evaluation panels to enhance research supported by the *Special Diabetes Program*. The input received at these meetings continues to be invaluable as the government makes plans for future research directions.

Evaluation Process: The public laws providing funds for the *Special Diabetes Program* also mandate interim and final evaluation reports on the use of the funds. Initiatives pursued with the P. L. 105-33 funds were described in a 2000 report to the Congress.[10] An interim report that describes research progress and opportunities that resulted from the *Special Diabetes Program* from FY 1998 through 2003 was published in April 2003.[11] Results from an evaluation of the *Special Diabetes Program* for FY 1998-2005 were submitted to the Congress in 2007.[12] The 2007 *"Evaluation Report"* described the collaborative, trans-HHS planning process that guides the use of the funds; the progress that had been achieved to date and the expected future accomplishments of the research programs and resources that had been established; and emerging research opportunities that resulted from the *Special Diabetes Program*. The final *"Evaluation Report"* presented here builds on the results reported in the 2007 *"Evaluation Report"* and describes advances, research programs, resources, and emerging opportunities that have resulted from the *Special Diabetes Program*.

Critical assessments of the planning and implementation processes, and of the scientific merit of the *Special Diabetes Program*, have been garnered through an evaluation process involving the external diabetes research community, as well as an internal review of archival data. Evaluation metrics used in this report include:

- *Research Accomplishments*: Review of scientific advances and technological developments that have had positive impacts on patients or enabled future

basic and clinical research. These data are primarily obtained from research publications, as well as from research advances included in *"Advances and Emerging Opportunities in Diabetes Research: A Strategic Planning Report of the DMICC."*

- *Professional Assessment*: Scientific judgment of external experts in the type 1 diabetes or related fields garnered from specific assessments of clinical and pre-clinical consortia supported by the *Special Diabetes Program* (see box earlier in chapter). Additionally, each individual consortium or project has ongoing assessment.

- *Bibliometric Analysis*: Compendium of *Special Diabetes Program*-associated publications in peer-reviewed scientific journals and the impact of these publications as determined by a citation analysis.

- *Grant Portfolio Analysis*: Use of NIH archival databases to determine program effectiveness in terms of dimensions such as recruitment of new investigators and stimulation of clinical research.

- *Input from Consortia Investigators*: Sample consortia investigators provided input on the importance and value of consortia supported by the *Special Diabetes Program*.

- *Other Metrics of Progress*: Outcome measures including patents, research resources (*e.g.*, microarray chips, antibodies, genetic and tissue samples, Internet-accessible data sets, animal models), and progress toward patient recruitment goals. These data are primarily obtained from annual progress reports or meetings of external review committees.

---

[10] www.niddk.nih.gov/federal/initiative.htm
[11] http://www2.niddk.nih.gov/AboutNIDDK/ReportsAndStrategicPlanning/Type_1_Diabetes_April_2003.htm
[12] www.t1diabetes.nih.gov/evaluation

ASSESSMENT MEASURES INDICATE THAT THE *SPECIAL DIABETES PROGRAM* HAS:

- Produced significant scientific advances with respect to each of the six overarching scientific Goals (see "Highlights of Scientific Accomplishments" earlier in this chapter), many of which were highlighted in *"Advances and Emerging Opportunities in Diabetes Research: A Strategic Planning Report of the DMICC"* as major advances in diabetes research.

- Yielded robust scientific output with at least 2,793 scientific publications. A citation analysis found these papers cited at least 52,739 times in other publications (prior to January 1, 2010), demonstrating that research supported by the *Special Diabetes Program* is having far-reaching effects, and accelerating progress in type 1 diabetes research.

- Led to at least 38 issued patents, many of which have enabled new lines of research or have been further developed by industry for use in medical practice.

- Promoted development of resources for use by the broad scientific community, including over 40 animal models of type 1 diabetes that closely mimic various aspects of human complications of diabetes; 50 new lines of genetically engineered mice or mouse embryonic stem cells for the study of beta cell biology; 110 antibodies against markers expressed at different stages of stem cell to beta cell maturation; invaluable collections of human biological samples; databases; and protocols.

- Attracted new investigators to pursue research on type 1 diabetes: 38 percent of new research project grants (R01, R21, and DP2 mechanisms) went to new investigators, which is comparable with NIH-wide data for grant applications from new investigators.

- Fostered clinical research—over 63 percent of *Special Diabetes Program* funding supported clinical research—and propelled research progress to a point where several human clinical trials are being conducted through the infrastructure created by the *Special Diabetes Program*. Twenty-three grants supported by the *Special Diabetes Program* involved Phase III clinical trials, the final stage required before a therapy can be approved by FDA.

- Established key research programs that have been successful in providing new insights into the understanding of type 1 diabetes and its complications.

- Promoted translation of promising therapeutic agents from the bench to bedside.

- Developed innovative funding mechanisms to bring together a diverse range of researchers to tackle interdisciplinary problems.

- Balanced a research portfolio of large-scale, collaborative projects with long time horizons with flexible, short-term projects that provide a rapid response to emerging research challenges of critical importance.

GOAL I

IDENTIFY THE GENETIC AND ENVIRONMENTAL CAUSES OF TYPE 1 DIABETES

The *Special Statutory Funding Program for Type 1 Diabetes Research* has enabled the establishment of large-scale, long-term clinical research studies and clinical trials that are essential for identifying the genetic and environmental causes of type 1 diabetes and testing interventions to prevent the disease. In addition to the significant research progress described in this chapter, information on the program evaluation related to Goal I can be found in Appendix A (Allocation of Funds), Appendix B (Assessment), and Appendix C (Evaluation of Major Research Consortia, Networks, and Resources).

Type 1 diabetes results from an interaction of genetic and environmental factors that triggers the autoimmune destruction of insulin-producing pancreatic beta cells. Discovering those genetic and environmental risk factors and determining how they interact to cause disease are key steps toward being able to identify individuals who are at risk for type 1 diabetes and accurately assess their specific level of risk. Moreover, research on type 1 diabetes triggers can reveal the molecular mechanisms associated with the development of autoimmune disease and aid in the development of new therapies to delay, prevent, or reverse type 1 diabetes.

The *Special Statutory Funding Program for Type 1 Diabetes Research (Special Diabetes Program or Program)* has invested significant resources into multiple large-scale, long-term clinical research studies aimed at identifying the genetic and environmental causes of type 1 diabetes or testing interventions to prevent the disease. Collectively, these studies are recruiting and intensively monitoring thousands of families and individuals affected by type 1 diabetes. This substantial investment of financial resources, along with the considerable time and effort of researchers and patients, has already led to new scientific advances. As a result of these studies, we now know how many children in the United States have diabetes, and are poised to see how rates of childhood diabetes are changing over time. Nearly 50 genetic regions that influence risk for type 1 diabetes are now known—up from three genes known a decade ago. Genetic evidence linking type 1 diabetes with other autoimmune diseases, such as celiac disease, suggests that research on the environmental risk factors for type 1 diabetes may benefit a larger patient group than originally anticipated. These and other findings represent only a fraction of the knowledge that is expected to accrue from the long-term investment in research on genetic and environmental risk factors of type 1 diabetes supported by the *Special Diabetes Program*.

Graphic: Drawing of DNA double helix. Image credit: National Human Genome Research Institute, NIH.

HIGHLIGHTS OF RECENT RESEARCH ADVANCES RELATED TO GOAL I

Identification of Genetic Regions Involved in Type 1 Diabetes Susceptibility: Researchers have analyzed data from the Type 1 Diabetes Genetics Consortium (T1DGC) collection and other genetic studies to identify over 40 genetic regions that are associated with type 1 diabetes risk. Most of the newly identified genes seem to be associated with T cells or other components of the immune system. For example, the genes *SH2B3, IL2RA, PRKCQ, TAGAP,* and *UBASH3A* are all implicated in T cell activation, and *IL2* and *IL27* are involved in T cell proliferation and differentiation, respectively. Another gene, *GLIS3,* is associated with development of the insulin-producing beta cells of the pancreas. Mutations in *GLIS3* have also been found in people who have a form of neonatal diabetes. Other implicated regions contain genes of unknown function, and further research on these genes may uncover new biochemical pathways involved in the pathogenesis of type 1 diabetes.

Completion of Recruitment for TEDDY and TRIGR: Major research accomplishments have been the completion of recruitment for The Environmental Determinants of Diabetes in the Young (TEDDY) study to find environmental triggers of type 1 diabetes and the Trial to Reduce IDDM in the Genetically At-Risk (TRIGR) study to test a dietary intervention to prevent type 1 diabetes. In TEDDY, over 425,000 infants were screened and over 8,000 children were enrolled for long-term monitoring. TRIGR recruited over 5,600 pregnant women and enrolled 2,160 eligible newborns. Recruitment of the TEDDY and TRIGR cohorts sets the stage for successful completion of these important clinical studies that could have great impact on public health efforts to prevent type 1 diabetes.

Epidemiology of Childhood Diabetes in the United States: The SEARCH for Diabetes in Youth study (SEARCH) is providing data on how many children and youth in the United States have diabetes and how those rates are changing over time. SEARCH found that in children under the age of 10 years, type 1 diabetes was the most common form of diabetes in all racial/ethnic groups examined. Type 2 diabetes was rarely diagnosed in this age group. Among youth under the age of 10 years, the rate of new cases was 19.7 per 100,000 each year for type 1 diabetes and 0.4 per 100,000 for type 2 diabetes. Among youth 10 years of age and older, the rate of new cases was 18.6 per 100,000 each year for type 1 diabetes and 8.5 per 100,000 each year for youth with type 2 diabetes. Non-Hispanic white youth had the highest rate of new cases of type 1 diabetes. While still infrequent, rates of type 2 diabetes were greater among youth aged 10 to 19 years compared to younger children, with higher rates among U.S. minority populations compared with non-Hispanic whites. Among non-Hispanic white youth aged 10 to 19 years, the rate of new cases was higher for type 1 than for type 2 diabetes. For Asian/Pacific Islander and American Indian youth aged 10 to 19 years, the opposite was true—the rate of new cases was greater for type 2 than for type 1 diabetes. Among African American and Hispanic youth aged 10 to 19 years, the rates of new cases of type 1 and type 2 diabetes were similar.

Increasing Role of Environmental Triggers in Type 1 Diabetes: A SEARCH site in Colorado found that the incidence of type 1 diabetes has increased 1.6-fold among non-Hispanic white and Hispanic youth aged 0-17 years from 1978-1988 to 2002-2004. Emerging evidence indicates that increasing environmental exposures might account for trends in the diagnosis of type 1 diabetes over time. For example, non-Hispanic white and Hispanic children diagnosed with type 1 diabetes between 2002 and 2004 were found to be less likely to have the highest risk Human Leukocyte Antigen (HLA) class II genotypes than those diagnosed between 1978-1988. This observation suggests that environmental factors might now be able to trigger disease in individuals who have lower genetic susceptibility to type 1 diabetes. SEARCH investigators also found that the age of type 1 diabetes diagnosis in Colorado children decreased by 9.6 months from the period 1978-1983 to 2002-2004. An increase in the height of children over this time period accounted for about 15 percent of the decreasing age of diagnosis, but the major environmental pressures affecting risk of type 1 diabetes remain unknown.

Diabetes Control in Youth with Type 1 Diabetes: In addition to providing the first national data on rates of childhood diabetes, SEARCH also provides information on the health status of children with diabetes. SEARCH investigators found that 17 percent of youth with type 1 diabetes have hemoglobin A1c (HbA1c) levels greater than 9 percent that reflect poor glycemic control. African American, American Indian, Hispanic, and Asian/Pacific Islander youth with type 1 diabetes were significantly more likely to have higher HbA1c levels than non-Hispanic white youth (rates for poor glycemic control of 36 percent, 52 percent, 27 percent, and 26 percent versus 12 percent respectively). Another analysis showed that insulin pump use, which is associated with the lowest HbA1c levels in all age groups, was more frequently used by older youth, females, non-Hispanic whites, and families with higher incomes and education. These findings point to the need to develop more effective treatment strategies to improve metabolic control in all youth with type 1 diabetes.

COMPLEXITY OF TYPE 1 DIABETES SUSCEPTIBILITY

By 1998, at the start of the *Special Diabetes Program*, scientists had long been studying patterns of type 1 diabetes in families and groups around the world to look for the causes of this disease. Their research efforts uncovered wide variations in an individual's chance of developing type 1 diabetes and suggested that complex interactions of multiple genetic and environmental factors might be involved in disease onset.

Studies of Large Populations Provide Insight into Type 1 Diabetes: By studying large populations,

researchers noted a significant geographical variation in the rate of type 1 diabetes. Several decades ago wide variation in the rates of type 1 diabetes around the world were recognized ranging from more than 20 cases diagnosed per 100,000 persons per year to fewer than 3 cases diagnosed per 100,000 persons per year.[13] In the United States, based on limited local data, rates were thought to be intermediate between those extremes.[14] More recent data on incidence of type 1 diabetes worldwide is presented in Figure 2. This great variability in disease incidence across national borders could reflect genetic differences among diverse racial and ethnic

---

[13] Dorman JS , McCarthy BJ, O'Leary LA, et al.: Risk Factors for Insulin-Dependent Diabetes. In *Diabetes in America* (pp. 165-178). Bethesda, MD: National Diabetes Data Group, NIH, 1995.

[14] *Ibid.*

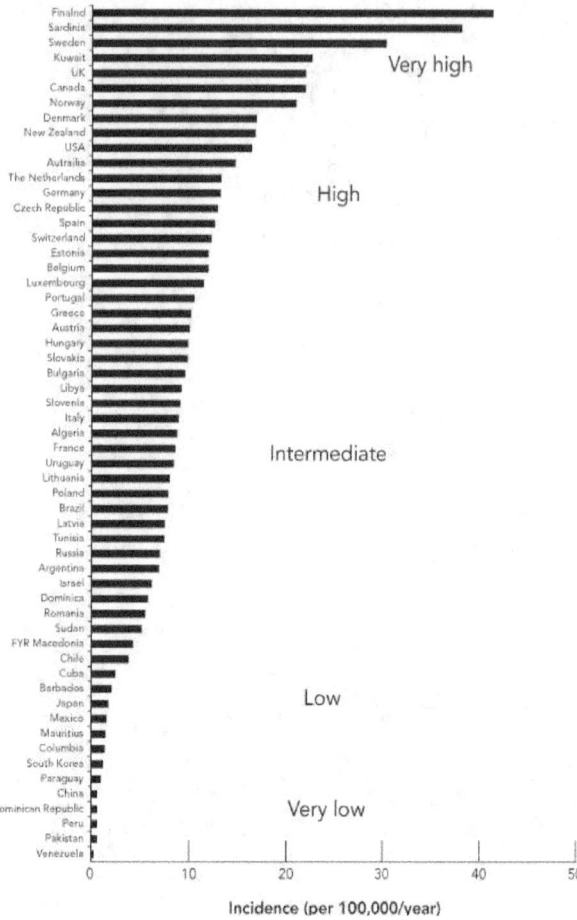

Very high

High

Intermediate

Low

Very low

Finland
Sardinia
Sweden
Kuwait
UK
Canada
Norway
Denmark
New Zealand
USA
Australia
The Netherlands
Germany
Czech Republic
Spain
Switzerland
Estonia
Belgium
Luxembourg
Portugal
Greece
Austria
Hungary
Slovakia
Bulgaria
Libya
Slovenia
Italy
Algeria
France
Uruguay
Lithuania
Poland
Brazil
Latvia
Tunisia
Russia
Argentina
Israel
Dominica
Romania
Sudan
FYR Macedonia
Chile
Cuba
Barbados
Japan
Mexico
Mauritius
Columbia
South Korea
Paraguay
China
Dominican Republic
Peru
Pakistan
Venezuela

Incidence (per 100,000/year)

Figure 2: Worldwide Incidence of Type 1 Diabetes in Children
Standardized rates (per 100,000/year) of type 1 diabetes in children aged 14 years or under worldwide 1990-1999. Countries are arranged in descending incidence rate. Reprinted with permission from the DIAMOND Project Group and *Diabetic Medicine* 23: 857-866, 2006, John Wiley and Sons Inc. publisher.

populations; environmental differences, such as variations in dietary practices or the level of exposure to sunlight; or a combination of genetic and environmental risk factors.

Insights from Individual Families with Type 1 Diabetes: Results from studies of individuals with type 1 diabetes and their families, as well as individuals without diabetes, strongly support the hypothesis that genetic susceptibility in combination with environmental factors is required for disease onset. Researchers found that a person who has a close relative with type 1 diabetes has up to a 15-fold higher[15] risk of developing the disease than someone with no close relative with type 1 diabetes. If an identical twin has type 1 diabetes, then his or her twin has a substantially greater risk of developing type 1 diabetes.[16] The second twin, however, still only develops type 1 diabetes about 40 percent of the time,[17] even though identical twins have the same genetic make-up. Importantly, more than 80 percent of people with type 1 diabetes have no close relative with the disease.[18] Together, these research findings indicated that genetic factors have a significant effect on disease susceptibility, but the autoimmune process leading to type 1 diabetes seems to also require an as-yet unknown environmental triggers.

Investing in Critical Infrastructure for Research on Genetic and Environmental Risk Factors for Type 1 Diabetes: The *Special Diabetes Program* has enabled the creation of large-scale research efforts to identify the genes that confer increased susceptibility to or protection from type 1 diabetes, as well as the environmental factors that trigger the autoimmune process in genetically susceptible individuals. With support from the *Special*

---

[15] Tillil H and Köbberling J: Age-corrected empirical genetic risk estimates for first-degree relatives of IDDM patients. Diabetes 36: 93-99, 1987.
[16] Kyvik KO, Green A, and Beck-Nielsen H: Concordance rates of insulin dependent diabetes mellitus: a population based study of young Danish twins. BMJ 311: 913-917, 1995.
[17] Rich SS: Mapping genes in diabetes: genetic epidemiological perspective. Diabetes 39: 1315-1319, 1990.
[18] Dorman JS, McCarthy BJ, O'Leary LA, et al.: Risk Factors for Insulin-Dependent Diabetes. In Diabetes in America (pp. 165-178). Bethesda, MD: National Diabetes Data Group, NIH, 1995.

Diabetes Program, T1DGC, TEDDY, SEARCH, and clinical trials to prevent type 1 diabetes, such as TRIGR, have begun a new era in research on the genetic and environmental causes of type 1 diabetes.

GENETIC CAUSES OF TYPE 1 DIABETES

A decade ago, scientists had identified three genetic regions that influence the risk for type 1 diabetes. As much as 50 percent of genetic susceptibility to type 1 diabetes is attributable to variations in the *HLA* class II regions of the Major Histocompatibility Complex. Proteins encoded by the *HLA* genes help a person's immune system distinguish their own cells from foreign cells, such as disease-causing bacteria. For reasons that are still being studied, some variations in the *HLA* genes make it more likely that the immune system will not recognize the body's cells as "self," and therefore launch an attack on these cells, triggering type 1 diabetes or another autoimmune disease. Other regions linked with type 1 diabetes included a portion of DNA that regulates the insulin gene and a gene called *CTLA4* that encodes a protein found in T cells of the immune system. While these three genetic regions together accounted for a large proportion of type 1 diabetes cases, it was clear that many genes for type 1 diabetes had yet to be discovered.

The search for genetic causes of type 1 diabetes is complicated by the fact that some genes might have small effects in many people across the population and other genes might have larger effects but only in a small group of individuals or families. In addition, some genetic risk factors might interact with each other such that increased risk in certain individuals might result from disease-associated variations in two or more genes. Scientists knew that identifying all genetic variants

that affect the risk of type 1 diabetes would require a large-scale, coordinated effort to systematically search the genomes of thousands of people with type 1 diabetes and their close relatives who do or do not also have the disease.

Coordinating and Implementing International Efforts To Discover the Genetic Causes of Type 1 Diabetes: In 2001, with support from the *Special Diabetes Program*, the T1DGC was established with the goal of organizing and implementing international efforts to identify genes that determine an individual's risk of type 1 diabetes. The Consortium is led by NIDDK in collaboration with NIAID, NHGRI, NICHD, and JDRF. The T1DGC established four international networks to coordinate the work of researchers across the globe.

The Consortium aimed to collect, store, and analyze DNA from 2,800 families with two or more siblings with type 1 diabetes. In populations with low rates of type 1 diabetes, families with only one child with type 1 diabetes, as well as individuals with or without type 1 diabetes, were also recruited to participate in the study. The T1DGC made significant efforts to collect DNA from non-Caucasian populations for which little information is available about the genetics of type 1 diabetes. The Consortium also created an extensive database containing clinical, genetic, and medical history information from each participant. With DNA samples and data from approximately 38,000 individuals, the T1DGC collection has amassed the statistical power needed to facilitate the search for type 1 diabetes genes and genetic interactions. To maximize scientific output from this unique genetic collection, the resources known as the NIDDK Central Repositories coordinate sharing of available T1DGC biosamples and data with qualified investigators for approved research studies. For more information on the T1DGC, please see the Investigator Profile of Dr. Stephen Rich in this chapter.

Newly Identified Genes Associated with Increased Susceptibility to Type 1 Diabetes: The T1DGC investment has already begun to pay off—researchers have used data gleaned from the T1DGC collection and other studies to identify nearly 50 genetic regions that are associated with type 1 diabetes risk. Most of these newly identified genes seem to be associated with T cells or other components of the immune system. More research is needed to understand how each of the genes associated with type 1 diabetes actually causes or contributes to the disease. The identification of these genetic regions sets the stage for new insights about type 1 diabetes. Because many of the genes that increase risk for type 1 diabetes are also associated with other autoimmune diseases, learning how the genes alter risk will shed light on multiple autoimmune disorders.

Fine-mapping Genetic and Genomic Variants that Contribute to Type 1 Diabetes: To build on the research resources made available by the T1DGC, the *Special Diabetes Program* is supporting new research to more finely map the newly identified susceptibility regions and to uncover the mechanisms by which the genes influence risk of type 1 diabetes. Researchers are taking a closer look at the susceptibility regions, each of which contain up to 27 genes, to identify the exact genes and sequence variants that are associated with disease risk. They are also exploring how variations in the *CTLA4* gene create subtle differences in the amount of protein that is produced from the gene and how those differences relate to the pathogenesis of type 1 diabetes, and testing the hypothesis that genetic changes that do not affect the DNA sequence can also influence type 1 diabetes

risk. By expanding knowledge of the pathogenesis of type 1 diabetes, this research could inform new strategies for prevention and treatment. It can also improve predictive abilities and enable the design of more specific clinical trials to test personalized interventions for patients with similar risk profiles.

ENVIRONMENTAL CAUSES OF TYPE 1 DIABETES

By the start of the *Special Diabetes Program* in 1998, scientists had garnered some clues to potential environmental causes of type 1 diabetes. Research uncovered an apparent seasonal pattern to type 1 diabetes onset with fewer cases diagnosed in warm summer months. This observation suggested to researchers that infectious agents, such as viruses, that are more common during colder months might be potential triggers of type 1 diabetes. Other studies found evidence of nutritional factors in disease onset. Breastfeeding was associated with a lower risk of type 1 diabetes in children, while early exposure to cow's milk or the introduction of cereal before 3 months or after 7 months of age were associated with a higher risk. Type 1 diabetes risk has also been linked to factors as diverse as levels of vitamin D in the blood, stress, maternal age, birth order, and socioeconomic status. Despite a wealth of research demonstrating significant associations between type 1 diabetes and a variety of potential risk factors, no single environmental factor has been definitively identified as a causative agent for type 1 diabetes.

Many early studies on the environmental causes of type 1 diabetes focused on individuals with existing type 1 diabetes and examined their history to try to determine potential environmental influences before or around the time of diagnosis. Such studies were limited by imprecision, recall bias, and failure to account for exposures early in life. Other studies enrolled too few children or followed participants for time periods that were too short to generate statistically significant results. Identifying environmental triggers of type 1 diabetes with certainty would require a prospective clinical study that allows for intensive observation of thousands of at-risk individuals before the onset of disease. Because the autoimmune process in type 1 diabetes can take years in some individuals, such a study would have to follow its participants over a long period of time.

Intensive Long-term Monitoring To Identify Environmental Triggers of Type 1 Diabetes: With support from the *Special Diabetes Program*, NIDDK, NIAID, NICHD, NIEHS, CDC, and JDRF established the long-term TEDDY study to provide a coordinated, multidisciplinary approach to understanding the infectious agents, dietary factors, or other environmental conditions that trigger type 1 diabetes in genetically susceptible individuals. TEDDY is an international consortium of six research groups located in the United States and Europe.

TEDDY investigators have screened over 425,000 newborns from the general population or who have either a parent or sibling with type 1 diabetes to identify infants with *HLA* gene sequences that predict an increased risk of type 1 diabetes. Over 8,000 high-risk infants are now being followed in the TEDDY study from birth through 15 years of age. For a decade and a half, investigators will regularly collect information on the child's diet, illnesses, vaccinations, and psychosocial stresses; biological samples, including blood, stool, and toenail clippings, will be collected and stored for future analysis as new

technologies and hypotheses are developed. In addition, TEDDY children will be frequently tested for evidence of the autoimmune process that characterizes type 1 diabetes, enabling researchers to study the very early stages in the development of the disease.

Because the study is scheduled to continue until 2023, TEDDY has been rigorously designed to maximize the probability of successfully identifying one or more environmental triggers of type 1 diabetes. Biosamples from TEDDY participants will be made available to researchers worldwide through the NIDDK Central Repositories so that innovative hypotheses related to the environmental causes of type 1 diabetes can be efficiently tested without the need to duplicate costly infrastructure and human resources. The substantial investment in TEDDY can reap major rewards and revolutionize the ability to prevent type 1 diabetes. For example, identification of a dietary or infectious cause of type 1 diabetes could have an enormously positive impact on public health through a diet change or vaccine for disease prevention.

Benefits of Research on Type 1 Diabetes for Other Autoimmune Diseases: Benefits of the TEDDY study are expected to extend more broadly to include people with celiac disease, a digestive disorder caused by autoimmunity directed at gluten proteins in wheat and other grains. Celiac disease and type 1 diabetes share some genetic susceptibility factors, and many people have both diseases. Celiac disease affects about 2 million Americans and, like type 1 diabetes, rates of the disorder are rising.[19] Because the newborns studied in TEDDY are at high risk of celiac disease, the researchers are studying the development of both autoimmune

---

[19] Fasano A, Berti I, Gerarduzzi T, et al: Prevalence of celiac disease in at-risk and not-at-risk groups in the United States. <u>Archives of Internal Medicine</u> 163: 268-292, 2003.

disorders. Thus, the intensive study of at-risk youth over many years to uncover environmental risk factors for type 1 diabetes will also identify factors that contribute to celiac disease and other autoimmune diseases.

Testing a Dietary Strategy for Type 1 Diabetes Prevention: While TEDDY represents an unbiased, prospective, long-term investment in finding the environmental causes of type 1 diabetes, scientists are also studying whether modification of specific potential triggers can prevent or reduce the incidence of type 1 diabetes. TRIGR, which is led by NICHD, is an international clinical trial testing whether weaning high-risk infants to a formula in which milk proteins have been broken down (hydrolyzed) into much smaller pieces can reduce the risk of diabetes-associated autoimmunity or type 1 diabetes compared to weaning to standard cow's milk formula. Families from 15 countries across North America, Europe, and Australia participate in TRIGR.

Research suggests that standard cow's milk proteins might interfere with the normal development of the immune system in genetically susceptible individuals and that hydrolyzed milk might be less likely to trigger that deleterious effect on the immune system. To test the hypothesis that hydrolyzed formula could reduce the risk of type 1 diabetes, TRIGR recruited over 5,600 pregnant women who have type 1 diabetes or have a relative with type 1 diabetes to participate in the early phases of the study. Ultimately, 2,160 of their infants were identified as being at high risk for type 1 diabetes and enrolled in TRIGR. Mothers of enrolled infants were encouraged to breastfeed for as long as possible. At weaning, infants were randomly assigned to receive either standard or extensively hydrolyzed formula. TRIGR investigators are monitoring these children for signs of diabetes-related autoimmunity or the development of type 1 diabetes

until they are 10 years of age. The last baby enrolled in TRIGR was born in 2007, so results from the trial are expected after 2017. If the TRIGR hypothesis is proven to be correct, a simple dietary intervention could have significant benefits for families that carry a high genetic risk of type 1 diabetes.

EPIDEMIOLOGY OF DIABETES IN AMERICAN YOUTH

A major challenge for understanding childhood diabetes in the United States has been the lack of reliable national information on the rates, types, and clinical course of diabetes in children and youth. With support from the *Special Diabetes Program*, CDC and NIDDK launched SEARCH, a multicenter epidemiologic study to identify cases of diabetes in children and youth under 20 years of age in six geographically dispersed regions across the United States. The SEARCH centers cover a large population of American youth with significant racial/ ethnic, socioeconomic, and geographic diversity.

Understanding the Complexity of Diabetes in Youth: SEARCH has revealed a more complicated picture of childhood diabetes than was previously assumed. In children under 10 years of age, type 1 diabetes represented the predominant form of new cases of diabetes in all racial/ethnic groups studied. Type 2 diabetes was only rarely diagnosed in this age group. In youth from 10 to 19 years of age, type 1 diabetes was the main form of newly diagnosed diabetes in non-Hispanic white children, while type 2 diabetes was more common in Asian/Pacific Islander and American Indian youth. New cases of diabetes were about equally split between type 1 and type 2 diabetes in older African American and Hispanic youth. Interestingly, SEARCH investigators found some diabetic youth had features of both forms of the disease. SEARCH is now leading efforts to better classify diabetes type in youth for both research and clinical purposes.

Discovering Risk Factors for Childhood Diabetes: SEARCH is contributing to the hunt for the genetic and environmental triggers of diabetes, which could inform new therapeutic strategies. SEARCH data showed that obesity—typically thought of as a risk factor for type 2 diabetes—might accelerate the onset of type 1 diabetes in children who already have reduced beta cell function. Ongoing investment in SEARCH will allow researchers to quantitate changes in the rates of childhood diabetes over time and better characterize the natural history and risk factors for all forms of diabetes in children and youth. For more information on SEARCH, please see the Investigator Profile of Dr. Dana Dabelea in Goal V.

SUMMARY

Research to identify the genetic and environmental causes of type 1 diabetes has profound implications for at-risk individuals, as well as those already living with the disease. Understanding the genetic risk factors will help scientists and clinicians better identify individuals with higher susceptibility for type 1 diabetes so that they can be offered enrollment in clinical trials of potential preventive strategies or be given interventions to prevent diabetes once such interventions are tested and validated. Even in the absence of prevention strategies, at-risk individuals can be closely monitored for early signs of autoimmunity. Research has shown that at-risk children who are monitored before diabetes onset have lower rates of diabetic ketoacidosis, a potentially fatal complication of untreated diabetes, and are less likely to be hospitalized at diagnosis. Similarly, identifying environmental risk factors might point to simple behavioral modifications—such as choosing a

different infant formula as is being tested in TRIGR—that can reduce the chance of developing type 1 diabetes. Defining the genetic and environmental risk factors could also reveal the biological pathways that go awry in type 1 diabetes and elicit autoimmune destruction of the beta cells. The design and development of drugs that correct those pathways could potentially reverse type 1 diabetes even in individuals with long-standing disease.

The *Special Statutory Funding Program for Type 1 Diabetes Research* has supported the establishment of unprecedented research infrastructure and resources that have already significantly advanced knowledge of the genetic and environmental causes of this complex disease. Nonetheless, the potential payoff from the investment in these large-scale, long-term studies is only beginning to be realized. All research consortia described in this chapter have invested substantial time, human resources, and effort to screen and enroll thousands of families and individuals affected by type 1 diabetes (see the Feature on "Critical Investment in Infrastructure for Type 1 Diabetes Research" later in this chapter). Likewise, the dedicated volunteers in these research studies have contributed significant amounts of time and effort toward the goal of attaining new knowledge about type 1 diabetes that would not otherwise be possible to attain without their participation. These efforts have set the stage for future research progress that is expected to be fully realized in the years to come. This important line of research could not be undertaken at all, or at least not at an unprecedented scale, without the financial and organizational resources of the *Special Diabetes Program* and the dedicated participation of the diabetes research and patient communities.

RESEARCH CONSORTIA AND NETWORKS RELATED TO RESEARCH ON THE GENETIC AND ENVIRONMENTAL CAUSES OF TYPE 1 DIABETES

Evaluation of research consortia and networks supported by the *Special Diabetes Program* and related to Goal I is found in Appendix C. Highlights of these programs are summarized below.

Type 1 Diabetes Genetics Consortium (T1DGC): The T1DGC coordinates and implements research to identify the genes that affect a person's risk for type 1 diabetes. Since its establishment in 2001, the T1DGC has collected DNA samples, as well as clinical, genetic, and medical history data, from 38,000 individuals, including members of 2,800 families with two or more siblings with type 1 diabetes. The T1DGC operates four clinical recruitment networks in Asia-Pacific, Europe, North America, and the United Kingdom. Because of the efforts of the Consortium and other studies, scientists have identified nearly 50 genetic regions that contribute to the risk of type 1 diabetes—up from only three susceptibility genes that were known a decade ago.

The Environmental Determinants of Diabetes in the Young Study (TEDDY): The TEDDY study provides a coordinated, multidisciplinary approach to understanding the infectious agents, dietary factors, or other environmental conditions that trigger type 1 diabetes in genetically susceptible individuals. Six clinical sites located in the United States, Finland, Germany, and Sweden screened more than 425,000 infants to determine their level of genetic risk for type 1 diabetes. Study investigators enrolled and will monitor over 8,000 infants who have been found to be at high risk for type 1 diabetes until 15 years of age to determine if and when diabetes-related autoimmunity or type 1 diabetes begin. This ambitious, long-term study is critically important for informing the development of new prevention strategies.

Trial To Reduce IDDM in the Genetically At-Risk (TRIGR): TRIGR is an international clinical trial testing a dietary intervention to prevent type 1 diabetes in children with a high genetic risk of developing the disease. More than 2,160 infants enrolled in TRIGR have been randomly assigned to receive either extensively hydrolyzed infant formula or standard cow's milk-based formula after weaning. Researchers will monitor these infants until 10 years of age for signs of diabetes-related autoimmunity or type 1 diabetes to determine whether hydrolyzed formula decreases the risk of developing type 1 diabetes.

SEARCH for Diabetes in Youth (SEARCH): SEARCH is a multicenter epidemiological study to identify cases of and characterize diabetes in children and youth less than 20 years of age in six geographically dispersed populations that encompass the ethnic diversity of the United States. SEARCH has defined prevalence and incidence of diabetes in youth, which has provided the most comprehensive picture to date of rates of childhood diabetes in the United States. SEARCH is now poised to evaluate how rates of diabetes are changing over time and better characterize the natural history and risk factors for all forms of diabetes in children and youth.

Feature:
Critical Investment in Infrastructure for Type 1 Diabetes Research

The goals of identifying the causes of type 1 diabetes, and determining strategies for curing, reversing, treating, and preventing the disease are challenging ones. Specific research questions in type 1 diabetes require large-scale team efforts to address and complement investigator-initiated studies. In particular, determination of the numerous genetic contributors to type 1 diabetes, discovery of environmental triggers that influence development of the disease, characterization and nationwide surveillance of diabetes in children, and the conduct of clinical trials, especially for prevention of the disease, necessitate significant, coordinated efforts and infrastructure. The *Special Statutory Funding Program for Type 1 Diabetes Research* has enabled the establishment of extensive, collaborative clinical research networks that are carrying out unprecedented studies to accelerate the pace of research on type 1 diabetes. As examples, the four research consortia described below each have unique requirements for a large infrastructure to achieve these important goals. Results from these vital projects have the potential to revolutionize the health and quality of life of people with and at risk to develop type 1 diabetes.

Type 1 Diabetes Genetics Consortium (T1DGC)

Type 1 diabetes is not caused by a single gene; rather, variations in many genes can affect susceptibility to the disease and these variants can be rare within a population. In addition, unique variants may be present in different ethnic/racial populations. Therefore, to identify comprehensively and confidently all of the variants that affect risk of type 1 diabetes, genomes from a large number of ethnically diverse individuals need to be screened. In 2001, the T1DGC, led by NIDDK, was established with the overarching goal of searching through the genome to identify the genes that determine an individual's risk of developing type 1 diabetes. To collect the significant number of samples necessary, the consortium includes four international clinical recruitment networks in Asia-Pacific, Europe, North America, and the United Kingdom, as well as a coordinating center, autoantibody laboratory, and Human Leukocyte Antigen genotyping laboratory that collectively represent more than 200 individual recruitment sites and nearly 350 Consortium members.

The T1DGC has used its clinical infrastructure to recruit, screen, and collect DNA from a large cohort of families and individuals affected by type 1 diabetes. As of spring 2010, the T1DGC has recruited and taken biosamples from 2,800 Caucasian families with two or more siblings with type 1 diabetes, 500 trios (father, mother, and a child with type 1 diabetes), 600 cases (people with type 1 diabetes), and 700 controls (people with no history of type 1 diabetes). The participation of minority populations is particularly valuable as little information is currently available on the genetic causes of type 1 diabetes in these populations. As many minority populations have a low prevalence of type 1 diabetes, it is difficult to achieve sufficient numbers of participants. Recruitment of trios, cases, and controls is ongoing in these populations, including African Americans and Mexican Americans. The approximately 38,000 DNA samples collected to date and samples currently being collected by the T1DGC should provide sufficient statistical power to find not only common genetic variants that influence type 1 diabetes risk in many people but also rare risk variants that affect few individuals.

In addition to its clinical infrastructure, the T1DGC requires substantial resources for biosample processing, information technology, and database storage capacity. Generation, analysis, and storage of sequence information from the 38,000 collected DNA samples are not trivial, and the productive T1DGC continues to generate more data from these valuable DNA samples as new technologies become available. Already, the investment in the T1DGC infrastructure is paying off. The T1DGC and its collaborators have identified over 40 genes or gene regions associated with type 1 diabetes, bringing the total number of known regions to near 50—up from only three genes that were known a few years ago. This remarkable explosion in knowledge opens exciting new opportunities for the development of improved strategies to identify and profile individuals at risk who could benefit from future prevention efforts, and novel avenues for the discovery of therapies to prevent or reverse the disease. For more information on the T1DGC, please see the Investigator Profile of Dr. Stephen Rich in this chapter.

The Environmental Determinants of Diabetes in the Young (TEDDY)

Several potential environmental triggers of type 1 diabetes have been suggested, but none have been demonstrated conclusively to cause the disease. These, or any number of unknown environmental triggers, might interact with specific genetic factors to induce development of type 1 diabetes. Identifying the environmental factors that trigger the disease in genetically susceptible individuals requires a herculean effort of large numbers of volunteers, over 2 decades of dedication, and significant quantities of collected biosamples and data. The thousands of participants are needed to ensure that any observed links between environmental exposure and disease development are meaningful and not coincidence. Also, it is not known if or when the genetically susceptible participants will develop the disease; therefore, they are being followed in large numbers from newborn to 15 years of age. Finally, great quantities of biosamples and data are being collected to capture every potential exposure to an environmental trigger as it is unknown where this exposure will appear.

Launched in 2002, TEDDY, led by NIDDK, represents a coordinated, multidisciplinary effort to unravel this complex puzzle. It is an international consortium of six clinical centers located in the United States and three countries in Europe, as well as a data coordinating center. More than 45 staff members, including principal investigators, project managers, and study coordinators, are involved in this intensive, 20-year effort. To identify potential participants with specific genetic markers indicating a high risk of type 1 diabetes, TEDDY investigators drew a blood sample and sequenced DNA of nearly 419,000 newborns from the general population, as well as over 6,000 newborns who have a first degree relative with type 1 diabetes. Screening these 425,000 newborns identified over 20,000 genetically at-risk infants; the parents of over 8,000 of these infants chose to enroll their child in TEDDY. TEDDY completed enrollment in 2010 and is anticipated to continue through 2023.

Participation in TEDDY requires families to dedicate a significant investment of time and effort. Parents keep regular, detailed records of their child's diet, illnesses, allergies, and other life experiences. Every 3 months for 4 years, parents bring their child to a TEDDY clinic for a 60 to 90 minute visit that includes a blood draw. After 4 years, children are seen at the clinic every

6 months until the child turns 15 years of age or develops type 1 diabetes. Other biosamples, such as stool and nail clippings, are also collected by parents at regular intervals and shipped to the study sites. Some biosamples are analyzed immediately for evidence of autoantibodies that indicate the early stages of type 1 diabetes. Other specimens and data are being stored for future analysis after the investigators learn which children develop type 1 diabetes and which do not. This consortium is creating an unparalleled and invaluable collection of data and biosamples that has the potential to transform research on the causes and progression of type 1 diabetes and have an enormous impact on public health efforts to prevent the disease.

SEARCH for Diabetes in Youth (SEARCH)

Research and public health efforts on childhood diabetes have been hampered in the United States by the lack of national epidemiologic data. This type of data requires a large sample size to collect accurate information. It is necessary to collect this information from diverse populations as these data are likely to vary among racial/ethnic groups. To generate these critical data, the SEARCH study, led by CDC and co-supported by NIDDK, was initiated in 2000 with the overarching goal of characterizing diabetes in individuals less than 20 years of age. SEARCH collects data in six geographically dispersed locations across the country from a racially and ethnically diverse population that includes non-Hispanic white, Hispanic, African American, American Indian, and Asian/Pacific Islander children and youth.

Over 5 million individuals are under surveillance by SEARCH as they reside within a geographic area or participate in a health plan covered by one of the research centers. Children newly diagnosed with diabetes or their parents are invited to fill out an initial patient survey that requests basic information on the child's diagnosis, processes of care, and quality of life. To date, more than 12,000 youth or families have completed this 20-minute survey, and over 6,000 also participated in baseline in-person visits at SEARCH clinics. Each 1 to 3 hour visit included a physical exam, collection of blood and urine samples, measurement of C-peptide levels, and collection of data related to family medical history, quality of life, depression, diet, and other issues. Children are asked to return for follow-up clinical visits 1, 2, and 5 years later. It is necessary for SEARCH investigators to observe the same individuals over a substantial period of time to monitor disease progression and long-term outcomes in these children. Therefore, mailings are sent periodically to maintain contact with SEARCH participants and encourage them to remain in the study. The SEARCH study is being conducted by staff at six research centers, a coordinating center, and a central laboratory.

Through the committed efforts of its investigators and participants, SEARCH has generated an unprecedented understanding of type 1 and type 2 diabetes in children and youth in the United States. SEARCH has generated incidence and prevalence data for diabetes in children, including racial/ethnic data, and findings from SEARCH point to the need for better treatment strategies and technologies to improve diabetes management in children and youth. Investigators are capitalizing on the data collected by SEARCH to conduct 11 ancillary studies on novel research questions. For more information on the use of SEARCH data to inform understanding of heart-related complications of diabetes, see the Investigator Profile of Dr. Dana Dabelea in Goal V. The investment in large-scale infrastructure for SEARCH has produced substantial contributions to characterizing diabetes in American children and will continue to lead to a better understanding of the natural history, complications, and risk factors of diabetes in childhood and adolescence.

Type 1 Diabetes TrialNet (TrialNet)

TrialNet, led by NIDDK, supports the development and implementation of clinical trials of agents aimed at preventing type 1 diabetes in people at risk for the disease and slowing disease progression in people who are newly diagnosed. TrialNet's mission is carried out by a large, multidisciplinary network consisting of 18 clinical centers in North America, Europe, and Australia; more than 150 additional patient recruitment sites; a biostatistical coordinating center; a Chairman's office; and various core facilities including six laboratories and a central pharmacy. Without the TrialNet infrastructure, every investigator wanting to evaluate a new potential type 1 diabetes prediction model, screening methodology, or therapy for prevention or treatment would have to create and support a framework for recruiting, screening, treating, and monitoring hundreds (for new-onset trials) or tens of thousands (for prevention trials) of individuals. This approach would be prohibitively expensive and duplicative, and would possibly limit the comparison of scientific outcomes across studies due to the absence of standard laboratory procedures. The TrialNet infrastructure ultimately saves time and resources by facilitating the efficient and timely conduct of clinical trials.

The TrialNet Natural History Study (NHS) was created to identify risk factors for type 1 diabetes and document disease characteristics and progression. As of mid-2010, over 79,000 individuals with a close relative with type 1 diabetes have participated in the NHS by consenting to a blood test for the presence of autoantibodies predictive of the disease. TrialNet expects to screen about 20,000 individuals per year in the future. So far, nearly 2,000 individuals have been found to be autoantibody positive. At-risk individuals are invited to continue in the NHS by visiting a TrialNet clinic every 6 months. At each visit, researchers conduct a series of tests to evaluate the individual's risk factors and monitor progression to type 1 diabetes. The number of autoantibody-positive individuals (2,000) compared to the total number screened (79,000) underscores the need for large-scale infrastructure to implement the NHS. Only 3 to 4 percent of relatives of people with type 1 diabetes have autoantibodies in their blood, and some autoantibody positive individuals never progress to diabetes. So, many geographically dispersed sites are needed to recruit, screen, and monitor the at-risk population—this research could not be done by an individual site.

At-risk or newly diagnosed individuals are invited to participate in clinical trials of new therapies for prevention or new-onset intervention. To date, approximately 200 individuals identified through the NHS and over 700 additional individuals with type 1 diabetes (mostly new-onset) have enrolled in TrialNet intervention trials. TrialNet has supported five trials of promising interventions in people newly diagnosed with type 1 diabetes and two prevention trials in individuals at risk for the development of the disease. TrialNet plans to launch one additional intervention trial in newly diagnosed individuals and two additional prevention trials in at-risk individuals in 2010 and 2011. In 2009, TrialNet reported that a drug targeting B lymphocytes in the immune system preserved the function of insulin-producing beta cells in people newly diagnosed with type 1 diabetes. The finding suggests that targeting these immune cells can be used as a strategy to prevent or treat type 1 diabetes. For more information on this study, see the

Investigator Profile of Dr. Mark Pescovitz in Goal II. The infrastructure developed by TrialNet allows clinical trials to be launched quickly and conducted efficiently. This ensures that promising therapies and preventative strategies are tested, and that the investment in basic research, as well as the investment in TrialNet, is fully maximized.

Coordination of Infrastructure and Resources for Type 1 Diabetes Research

To extend and capitalize on research infrastructure and resources supported by the *Special Diabetes Program*, NIH and CDC have made a concerted effort to promote collaboration and coordination across research groups. These interactions have been particularly important and fruitful among the consortia charged with understanding the etiology and epidemiology of type 1 diabetes. For example, TEDDY and the Trial to Reduce IDDM in the Genetically at-Risk (TRIGR) both required massive international screening programs to identify newborns with a high degree of genetic risk for type 1 diabetes. Thus, TEDDY and TRIGR implemented similar standards for data collection, quality control, and analysis so that results obtained in each study can be directly compared. In another example, all TrialNet sites and four SEARCH centers served as recruitment centers for T1DGC, allowing eligible individuals with type 1 diabetes to contribute to multiple research studies. Additional information on collaboration across consortia can be found in Appendix D.

Conclusion

In 1983, the NIH began the 10-year landmark Diabetes Control and Complications Trial (DCCT) with 1,441 volunteers. The DCCT ultimately demonstrated that intensive insulin therapy to control blood glucose could dramatically reduce the risk of complications of the eyes,

kidneys, and nerves in people with type 1 diabetes. Since 1994, researchers have continued to monitor the health of about 95 percent of the DCCT participants in the follow-up Epidemiology of Diabetes Interventions and Complications (EDIC) study to determine the impact of intensive insulin therapy on complications that take longer to manifest. The long-term duration of this effort enabled EDIC to show, among other results, that intensive blood glucose control reduces the risk of cardiovascular complications of type 1 diabetes and that the benefits of intensive control in reducing eye, nerve, and kidney disease extended long after the trial was completed. Moreover, insights from this trial established biomarkers that the U.S. Food and Drug Administration has used to approve multiple classes of medications for type 2 diabetes and is considering for approval of new therapeutics to preserve beta cell function in type 1 diabetes. Thus, for more than a quarter of a century, NIH investment in the DCCT/EDIC studies has continued to yield unique and important scientific insights that have changed the standard of care for daily management of type 1 diabetes. Because type 1 diabetes is a chronic disease that progresses at variable rates in individuals over the course of decades, these landmark discoveries would not have been possible without NIH's commitment to long-term support of DCCT/EDIC at a scale that permitted statistically significant outcomes to be achieved.

Likewise, the T1DGC, TEDDY, SEARCH, and TrialNet consortia, all supported by significant resources and investment from the *Special Diabetes Program*, offer exceptional opportunities to accelerate the pace of scientific discovery related to type 1 diabetes. These challenging projects require large scales, long durations, and substantial efforts to complete. The investment in infrastructure by the *Special Diabetes Program* is not limited to clinical research, but also includes basic research studies critical to the development of new therapeutics. For example, the Beta Cell Biology Consortium (BCBC) brings together over 50 multidisciplinary principal investigators and over 200 affiliates to work collaboratively toward the development of cell replacement therapy as a potential cure for type 1 diabetes. The goal of cell replacement therapy requires addressing both the developmental biology of the insulin-producing beta cell as well as modulation of the immune system to prevent an immune attack on the newly introduced cells and therefore benefits from a multidisciplinary team approach (more information on the BCBC can be found in Goal III and Appendix C).

The investment to date in these infrastructures ensures that this research can be carried out in the most scientifically productive manner. Benefits of the NIH investment in these consortia have already been realized and are expected to accrue for years to come as new technologies are developed and new insights emerge. Importantly, the time and efforts of tens of thousands of dedicated volunteers affected by type 1 diabetes have been instrumental to the success of these consortia. With sustained involvement by NIH, researchers, and volunteers, T1DGC, TEDDY, SEARCH, and TrialNet have the potential to shift existing paradigms of type 1 diabetes prediction, prevention, and treatment, benefitting individuals who are living with or at risk for type 1 diabetes and improving public health.

Investigator Profile

Stephen S. Rich, Ph.D.

Making Unprecedented Contributions to the Genetics of Type 1 Diabetes

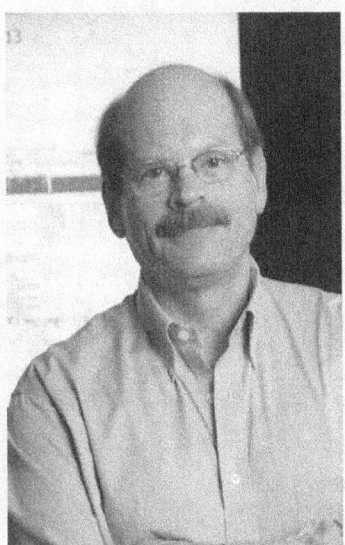

Stephen S. Rich, Ph.D.

Stephen S. Rich, Ph.D., is a Professor of Public Health Sciences at the University of Virginia School of Medicine. Since 2002, Dr. Rich has served as Chair of the Steering Committee and Director of the coordinating center of the Type 1 Diabetes Genetics Consortium (T1DGC), which is led by NIDDK and supported by the Special Statutory Funding Program for Type 1 Diabetes Research. The T1DGC aims to organize and implement international efforts to identify genes that determine an individual's risk of developing type 1 diabetes. This profile describes the unparalleled resources created by the T1DGC and how those resources are being used by Dr. Rich and other investigators to uncover the genetic causes of type 1 diabetes.

A 30-Year Commitment to Research on the Genetics of Type 1 Diabetes

In 1980, Dr. Rich began his academic career as a faculty member at the University of Minnesota working on a project related to the genetics of type 1 diabetes. At the time, Dr. Rich notes, "We knew very little about the disease and the genetics of it. So, this was a very new, emerging field." Researchers had shown through studies of twins that the risk of developing type 1 diabetes is heavily influenced by genes—identical twins have about a 40 percent risk[20] of developing type 1 diabetes if their twin already has the disease compared to about 0.2 percent risk[21] in the general population. In the mid-1970s, other scientists had found that type 1 diabetes is triggered by an autoimmune reaction and that genes of the HLA (Human Leukocyte Antigen) system are associated with risk for type 1 diabetes. Over roughly the next 15 years, Dr. Rich and other genetics researchers identified other genes involved in type 1 diabetes risk—namely, the *insulin*, *CTLA4*, and *PTPN22* genes. Still, researchers knew that many more genes affecting type 1 diabetes risk had yet to be discovered.

A turning point in the field of type 1 diabetes genetic research occurred in the late 1990s. Scientists from around the world with an interest in this subject met in Denmark at a meeting sponsored, in part, by NIDDK and JDRF. "We realized that part of our problem was lack of available clinical resources, data resources, and the ability to leverage emergent technology," says Dr. Rich. "We decided that instead of a group of investigators working individually and perhaps in competition with each other with limited resources, why not form a group of investigators working along the same path?" Dr. Rich

---

20 Rich SS: Mapping genes in diabetes: genetic epidemiological perspective. <u>Diabetes</u> 39: 1315-1319, 1990.
21 SEARCH for Diabetes in Youth Study Group, et al: The burden of diabetes mellitus among US youth: prevalence estimates from the SEARCH for Diabetes in Youth Study. <u>Pediatrics</u> 118: 1510-1518, 2006.

accepted primary responsibility for writing the grant application that resulted in funding for and creation of the T1DGC. Subsequently, as chair of the T1DGC Steering Committee, Dr. Rich has worked to build consensus on the scientific directions and methods of the Consortium and overseen general operations.

Scientists and Families Working Together To Combat Type 1 Diabetes

The T1DGC represented a new paradigm of collaboration in the field of genetics research for type 1 diabetes. Dr. Rich points out that the Consortium made it possible to conduct research studies that could not have been accomplished in individual laboratories. He emphasizes, "No one investigator typically has the resources to collect an adequate number of samples to robustly investigate [genetic] risk. No one investigator typically has sufficient numbers of people who can clinically phenotype patients or perform the genetic analyses in a genome-wide, robust, unbiased way. No individual investigator typically would have the analytic, bioinformatic, and informatic infrastructure to handle this type of data." Moreover, the collaborative nature of the T1DGC gave researchers an opportunity to openly discuss complex problems with other leaders in the field without concerns about scientific competition.

T1DGC investigators recognized early on that the success of the Consortium's mission would rely not only on the willingness of scientists to work together but also on the voluntary participation of sufficient numbers of families affected by type 1 diabetes. Researchers estimated that genetic material would need to be collected from 4,000 families with at least two siblings affected by type 1 diabetes ("affected sib-pair families") in order to identify all genes that have a major effect on type 1 diabetes risk. After pooling samples that some investigators had

already collected, the T1DGC would need to recruit at least 2,800 additional affected sib-pair families from around the world.

From the beginning, the T1DGC was sensitive to the concerns that potential participants in a genetics study might have regarding ethics, social and legal issues, and protection of their individual rights. Because those concerns differ not only across the United States, but also among different countries, the international T1DGC made a concerted effort to be transparent about the nature of the study and the rights of individual participants. Dr. Rich observes that these efforts paid off in terms of families' willingness to contribute their DNA to the T1DGC study, noting that "The overall impact on the research by the participation of these individuals has been phenomenal. Even though it was an extraordinarily hard task to identify 2,800 families to provide this [T1DGC] resource, whenever they've been identified, they've been willing to participate. And, I think part of this is the transparency and the understanding of the [participants'] needs and expectations."

A New Resource for Research on the Genetics of Type 1 Diabetes

According to Dr. Rich, a major accomplishment of the T1DGC has been the assembly of an unprecedented collection of material and data for research on the genetic causes of type 1 diabetes. In addition to the newly collected 2,800 sib-pair families, the Consortium has collected genetic materials from a large number of unrelated individuals with type 1 diabetes, as well as from individuals without the disease. Importantly, materials have been collected in populations that are thought to be at lower risk for type 1 diabetes, such as those of African American or Mexican American ancestry, in which little is known about the genetic causes of type 1 diabetes.

These materials, along with data from the genetic analyses conducted with the samples, are all available to the scientific community through the NIDDK repositories. In this way, Dr. Rich says, "The funding of the T1DGC is exponentially multiplied in terms of the leverage and the use of the materials that the [NIH] provided. People can access collections of DNA, plasma, and serum to perform additional studies without their having to invest in [collecting their own samples]."

The rapid evolution of technologies for genetic and genomic research that occurred over the past decade has made the T1DGC collection even more valuable than originally envisioned. Better technology, accompanied by a dramatic reduction in the cost of genotyping, allowed T1DGC researchers to accomplish their original goal of identifying all genes or gene regions that have a major effect on type 1 diabetes risk and also to search for genes that have a modest or small effect on risk. To date, the T1DGC and its collaborators have identified over 40 genes or gene regions associated with type 1 diabetes, bringing the total number of known regions to near 50—a far cry from the 3 genes that were known a decade ago when the Consortium was first envisioned.

"My feeling personally is that by having a type 1 diabetes genetics consortium, we've probably reduced the time that it may take to really identify the genetic bases of type 1 diabetes not by the 5-10 years that the consortium has been in existence, but probably by 20 years simply because we've been able to assemble the resources and make them available to everyone," stresses Dr. Rich.

Looking to the Future

The T1DGC directly examined differences at individual base pairs—called single nucleotide polymorphisms—to identify genes that influence type 1 diabetes risk. In addition, NIH solicits and supports research proposals from individual investigators to make use of the T1DGC collection for novel genetic studies. In fiscal year 2009, Dr. Rich and his collaborators were awarded two of five grants from NIDDK and with support from the *Special Diabetes Program* aimed at building on the T1DGC findings by fine-mapping and functional analysis of genetic and genomic contributors to type 1 diabetes risk. Dr. Rich's group is looking for structural variations in the genome, such as duplications, insertions, deletions, or rearrangements of DNA segments, that could contribute to risk. Other funded investigators are exploring the role of variants in gene expression or epigenetic modifications to the DNA in type 1 diabetes risk. Now that the T1DGC and its collaborators have identified the genes and genetic regions involved in type 1 diabetes, this new research will help us to understand how they exert their effects.

The T1DGC collection contains a renewable resource—existing clinical and genetic data as well as immortalized cell lines created for most participants supply unlimited amounts of DNA for analysis. Thus, valuable scientific insights resulting from the T1DGC collection will continue to accrue in the future as technologies for genetic research evolve. As Dr. Rich observes, "The T1DGC has been extraordinarily successful in performing genetic studies and providing resources to the scientific community. But, the resources themselves are not finite in their utility. They are going to be critically important for the next phase of genetic research in type 1 diabetes." Thus, the collaboration and vision of the T1DGC investigators, coupled with the willing participation of thousands of people affected by diabetes, have transformed type 1 diabetes genetics research from the emerging, undeveloped field that Dr. Rich first entered 30 years ago to a vibrant field of research that continues to expand our understanding of the genetic risk factors and biochemical pathways involved in type 1 diabetes.

Patient Profile

Nilia Olsen

Participating in TEDDY To Identify What Triggers Type 1 Diabetes in Children

Four-year-old Nilia Olsen has no idea she's participating in a study that has determined she has an elevated risk for developing type 1 diabetes. She just knows that, every 3 months, she goes to the doctor's office to have her blood drawn, and, of all things, "she loves it," says her mom, Sonya.

"She likes the different colors on the tops of the vials," says Sonya, referring to the collection vials for blood samples. "Her favorite color is pink, so she likes to fill that one up first."

Nilia is one of over 8,000 children participating in The Environmental Determinants of Diabetes in the Young study, otherwise known as TEDDY. TEDDY is led by the NIDDK and supported by the *Special Statutory Funding Program for Type 1 Diabetes Research*. The international study's long-term goal is to try to identify infectious agents, dietary factors, or other environmental agents, including psychosocial factors, that trigger type 1 diabetes in genetically susceptible individuals or protect against the disease.

But such details don't concern Nilia right now. She's a typical little girl who attends pre-school, likes to dress up—as well as dig for worms. "She's high energy," her mother laughs.

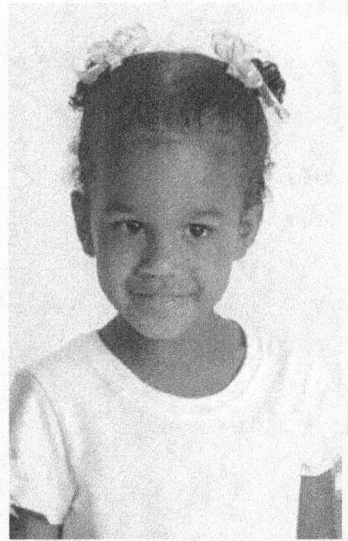

Nilia Olsen

About the TEDDY Study

Researchers have discovered that children who develop type 1 diabetes have certain kinds of "high-risk" genes. Analyzing DNA from Nilia's blood shortly after she was born indicated that she was genetically at high risk to develop the disease. Researchers also know that some children with high-risk genes develop type 1 diabetes, while others don't. This has led them to think that something in the environment "triggers" or causes a child with high-risk genes to actually get type 1 diabetes. The purpose of TEDDY, therefore, is to try to identify the environmental triggers that cause children to get the disease. TEDDY has enrolled genetically susceptible newborns into the study from two populations: those with a sibling or parent with type 1 diabetes, and those from the general population with no family history of the disease. Nilia falls into the general population group because she has no family history of type 1 diabetes.

Like Nilia, the other children in this study, all of whom were identified within 3 months of their birth as being at high genetic risk for developing type 1 diabetes, will be followed until age 15. During that time, information will be collected about their diets, illnesses, allergies, and other life experiences. Blood samples will be collected every 3 months and stool samples will be collected monthly for the first 4 years. After 4 years, these samples will be collected every 6 months until the children turn 15 years old. Parents are also asked to fill out questionnaires at regular intervals, and to record events, such as illnesses, in the child's "TEDDY Book."

From these numerous samples and other information collected about the children, researchers hope to identify a factor or factors that lead some genetically predisposed children to develop type 1 diabetes while others do not. This information is critically important for identifying strategies for disease prevention. For example, if a virus were found to trigger type 1 diabetes, a vaccine could possibly be developed. If a dietary factor were found to be causative, then changes to children's diets could be made.

It is only through the dedicated efforts of families, such as the Olsen family, that the TEDDY study could be conducted. Responsibilities such as making regular doctor's visits for blood draws, taking monthly stool samples for 4 years, and keeping detailed notebooks with information about their child's health is no small task. It is clear that TEDDY families are dedicated to the study and its goals. This commitment can reap major rewards if an environmental trigger is discovered, which could pave the way toward being able to prevent type 1 diabetes and help future generations of children.

One Family's Experience with the TEDDY Study

The day after Nilia was born, Sonya was asked if her daughter's blood could be sampled for a study to see if the child had an elevated risk for type 1 diabetes. Although there is no history of type 1 diabetes in the family, Sonya was aware that nearly all of the women on her father's side have type 2 diabetes (formerly called adult-onset diabetes). Sonya immediately agreed and enrolled Nilia into TEDDY when researchers found that Nilia carried high-risk genes for type 1 diabetes.

"I don't have diabetes, and neither does my husband, Thomas," says Sonya. Thomas is in the military and was deployed to Iraq on his second tour of duty in October 2009. Beyond her daughter's increased genetic risk for type 1 diabetes, Sonya says that an additional motivation for her to enroll Nilia into TEDDY was "knowing that type 2 diabetes runs on my father's side of the family." Both forms of diabetes can lead to serious health complications.

At the time this profile was written, it's been 4 years since Nilia's blood was originally sampled, and although it was discovered that she has an elevated risk for developing type 1 diabetes, fortunately she remains diabetes-free. Sonya says that knowing Nilia has an elevated risk "was something that as a family we knew we would take in stride." Not only have they taken it in stride, they have remained dedicated to contributing to an important research study that can lead to new ways to prevent type 1 diabetes. According to TEDDY staff, Sonya has always gone the extra mile to do everything she could for TEDDY research, including participating in optional fun events designed to build community among local TEDDY families. However, the Olsen family lived in Augusta, Georgia, when Nilia first entered the study. Since then, the family has been transferred by the military to Alabama. "The study staff has been very flexible," says Sonya. "We do everything through the mail. Every time Nilia's blood and stool samples get tested, they mail us the results. It's great. The continuity provides us with a sense of peace."

"I would strongly encourage other families to participate in clinical trials like TEDDY," says Sonya. "Knowing that our daughter is in a trial like TEDDY gives us a great deal of peace of mind."

As with all other study participants, the Olsen family was provided a calendar, "and we record whenever Nilia goes to the doctor," says Sonya. "We write down when she's sick and what kind of medication she may be taking. We record if she goes to the hospital." But so far, according to Sonya, Nilia has not had any hospitalizations or health issues related to diabetes. As for filling out the calendar and other paperwork related to the study, "It's not difficult, at all," says Sonya. "It just takes a few minutes to record."

Nilia may be a big reason the family is able to cope so well. At age 4, she is proving to be a real trooper when it comes to participating in the study. "Whenever she goes to the bathroom, she asks if she needs to poop in the cup," Sonya says, with a slight laugh. "And she's really good at having her blood drawn. She never cries about it and never has." In fact, Nilia is so good about having her blood drawn that she is featured in a video about blood draws for TEDDY that has been distributed to other TEDDY sites.

"I would strongly encourage other families to participate in clinical trials like TEDDY," says Sonya. "Knowing that our daughter is in a trial like TEDDY gives us a great deal of peace of mind."

Nilia's father, Thomas, calls home once a week from Iraq and asks how Nilia is doing. "It pleases me to be able to tell him she's doing well."

EMERGING RESEARCH OPPORTUNITIES RESULTING FROM THE *SPECIAL DIABETES PROGRAM*

The *Special Statutory Funding Program for Type 1 Diabetes Research* has fueled the emergence of a wide range of research opportunities. These opportunities were identified in a strategic planning process as being critically important for overcoming current barriers and achieving progress in diabetes research. Key questions and research opportunities relevant to type 1 diabetes, including those related to identifying the genetic and environmental causes of type 1 diabetes, are outlined in Appendix F.

GOAL II

PREVENT OR REVERSE TYPE 1 DIABETES

The *Special Statutory Funding Program for Type 1 Diabetes Research* has enabled the establishment of large-scale, collaborative research groups and clinical trials networks that are identifying and testing novel type 1 diabetes prevention and reversal strategies. In addition to the significant research progress described in this chapter, information on the program evaluation related to Goal II can be found in Appendix A (Allocation of Funds), Appendix B (Assessment), and Appendix C (Evaluation of Major Research Consortia, Networks, and Resources).

Attempts have been made for nearly 3 decades to turn advances in understanding the autoimmune basis for type 1 diabetes into a cure. Progress in the last decade has been fueled by support from the *Special Statutory Funding Program for Type 1 Diabetes Research (Special Diabetes Program* or *Program)*. In just the past several years, scientists have learned a great deal about the immune system and how its normally protective functions go awry in type 1 diabetes and other autoimmune diseases. New discoveries and technologies have led to better understanding of beta cell development and biology (Goal III), steps forward toward imaging beta cells and autoimmunity in living animals and potentially people (Goal VI), and more effective and safer ways to intervene in the autoimmune process (Goal II). These advances have accelerated other clinical efforts to develop therapeutic approaches to prevent or reverse type 1 diabetes, as discussed in this chapter.

Type 1 diabetes is an autoimmune disease that results when the body's own immune system launches a misguided attack on the insulin-producing beta cells in the pancreas. Harmful immune system cells, including some T cells, are normally eliminated during their maturation or regulated thereafter. However, in susceptible individuals, these disease-causing T cells evade elimination or regulation and initiate an inflammatory process in the pancreas that eventually leads to the destruction of beta cells. The initiation of autoimmunity is marked by the appearance of pancreas protein-specific antibodies made by autoreactive B cells. These "autoantibodies" are well-established markers that predict a person's risk of developing type 1 diabetes. Tests of these antibodies together with tests for genes affecting type 1 diabetes risk in the siblings or offspring of people with type 1 diabetes can predict with great reliability whether the unaffected relatives will develop the disease. This predictive tool, coupled with other new technologies, has given researchers the remarkable ability to design and conduct primary prevention clinical trials.

Graphic: Computer model image of antibodies—proteins that the body's immune system produces to protect itself from foreign substances. In people with type 1 diabetes, the immune system produces antibodies against insulin-producing cells in the pancreas. Image credit: Kenneth Eward/Photo Researchers, Inc.

HIGHLIGHTS OF RECENT RESEARCH ADVANCES RELATED TO GOAL II

Rituximab Slows Progression of Type 1 Diabetes in Newly Diagnosed Patients: Researchers in Type 1 Diabetes TrialNet (TrialNet) reported that the drug rituximab slowed the decline of the function of insulin-producing beta cells in people newly diagnosed with type 1 diabetes. Rituximab destroys B cells of the immune system and has been approved by the U.S. Food and Drug Administration (FDA) for treatment of B cell non-Hodgkin's lymphoma and some autoimmune disorders, such as rheumatoid arthritis. Because B cells are thought to play a role in type 1 diabetes, scientists tested whether four separate infusions of rituximab shortly after diagnosis could slow disease progression. After 1 year, people who had received the drug produced more insulin, had better control of their diabetes, and did not have to take as much insulin to control their blood glucose levels, compared to people receiving placebo. The finding will propel research to find drugs targeting the specific B cells involved in type 1 diabetes because drugs such as rituximab that broadly deplete B cells can increase the risk of infection.

***Deaf1* Gene May Play a Role in Type 1 Diabetes:** Scientists in the Cooperative Study Group for Autoimmune Disease Prevention identified a gene that may play a role in the development of type 1 diabetes. In a mouse model of the disease, scientists found that cells in the animals' pancreatic lymph nodes make two forms of a gene called *Deaf1*. One form encodes full-length, functional Deaf1 protein, while the other encodes a shorter, nonfunctional variant form. Additional experiments in mice suggested that the functional form of Deaf1 may control the production of molecules needed to eliminate immune cells that can destroy insulin-producing cells in the pancreas, thus preventing type 1 diabetes. Researchers also found that levels of the variant form of Deaf1 were higher in people with type 1 diabetes compared to levels in people without the disease. The research suggests that the development of type 1 diabetes may in part be due to increased levels of the Deaf1 variant protein in pancreatic lymph nodes, which may, in turn, lead to reduced production of molecules that are required to "educate" the immune system not to attack the body's own cells, including the insulin-producing cells of the pancreas.

New Markers Discovered for Identifying Type 1 Diabetes-susceptible Individuals Prior to Disease Onset: Scientists in the Beta Cell Biology Consortium (BCBC) discovered a new autoantibody that is an excellent additional marker for identifying pre-clinical type 1 diabetes, and improves the ability to predict disease when combined with previously known autoantibodies. With the discovery of this fourth major autoantibody, called ZnT8, and analysis of large cohorts of children, autoantibody prediction of type 1 diabetes risk continues to gather strength, with increasing evidence for its feasibility both for relatives and, more importantly, for the general population. Approximately 1 million Americans express multiple autoantibodies targeting islet proteins and are at high risk of progression to type 1 diabetes. Prediction using autoantibodies, combined with increasing refinement of genetic and metabolic prediction, sets the stage for prevention trials at multiple stages of the disease.

Elucidating Mechanisms Underlying Tolerance: Type 1 diabetes is thought to arise from a defect in immune tolerance, the "normal" state in which the immune system is non-reactive to healthy cells and tissues. Scientists have learned much about the cellular and molecular mechanisms controlling tolerance induction in recent years. In particular, some gene expression regulators (transcription factors, *e.g.*, Foxp3) are important for the proper function of regulatory T cells, which suppress misdirected immune responses, while other transcription factors (*e.g.*, Aire) function to allow the removal of autoreactive T cells during development. Other factors known to be important for tolerance induction or maintenance include those involved in immune cell signaling or modulating immune responses (co-stimulatory molecules and cytokines); the biology of regulatory T cells; and the function of dendritic cells, a type of antigen presenting cell, in the process. This knowledge has enabled the design of several successful strategies for imposing a state of tolerance for example, to transplantation antigens in normal rodents, but this has proven to be much more challenging for restoring self-tolerance in rodent models of diabetes. Numerous observations suggest that similar deficiencies in tolerance induction play an important role in human type 1 diabetes, including the association between alleles of the gene encoding insulin (Ins gene), their expression level in the thymic stroma (where removal of autoreactive T cells takes place), and diabetes incidence; the development of diabetes in patients with mutations in the *AIRE* and *FOXP3* genes; and the observations of defective regulation of activated T cells by regulatory T cells in type 1 diabetes patients. These findings are helping pave the way to future approaches that could restore a state of immune tolerance in people with type 1 diabetes.

Development of Sophisticated Mouse Models of Human Disease for Study of Type 1 Diabetes: Increasingly sophisticated stocks of mice modeling human disease have been developed that could provide the means to understand clinically relevant components of type 1 diabetes pathogenesis. These particular mouse models are mice that are either engrafted with functional human cells or tissues, genetically engineered to express human genes, or both, and can recapitulate aspects of the pathogenic process. These mice have been used to identify targets of the human immune response against transplanted islet cells, and have led to insights into the destructive cell populations that are important to this process. Mice engrafted with functional human immune systems may permit certain human immune responses, including autoimmune responses, to be manipulated in small animal models. As these types of studies cannot be done in people, such mouse models could facilitate the conduct of important translational research, providing insights into safety and efficacy before enrolling participants into clinical trials.

PREVENTING TYPE 1 DIABETES

A major goal of type 1 diabetes research is to identify strategies to prevent the disease. Ideally, effective interventions to prevent type 1 diabetes should selectively inhibit harmful immune processes, without the need for lifelong suppression of the patient's entire immune system. One major trial that tested a novel prevention strategy and laid the foundation for future clinical trials was the Diabetes Prevention Trial–Type 1 (DPT-1), which was conducted from 1994 to 2003. The trial tested whether insulin administered orally or by injection could prevent type 1 diabetes in relatives of people with the disease. Although the DPT-1 prevention strategies did not prove generally effective, a subset of trial participants who had higher levels of insulin autoantibodies seemed to benefit from oral insulin treatment, though this result was not definitive.

Importantly, the researchers' estimates of risk for disease based on genetic and antibody tests proved to be remarkably accurate. DPT-1 thus demonstrated that it is possible to identify people at risk for type 1 diabetes based on genetic evaluation and tests of antibodies in blood. It also showed that trials requiring massive screening efforts—tens of thousands of people— and involving intensive treatment regimens could be efficiently accomplished.

Testing Prevention Strategies in Type 1 Diabetes TrialNet: The accomplishments of the DPT-1 laid the foundation for current research efforts to prevent the disease. DPT-1 served as the prototype for the present-day Type 1 Diabetes TrialNet, which completed the oral insulin arm of the DPT-1. TrialNet is a large, multidisciplinary, international network established to screen relatives of people with type 1 diabetes for their risk of developing disease and to support the creation and implementation of clinical trials of agents to slow progression of and/or prevent the disease. TrialNet receives support from the *Special Diabetes Program* and is led by NIDDK in collaboration with NIAID, NICHD, NCRR, NCCAM, JDRF, and ADA.

TrialNet is building on the results of the DPT-1 that suggested that oral insulin may prevent or delay type 1 diabetes in people with high levels of insulin autoantibodies. TrialNet developed a new clinical trial to test oral insulin administration in this subset of people. The trial, which requires screening large numbers of people, was started in 2007. Because of the huge effort and expense involved in finding high-risk individuals for prevention studies, a promising strategy is to study the prevention potential of drugs that slow disease progression in individuals newly diagnosed with type 1 diabetes. Thus, TrialNet is developing a prevention trial

with an agent called anti-CD3, which targets the immune system and previously has been shown to slow disease progression in people newly diagnosed with type 1 diabetes. Another prevention trial plans to test whether injections of a bioengineered form of a protein made by the insulin-producing beta cells, called glutamic acid decarboxylase (GAD), could prevent the disease in at-risk people. This trial is under development and anticipated to start after more safety data are available in children newly diagnosed with type 1 diabetes. TrialNet also completed a pilot trial testing whether omega-3 fatty acid supplements could affect an immune marker in babies who have a relative with type 1 diabetes. While measurable differences in omega-3 fatty acids were achieved, there was no difference in the immune marker studied, so a full trial will not be launched.

Testing Dietary Intervention To Prevent Type 1 Diabetes: Another important prevention trial supported by the *Special Diabetes Program* is the Trial to Reduce IDDM in the Genetically At Risk, or TRIGR, which began in 2001 and is expected to be completed in 2017 (also see information about TRIGR in Goal I). TRIGR is led by NICHD in collaboration with NIDDK, as well as the JDRF and several other non-federal sources. TRIGR has completed recruitment of newborns into this study, which is testing whether weaning infants to an extensively hydrolyzed formula, as compared to standard cow's milk formula, will reduce the risk of developing type 1 diabetes-predictive antibodies and, ultimately, type 1 diabetes. The design of the TRIGR study was based on both animal studies and a pilot study in humans. The pilot study included 242 children at high risk for the development of type 1 diabetes; data from the study showed that levels of autoantibodies predictive of type 1 diabetes were lower in children who received the intervention formula—the extensively hydrolyzed formula—compared to children fed conventional formula. Based on those results, and on similar observations made in animal studies, the large-scale TRIGR trial was launched. If TRIGR shows that a dietary modification in infancy could reduce type 1 diabetes, it would have a significant positive impact on patient care.

PRESERVING FUNCTION OF INSULIN-PRODUCING BETA CELLS AND REVERSING TYPE 1 DIABETES

For people who have already developed type 1 diabetes, reversing or slowing beta cell loss is a key goal because prevention is no longer possible. It was historically thought that people diagnosed with type 1 diabetes did not have any functional beta cells, but research has demonstrated that, at disease onset, 10-20 percent of people's beta cells remain.[22] The basis for immune intervention in type 1 diabetes is to suppress autoimmunity in order to "rescue" the remaining beta cells from immune destruction. The goal of preserving beta cell function is very important because data from NIDDK's landmark Diabetes Control and Complications Trial (DCCT) showed that people whose pancreas continued to produce some insulin had better diabetes control, less hypoglycemia, and reduced rates of disease complications. Preserving remaining beta cells may also allow for the possibility for patients to regrow pancreatic tissue. Research supported by the *Special Diabetes Program* is also pursuing strategies to coax new beta cell formation in the pancreas (see Goal III).

Testing Therapies in Newly Diagnosed Patients in TrialNet: Because of the importance of preserving beta

cell function and possibly reversing disease, the *Special Diabetes Program* vigorously supports research toward these goals. For example, TrialNet has supported five trials testing therapies in newly diagnosed patients. In 2009, TrialNet reported the result that the drug rituximab preserved the function of insulin-producing beta cells in people newly diagnosed with type 1 diabetes. Improved insulin production was maintained 1 year after the drug was administered. This drug had been approved by FDA for treatment of certain cancers and autoimmune disorders. It was historically believed that therapies to combat type 1 diabetes should focus on the T cells of the immune system, which attack and destroy the insulin-producing beta cells. However, rituximab targets other cells of the immune system—B cells. Therapies targeting B cells had been tested in mouse models of type 1 diabetes, but they had not been tested in people. Thus, rituximab was the first drug targeting B cells to be tested in people. While the drug was only given transiently after onset of type 1 diabetes and the effect of rituximab had dissipated at 2 years, the observation that a therapy that targets B cells could preserve beta cell function in people is therefore a novel finding and suggests that other therapies to target B cells may be effective for type 1 diabetes prevention or early treatment.

In addition to testing rituximab, TrialNet is also testing the ability of other therapies to halt beta cell destruction in new-onset type 1 diabetes. Three clinical trials are ongoing testing a vaccine using a recombinant form of the beta cell protein GAD administered with the immune adjuvant alum; a drug called abatacept (which inhibits T cell activation); and early and intensive blood glucose

---

[22] Skyler JS and Marks JB: Immune Intervention. In *Diabetes Mellitus: A Fundamental and Clinical Text, 3rd Edition*, edited by LeRoith D, Taylor SI, and Olefsky JM (pp. 701-709). Philadelphia, PA: Lippincott Williams & Wilkins, 2004.

control using a closed-loop system shortly after disease onset. TrialNet also completed a trial testing the combination of two drugs (MMF/DZB) for treating newly diagnosed patients and found no effect on slowing beta cell loss.

Testing Therapies To Induce Tolerance in the Immune Tolerance Network: The *Special Diabetes Program* also supports the Immune Tolerance Network (ITN), which is an international group of researchers dedicated to evaluating therapies to reprogram harmful immune responses to reduce autoimmunity, allergy, and asthma; and to improve islet, kidney, and liver transplantation (see Goal III for ITN research related to islet transplantation). The ITN is led by NIAID in collaboration with JDRF and NIDDK through its oversight of the *Special Diabetes Program*; the Network also works closely with TrialNet. The ITN also carries out laboratory tests to understand how the body responds to treatments studied in clinical trials and to find better markers of immune function. The ITN is trying to move away from current approaches of suppressing the immune system, in which people take drugs for the rest of their lives and may encounter significant side effects. Rather, the ITN is looking to induce "tolerance," in which a short-term therapy re-educates the immune system so that it does not destroy the body's own cells. The focus of the ITN's current type 1 diabetes research portfolio is to preserve beta cell function in newly diagnosed patients. For example, the Network completed a Phase I clinical trial testing a novel vaccine (insulin-B chain peptide) and found that it elicited a detectable immune response in the patients. In addition, the ITN is building on the results of research showing that the anti-CD3 monoclonal antibody could preserve patients' beta cell function. The Network is testing whether multiple doses of anti-CD3 have

additional benefits. Other therapies being tested in newly-diagnosed patients include thymoglobulin, and IL-2 plus sirolimus.

CREATING A PIPELINE OF NEW THERAPIES FOR TYPE 1 DIABETES PREVENTION AND REVERSAL

The *Special Diabetes Program* has enabled the creation of a pipeline of therapeutic agents for testing in clinical trials and has also created the infrastructure to test them. As new knowledge is gained about the underpinnings of disease development, more strategies for disease prevention and reversal will be identified, which will feed into this critically important pipeline made possible by the *Program*. For example, the TEDDY study (see Goal I) is examining environmental triggers of type 1 diabetes. If scientists identify a possible environmental trigger, such as a dietary factor, then researchers in clinical trials networks, such as TrialNet, could test the ability of that factor to prevent disease in at-risk people. The *Special Diabetes Program* also supports pre-clinical research resources that foster translational research from the bench to the bedside. For example, the Type 1 Diabetes-Rapid Access to Intervention Development (T1D-RAID) program helps scientists ready agents for testing in clinical trials to bridge basic research discoveries with clinical trials in people.

This research pipeline has already resulted in the movement of therapies from discovery in the laboratory to clinical trials. For example, researchers in the Non-human Primate Transplantation Tolerance Cooperative Study Group (see Goal III), which is supported by the *Special Diabetes Program* and led by NIAID, demonstrated long-term survival of islets after transplantation when the animals were given a novel mixture of medicines that target the immune system. Based on those findings, the ITN approved a clinical trial to test this therapy in newly diagnosed type 1 diabetes patients, to determine if the medicines can slow progression of disease. The T1D-RAID program is generating the medicines for use in the trial. This example demonstrates how the *Special Diabetes Program* supports the discovery, manufacture, and testing of promising therapeutic agents—creating a robust pipeline of agents that can improve the health of people with type 1 diabetes.

IMPROVING PREDICTIVE ABILITIES AND THE ABILITY TO CONDUCT TRIALS ON TYPE 1 DIABETES PREVENTION AND REVERSAL

Clinical trials to test type 1 diabetes prevention strategies require screening large numbers of people to identify at-risk individuals. For example, scientists in the DPT-1 screened about 100,000 relatives of people with type 1 diabetes to enroll 372 into the study—an undertaking that was both time- and resource-intensive. In addition, TrialNet plans to screen 20,000 people annually to identify those who are eligible to enroll in prevention trials.

The *Special Diabetes Program* supports a broad range of research to streamline this process by improving methods to assess risk and identify people who may benefit from prevention therapies. Researchers have made progress in identifying novel markers of the disease process in order to improve the ability to identify people at risk. For example, scientists in the BCBC (see Goal III), which is supported by the *Special Diabetes Program*, discovered that antibodies to a protein called ZnT8 are an excellent marker for pre-clinical type 1 diabetes and

greatly improve predictive abilities when combined with previously identified disease markers. Some research studies supported by the *Special Diabetes Program* are now screening for the presence of these antibodies in people in their studies. Identification of new type 1 diabetes susceptibility genes by the Type 1 Diabetes Genetics Consortium (see Goal I) can also pave the way toward using those new genes to improve predictive abilities. The efforts to improve predictive abilities are not only important for enhancing the ability to conduct clinical trials with fewer people, but are also critical for identifying at-risk individuals in the general population, so that as many people as possible can benefit when new prevention strategies are proven effective.

Because clinical trials to prevent or reverse type 1 diabetes occur at various sites throughout the United States and the world, it is critically important to have standardized tests so that data can be combined and compared. C-peptide is a byproduct of insulin production and thus useful as a marker of beta cell function. Indeed, C-peptide is used as an outcome measure to indicate insulin production in clinical trials focused on type 1 diabetes prevention and reversal, including trials supported by industry to gain regulatory approval of new drugs. To standardize C-peptide measurement in clinical trials, the *Special Diabetes Program* supports the C-peptide Standardization Program, which is led by CDC in collaboration with NIDDK. The scientists have made progress toward optimizing measurement techniques and standardizing results of C-peptide tests conducted at laboratories throughout the world by developing a highly precise reference method.

Understanding the Regulation of the Immune System

While clinical trials are ongoing, parallel research efforts are continuing to investigate the underlying causes of type 1 diabetes. Significant research progress on understanding the underlying mechanisms of type 1 diabetes have laid the foundation for conducting the clinical trials already described in this chapter. Researchers are building on the success to date and are now vigorously trying to understand the interactions between the environment and the immune system, as well as the means by which genes influence immune responses resulting in autoimmunity. Scientists are also studying the roles that the less specific arms of the innate immune system may play as contributors to the complex underpinnings of type 1 diabetes. Recent research has also suggested that inflammatory cells, such as mast cells and neutrophils, and cells of the innate immune system, such as natural killer cells, may play a role in type 1 diabetes. At the same time, scientists are studying the role of other important immune system cells, including dendritic cells, that control immune response and tolerance. Research to define the key components and the molecular defects that provoke the immune system to attack and destroy the beta cells is key to predicting, diagnosing, treating, and ultimately preventing this autoimmune process.

Cell-based Immune Modulation Therapy: Researchers supported by the *Special Diabetes Program* have made strides toward using dendritic cell therapy for preventing and treating type 1 diabetes in animal models. Some types of dendritic cells are involved in activating T cells, which are the cells that are central to the attack on the beta cells in type 1 diabetes, while others can induce tolerance to beta cells. Recent studies have tested approaches to modify dendritic cells to prompt the elimination of errant T cells to prevent the destructive immune attack. For example, scientists have modified dendritic cells in culture and then used them to successfully prevent or delay type 1 diabetes in a mouse model of disease. Other researchers have modified dendritic cells directly in the mouse. For instance, researchers used "microspheres" to deliver certain molecules to the animals that modify the dendritic cells in a way to make them suppress, rather than incite, T cell attacks on beta cells. A single injection of microspheres containing these suppressive molecules significantly delayed onset of diabetes in a mouse model of type 1 diabetes; several consecutive injections prevented the disease altogether. In mice that already had diabetes, the microsphere therapy reversed the disease. These studies demonstrate that modifying dendritic cells is a possible therapeutic approach for preventing, delaying, or reversing type 1 diabetes. Future research will help to determine if dendritic cell therapy might have the same dramatic benefits in people.

Identifying Targets of Autoimmune Attack in Type 1 Diabetes: For years, scientists have struggled to determine which beta cell proteins are key targets of autoimmune attack. A major advance in this area was made by the *Special Diabetes Program*-supported Cooperative Study Group for Autoimmune Disease Prevention (Prevention Centers), which is led by NIAID in collaboration with NIDDK and JDRF. The research group showed that they could prevent the disease in the non-obese diabetic (NOD) mouse model of type 1 diabetes by eliminating a primary sequence of insulin previously known to be a target of autoimmunity. Insulin is also known to be a key target in humans. These findings suggest that autoimmune reaction against insulin may be a critical initiator of the pathway toward beta cell destruction in humans.

Understanding How Risk Genes Cause Disease:
The Prevention Centers have made other significant contributions toward understanding the underpinnings of type 1 diabetes. For example, the Centers have spearheaded the "NOD Roadmap" project, which is generating a comprehensive time course of disease in the NOD mouse model and providing other key data. One important finding from this project was the identification of a gene that may play a role in the development of type 1 diabetes. Scientists found that cells in the animals' pancreatic lymph nodes make two forms of a gene called *Deaf1*. One form encodes full-length, functional Deaf1 protein, while the other encodes a shorter, nonfunctional variant form. Research suggested that the functional form of Deaf1 may control the production of molecules needed to eliminate immune cells that can destroy insulin-producing cells in the pancreas, thus preventing type 1 diabetes. Researchers also found that levels of the variant form of Deaf1 were higher in people with type 1 diabetes compared to levels in people without the disease. The research suggests that the development of type 1 diabetes may in part be due to increased levels of the Deaf1 variant protein in pancreatic lymph nodes, which may, in turn, lead to reduced production of molecules that are required to "educate" the immune system not to attack the body's own cells, including the insulin-producing cells of the pancreas.

Uncovering the Relationship Between Gut Bacteria and Type 1 Diabetes: Insights from research supported by the *Special Diabetes Program* has also found that the trillions of bacteria and other microbes that live in the gut can blunt the immune system attack that causes type 1 diabetes. During the past decades, researchers observed increased incidence (number of new cases) of type 1 diabetes in developed countries, which was thought to be due to changes in the environment, including the microbes that live in our bodies. Supporting this idea, previous studies found that the incidence of type 1 diabetes in mice susceptible to this disease can be affected by microbes in their environment. Thus, researchers supported by the *Special Diabetes Program* set out to further explore the possible connection between type 1 diabetes and microbes. They discovered that a complex interaction between the immune system and bacteria in the gut may help to lower the risk of developing type 1 diabetes in the mouse model of the disease. The widespread use of antibiotics and more aggressive cleanliness of modern society can alter the mix of microbes living in our body. This research suggests that an unexpected consequence of this environmental change may be an increased risk of autoimmune diseases like type 1 diabetes.

Promoting Translational Research: Researchers supported by the *Special Diabetes Program* have made progress in generating increasingly sophisticated stocks of mice with the expectation that they will show greater fidelity to human type 1 diabetes, and which may provide the means to understand clinically relevant components of type 1 diabetes pathogenesis. These mice are either engrafted with functional human cells or tissues, genetically engineered to express human genes, or both, and can recapitulate aspects of the pathogenic process. These mice have been used to identify targets of the human immune response against transplanted islets and have led to insights into the destructive immune cell populations that are important to this process. Mice that are engrafted with functional human immune systems may permit certain human immune responses to be manipulated in small animal models. As these types of studies cannot be done in people, such mouse models could facilitate the conduct of important translational research, providing insights as to safety and efficacy before enrolling people into clinical trials.

Summary

This chapter highlights some of the significant research progress that has been made possible by the *Special Diabetes Program* toward the goal of preventing and reversing type 1 diabetes. Without support from the *Special Diabetes Program*, it would not have been possible to establish large, collaborative networks, such as TrialNet, at an unprecedented scale. As basic research supported by the *Program* continues to identify possible new therapeutic targets, networks such as TrialNet and the ITN are poised to test these new therapies in people. Progress has already been achieved, and additional progress is expected in the future as new therapies are identified and tested in the people who could benefit from them.

RESEARCH CONSORTIA AND NETWORKS RELATED TO TYPE 1 DIABETES PREVENTION AND REVERSAL

Evaluation of research consortia and networks supported by the *Special Diabetes Program* and related to Goal II is found in Appendix C. Highlights of research progress are summarized below.

Type 1 Diabetes TrialNet: TrialNet is an international network that screens large numbers of people and conducts clinical trials of agents to prevent type 1 diabetes in at risk people and to slow progression of the disease in people who are newly diagnosed. TrialNet has screened over 74,000 people for type 1 diabetes risk to identify those eligible for participation in three ongoing or planned disease prevention trials. TrialNet also supports trials in people newly diagnosed with type 1 diabetes that hope to delay disease progression. TrialNet reported a novel finding that therapies targeting B lymphocytes of the immune system may be a strategy for preventing or reversing type 1 diabetes.

Immune Tolerance Network (ITN): The ITN is an international group of researchers dedicated to evaluating therapies to reprogram harmful immune responses to reduce autoimmunity, allergy, and asthma; and to improve islet, kidney, and liver transplantation (see Goal III for ITN research related to islet transplantation). ITN has developed eight clinical trials in people newly diagnosed with type 1 diabetes to test novel therapies to slow disease progression. In addition, the ITN completed the first multicenter study of islet transplantation in sites across North America and Europe, laying the groundwork for the Clinical Islet Transplantation Consortium (see Goal III).

Trial To Reduce IDDM in the Genetically At-Risk (TRIGR): TRIGR completed recruitment of 2,160 newborns for a trial examining whether hydrolyzed infant formula compared to standard cow's milk-based formula decreases the risk of developing type 1 diabetes in at-risk children. Researchers are now following the enrolled children.

Cooperative Study Group for Autoimmune Disease Prevention: The Prevention Centers engage in scientific discovery to advance knowledge toward the prevention and regulation of autoimmune diseases, such as type 1 diabetes, and create improved animal models of disease to better understand immune mechanisms. The Study

Group identified insulin as a primary target of the immune attack in a mouse model of type 1 diabetes, and also identified a gene (*Deaf1*) that may contribute to the development of type 1 diabetes and be a target for therapy.

Standardization Programs: Three different standardization programs are improving reliability in measurement of autoantibodies, C-peptide, and hemoglobin A1c (HbA1c) (also see Goal V). The ADA has built on the tremendous success of the HbA1c standardization program to set treatment goals for glucose control in all forms of diabetes based on the test and more recently recommended HbA1c as a more convenient approach to diagnose type 2 diabetes.

Type 1 Diabetes–Rapid Access to Intervention Development (T1D-RAID): This program provides services to scientists to help them ready agents for testing in clinical trials, thus bringing novel prevention and treatment approaches to people who could benefit from them. T1D-RAID has manufactured several agents that are being tested in ongoing clinical trials supported by the *Special Diabetes Program*. The Pre-clinical Testing Program associated with T1D-RAID has developed better methods for using rodent models for pre-clinical testing and has initiated testing of several new possible therapeutics. In addition to agents related to prevention and reversal of type 1 diabetes, the T1D-RAID and the Pre-clinical Testing Program are providing resources for agents related to preventing or treating diabetes complications (Goal V).

Investigator Profile

Mark D. Pescovitz, M.D.*

Leading a Clinical Trial Testing Rituximab in People with Newly Diagnosed Type 1 Diabetes

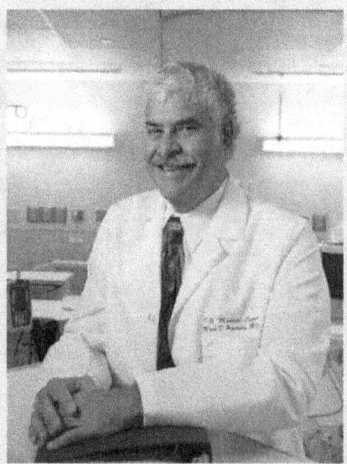

Mark D. Pescovitz, M.D.

Mark D. Pescovitz, M.D., is Professor of Surgery and Professor of Microbiology and Immunology at Indiana University School of Medicine, in Indianapolis, Indiana. Through his participation in Type 1 Diabetes TrialNet, which is supported by the Special Statutory Funding Program for Type 1 Diabetes Research, he leads a clinical trial testing the ability of a drug, called rituximab, to preserve the function of insulin-producing beta cells in people with newly diagnosed type 1 diabetes. This profile describes how he came to be involved in type 1 diabetes research, the origin of the rituximab trial, and how Type 1 Diabetes TrialNet facilitated the trial.

"I've always had a strong interest in immunology," says Dr. Pescovitz. "Because my father was a surgeon, I also had an interest in surgery. My combined interests in immunology and surgery led me to focus my career on being a transplant surgeon, but with a strong interest in immunology."

Upon his arrival as a faculty member at Indiana University in 1988, Dr. Pescovitz started a pancreas transplant program, beginning his long-standing interest in the management of type 1 diabetes. Because of the need to suppress people's immune systems after they undergo an organ transplant, Dr. Pescovitz was involved in developing several new immunosuppressive agents. He subsequently became interested in applying those agents to the treatment of type 1 diabetes, which results from the misguided attack of the immune system on the insulin-producing beta cells in the pancreas. Thus, therapies targeting the immune system could be a way to prevent or reverse the disease.

At about the same time that Dr. Pescovitz and a colleague were planning for a trial to test an immunosuppressive agent in new-onset type 1 diabetes, NIDDK was soliciting applications to establish a new collaborative clinical trials network, called Type 1 Diabetes TrialNet. Because the goals of the network dovetailed with his research interests, he and his colleagues at Indiana University applied and successfully competed to become a TrialNet clinical center, which began his involvement in the network. TrialNet is an international network of investigators, clinical centers, and core support facilities that recruits patients and develops and conducts clinical trials testing strategies for type 1 diabetes prevention and early treatment.

This profile is printed in honor and memory of Dr. Pescovitz whose death in 2010 was a major loss to the diabetes community.

A New Clinical Trial Concept

Rituximab destroys B lymphocytes (also called B cells). These are the part of the immune system that produce antibodies. The connection between rituximab and treating type 1 diabetes came when Dr. Pescovitz attended an annual B lymphocyte summit sponsored by Genentech, Inc., which markets Rituxan® (rituximab). At that time, most of the research discussed at the summit was focused on using rituximab to treat lymphoma; the drug had been approved by the U.S. Food and Drug Administration (FDA) in 1997 for the treatment of B cell non-Hodgkin's lymphoma. However, Dr. Pescovitz recalls, "At one of the meetings, I heard a presentation about rituximab being used successfully in early studies for the treatment for rheumatoid arthritis. Rheumatoid arthritis is similar to type 1 diabetes in that they are both autoimmune diseases thought to be T cell mediated and associated with autoantibodies that are not necessarily pathogenic. It was an easy leap for me to think that, if rituximab works for rheumatoid arthritis, maybe it will work for type 1 diabetes." With that thought, a new clinical trial concept was born.

Launching a Clinical Trial Through Type 1 Diabetes TrialNet

While there was research being done testing B lymphocyte therapies in mouse models of type 1 diabetes, "there was nothing being done in humans," says Dr. Pescovitz. In fact, immune therapies being tested in people targeted other cells in the immune system, called T cells, which attack and destroy insulin-producing beta cells. Thus, rituximab, which targets B lymphocytes, was a novel approach for treating people with type 1 diabetes.

TrialNet requires researchers both inside and outside of the project to submit clinical trial proposals for consideration by the network. Thus, Dr. Pescovitz submitted his clinical trial proposal to TrialNet, which would provide the funding and infrastructure for the trial, as well as to Genentech, which would provide the drug. Both groups approved the concept to test rituximab in people newly diagnosed with type 1 diabetes. The trial enrolled 87 patients who received four separate infusions of either rituximab or a placebo. In November 2009, Dr. Pescovitz and his colleagues published the results of the trial in the New England Journal of Medicine. The trial showed that, after 1 year, the people receiving rituximab produced more insulin, had better control of their diabetes, and did not have to take as much insulin to control their blood glucose levels, compared to people receiving placebo. The patients are now being followed to assess longer-term outcomes. The exciting results suggest that rituximab delays progression of type 1 diabetes; additional research is needed before the drug would be approved for treating patients. The success of the trial also suggests that other therapies to target B lymphocytes may be useful for treating or preventing the disease—knowledge that could inform future clinical trials.

Dr. Pescovitz stressed that the trial did not happen overnight. "It took 5 years from concept proposal to looking at the results, and 6 years from concept proposal to publication," he explains. "It takes a long time to do these trials, and you cannot expect instantaneous answers. Clinical research, in particular, takes long time horizons to pursue and to see results." Because of ethical considerations to the dedicated patients involved in trials, and the long timeframes necessary to conduct trials and adequately follow participants, Dr. Pescovitz says, "These trials also require a long time horizon in terms of funding." If there had been uncertainty as to whether there would be sufficient funds to complete the trial, "I couldn't have started the study," he says.

The Benefits of Type 1 Diabetes TrialNet

Rituximab was an FDA-approved drug for the treatment of B cell non-Hodgkin's lymphoma and subsequently for rheumatoid arthritis and chronic lymphocytic leukemia. However, Dr. Pescovitz notes that, "Industry did not have an interest in developing the drug for the treatment of type 1 diabetes. So if it hadn't been for someone like me, industry would not have moved forward on their own. They were happy to provide the drug to be used in the trial, but I needed to have support and patients."

The support and patients came in the form of TrialNet. "TrialNet was the perfect fit because it had the large infrastructure that provided access to patients and it had the clinical support structure in place. It was a perfect combination," says Dr. Pescovitz. Dr. Pescovitz could have applied for NIH funding for the trial through an investigator-initiated R01 grant mechanism. However, in this case, he explains that, "Using an R01 mechanism would have been more cumbersome, difficult, and taken a longer period of time. TrialNet was the perfect fit for this type of trial."

Dr. Pescovitz also says that his research has benefited from interactions and collaborations with other scientists in TrialNet. "I am a transplant surgeon and an expert in immunology, but not a diabetes guy," he says, "and I think there is great synergism in having people like me interacting with people who are experts in diabetes." He also stressed the importance of collaborations on mechanistic studies. "There are a group of top diabetes immunologists from around the world who sit at a table and provide ideas as to how to look at mechanism—not just whether a therapy works or not, but how or why it works. Those are collaborations facilitated by TrialNet." Understanding the mechanism by which a drug works could shed light on the molecular underpinnings of disease and open up new avenues for therapy.

The rituximab trial tested the drug in newly diagnosed patients, but TrialNet also conducts clinical trials to prevent the disease in at-risk individuals. Dr. Pescovitz explains, "Prevention trials are an entirely different type of trial that only an organization like TrialNet can do because you have to screen large numbers of patients to find those who are eligible." Indeed, TrialNet has screened over 70,000 people to date to identify those eligible for prevention trials and screening is ongoing. Dr. Pescovitz also notes that industry is unlikely to undertake such a large-scale effort to study type 1 diabetes prevention. Thus, TrialNet provides a unique infrastructure—made possible by the *Special Diabetes Program*—to conduct these important studies.

Through TrialNet, Dr. Pescovitz was able to move forward a new idea for type 1 diabetes treatment to testing it in people. TrialNet enabled the conduct of this trial in a more streamlined timeframe than would otherwise have been possible. The trial not only identified a potential new therapy to slow progression of type 1 diabetes, but also suggested that other therapies targeting B lymphocytes may be effective. TrialNet remains critically important for testing these and other new and emerging therapies to improve the health of people with type 1 diabetes, and the creativity and innovation of scientists, such as Dr. Pescovitz, remains a cornerstone of realizing progress in type 1 diabetes research.

Patient Profile

The Gould Family

Dedicated To Participating in Research To Be Part of a Cure for Type 1 Diabetes

Dave and Ellen Gould of Nashville, Tennessee have eight children ranging in age from 2 to 17. Within the last 5 years, four of their children have been diagnosed with type 1 diabetes. Even though their lives are busier than most people can imagine, the Goulds make time not only to participate in clinical research studies, but also to tell others about the importance of research toward combating type 1 diabetes and finding a cure.

Their passion and dedication was evident when Ellen testified in Congress at a hearing held in conjunction with the Juvenile Diabetes Research Foundation's 2009 Children's Congress. In her testimony, Ellen related how, on a Saturday morning several months earlier, the family was awakened by then 12-year-old son, Sam, who collapsed in his room, incoherent, because of a dangerously low blood sugar level. "It took us 20 minutes to get him back to normal," Ellen said. "But what happens the next time if we don't hear him? As their mother, I just want to reach out and make it better—but I can't. I can't cure this disease; I can't make it better for my kids. I need help. Finding a cure means everything to my family, and we are willing to be part of the solution."

To that end, the Goulds are participating in NIDDK's Type 1 Diabetes TrialNet, an international network of researchers exploring new strategies to prevent, delay, and reverse type 1 diabetes. TrialNet is also supported by the *Special Statutory Funding Program for Type 1 Diabetes Research.*

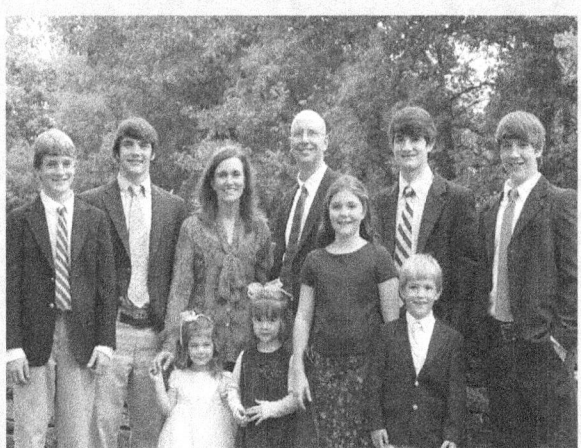

The Gould family.
Back row, left to right: Sam, Patrick, Ellen, Dave, Andrew, and Nicholas.
Front row, left to right: Maggie, Annie, Sarah, and Oliver.
Photo credit: Amy McIntyre

"Finding a cure means everything to my family, and we are willing to be part of the solution," said Ellen.

"There are a lot of smart people working on a cure for this disease," Dave said in a later interview. "I'm an optimist. I believe a cure is coming, and if my family can help speed it up a bit by being part of an important study, all the better."

"Diabetes Is Part of Our Family"
Type 1 diabetes is a chronic disease in which the body's immune system launches a misguided attack and destroys the insulin-producing cells of the pancreas. People with the disease need daily administration of insulin, either by injection or with a pump, and must monitor their blood sugar levels vigilantly.

"Diabetes is part of our family," Ellen said. "We're constantly filling prescriptions, scheduling doctors' appointments, filling out forms for school and various activities, educating others—and making sure our kids are safe," she added.

For the Goulds, the beginning of a life dominated by type 1 diabetes started 5 years ago when their oldest son, Patrick, then 12 years old, was diagnosed with the disease.

"I was watching him lose weight, and as a mother, I knew something was wrong," Ellen said. "I even asked Dave, 'do you think it could be diabetes?'"

As fate would have it, the family was on vacation when Ellen came upon a 1974 edition of Life Magazine at a flea market. The cover story just happened to be "Does Your Child Have Diabetes?" It was all the impetus she needed. As soon as the vacation ended, Ellen brought Patrick to their pediatrician where a blood test revealed that he had the disease. "Patrick's diagnosis came as a complete shock," Ellen said. "There's no history of diabetes in Dave's or my families."

Eighteen months later, their daughter Sarah, then 6 years old, began losing weight and urinating frequently at night. She too was diagnosed with type 1 diabetes. "Sarah took it very cavalierly, just like a trooper," says Ellen. But when Ellen and Dave told Patrick of his sister's diagnosis, "he just broke down and cried. Since having been diagnosed, Patrick had always dealt with his diabetes well and never really complained. But at that moment we knew how bad it was for him," said Ellen.

Shortly after Sarah was diagnosed, the family's endocrinologist told them about TrialNet, in which researchers were looking for children whose siblings had type 1 diabetes to see if other children in the family were at risk for developing the disease.

Dave said that at first he and Ellen didn't want to have their other children screened for the disease. "We just didn't want that cloud hanging over our heads," Ellen added. However, the more they thought about it, the more they began to realize that "maybe we can learn something from this. We also felt strongly that we needed to be part of this search for a cure, and the more we thought about it the more enthusiastic we became," said Dave. It was through a TrialNet screening that the Goulds learned that then 10-year-old Sam also had type 1 diabetes.

Participating in a Clinical Trial To Prevent Type 1 Diabetes

A clinical trial being conducted by TrialNet is building on the results of a previous NIDDK-supported clinical trial, called the Diabetes Prevention Trial-Type 1 (DPT-1). The DPT-1 studied whether injected or oral insulin administration could prevent or delay type 1 diabetes in persons at high- or moderate-risk for the disease. While the DPT-1 did not find an overall protective effect of injected or oral insulin, a subset of trial participants who had higher levels of a certain predictive marker of the disease (insulin autoantibodies) seemed to benefit from oral insulin treatment, though this result was not definitive. TrialNet is now building on these observations, and has launched a clinical trial to determine if oral insulin therapy could prevent the disease in people with elevated insulin autoantibodies.

Through a TrialNet screening, the Goulds learned that 4-year-old Oliver had elevated levels of insulin autoantibodies, which made him eligible to enroll in the TrialNet oral insulin prevention study. The Goulds enrolled Oliver into the study, which randomly assigns participants to receive either an insulin pill or a placebo (inactive pill without insulin). Those participating in the trial do not know whether they are getting the insulin or the placebo. This randomization allows researchers to compare the two groups to determine if oral insulin could prevent or delay the development of type 1 diabetes.

Oliver has since developed type 1 diabetes—the fourth of the Goulds' children to be diagnosed with the disease—and, until the study is over, the family will not know whether he received insulin or placebo. "When we decided to enroll Oliver in the study, friends would ask, 'if you don't know whether he's receiving insulin or placebo, why did you enroll him?'" said Dave. "Ellen's and my response to them is: that's what research is. You have to be willing to accept that when you get into a study like this." He quickly added that, "We would be ready, willing, and able to do it all again. The best thing about TrialNet is that it's helping all of us move closer to preventing or delaying type 1 diabetes."

Likewise, significant knowledge will be gained no matter the outcome of the trial—it is only through a rigorous clinical trial that researchers definitively learn which therapies work and which ones don't. When effective therapies or preventative approaches are found, other patients and people at risk can benefit from them. If a potential intervention turns out to be ineffective, then scientists know to explore other avenues to find therapies that work. It is thanks to the dedication of the Goulds and other families that this important new knowledge can be gained.

"When we decided to enroll Oliver in the TrialNet study, friends would ask, 'if you don't know whether he's receiving insulin or placebo, why did you enroll him?'" said Dave. "Ellen's and my response to that is: that's what research is. You have to be willing to accept that when you get into a study like this." He quickly added that, "We would be ready, willing, and able to do it all again."

Fortunately, the Goulds' other four children—Maggie, Annie, Nicholas, and Andrew—so far have tested negative for early markers of type 1 diabetes. But that doesn't mean that they are not affected by the disease. According to Ellen, 3-year-old Annie asks "When I am I going to get diabetes?" and 2-year-old Maggie tries putting Patrick's glucose meter on her finger to test herself. Describing his perspective on this disease, 13-year-old Nicholas said, "I'm really glad I don't have it. I see what my brothers and sister have to go through every day. I try to help as best I can, but I'm worried about them."

But Dave lays claim to being the family's ultimate worry-wart. "Ever since Sam's low blood sugar episode, I'm up with every bump I hear during the night, checking their bedrooms."

Through another study being conducted by TrialNet—the Natural History Study—the Goulds' four children who don't have type 1 diabetes will continue to be screened annually. For the four who do have the disease, the best news to date is that they are all doing well and show no signs of complications from the disease.

"When I was first diagnosed," Patrick said, "I got a note from someone in the Juvenile Diabetes Research Foundation, and it said 'Hang in there. There's a cure coming. Take as good care of yourself as you can; you're not going to have to do this much longer.' My message to others with type 1 diabetes is the same: There's a cure coming. Hang in there."

As for his mother's testifying in front of Congress with her urgent message for finding a cure for her children and all the others who must deal with type 1 diabetes every minute of every day, Patrick said: "She was awesome!"

For information about participating in Type 1 Diabetes TrialNet, please call 1-800-HALT-DM1 or visit www.diabetestrialnet.org

EMERGING RESEARCH OPPORTUNITIES RESULTING FROM THE *SPECIAL DIABETES PROGRAM*

The *Special Statutory Funding Program for Type 1 Diabetes Research* has fueled the emergence of a wide range of research opportunities. These opportunities were identified in a strategic planning process as being critically important for overcoming current barriers and achieving progress in diabetes research. Key questions and research opportunities relevant to type 1 diabetes, including those related to type 1 diabetes prevention and reversal, are outlined in Appendix F.

GOAL III

DEVELOP CELL REPLACEMENT THERAPY

The *Special Statutory Funding Program for Type 1 Diabetes Research* has laid the foundation for, and contributed to, major advances toward developing cell replacement therapies for type 1 diabetes. Collaborative research consortia supported by the *Special Diabetes Program* have played a central role in advancing pancreatic islet transplantation and other potential cell replacement therapies while opening a range of new scientific avenues. In addition to the significant research progress described in this chapter, information on the program evaluation related to Goal III can be found in Appendix A (Allocation of Funds), Appendix B (Assessment), and Appendix C (Evaluation of Major Research Consortia, Networks, and Resources).

Type 1 diabetes is characterized by the destruction of a person's beta cells by their own immune system. These insulin-producing cells of the pancreas are critical to the ability of the body to regulate uptake of dietary glucose (sugar) for energy into cells and tissues. Without insulin, the cells and tissues of people with type 1 diabetes are starved while blood glucose levels continue to rise. Patients are faced with requiring a lifetime of insulin replacement therapy, administered by injections or a pump, to control their blood glucose levels. While insulin helps people with type 1 diabetes control blood glucose levels, it is not a cure. Even the most diligent patients are at risk for sudden, acute episodes of dangerously low or high blood glucose levels, either of which can be life-threatening in extreme cases. Therefore, a major goal of research supported by the *Special Statutory Funding Program for Type 1 Diabetes Research* (*Special Diabetes Program* or *Program*) is to vigorously investigate methods to replace the destroyed beta cells—a potential cure for the disease.

One strategy for replacing beta cells is islet transplantation. As described in this chapter, at the beginning of the *Special Diabetes Program* in 1998, the potential of islet transplantation as a treatment for type 1 diabetes was as yet unrealized. Now, due largely to support from the *Special Diabetes Program*, the potential of islet transplantation has grown and critical efforts are under way to improve this experimental procedure and its outcomes. Scientists are also exploring other strategies to replace beta cells, such as coaxing any remaining beta cells in the pancreas to generate additional beta cells, expanding islets in culture, or directing other pancreatic cell types to become beta cells. The development of strategies to successfully generate beta cells from human embryonic stem (ES) cells,[23] and other stem/progenitor cell populations, such as induced pluripotent stem (iPS) cells holds great promise. Huge strides have been made in these areas and in the basic understanding of pancreas development due to research supported by the *Special Diabetes Program*. As described in this chapter, the *Special Diabetes Program* has supported many accomplishments that are accelerating progress toward the development of cell-based therapies as a cure for type 1 diabetes.

---

[23] The NIH supports research using human embryonic stem cells within the NIH Guidelines for Human Stem Cell Research.

Graphic: Image of human islet. Islets in the pancreas produce and secrete insulin to aid in metabolism. In people with type 1 diabetes, the insulin-producing beta cells in islets are destroyed by a misguided immune system attack. Image credit: Steve Gschmeissner/Photo Researchers, Inc.

HIGHLIGHTS OF RECENT RESEARCH ADVANCES RELATED TO GOAL III

Conducted First Multicenter Trial of Islet Cell Transplantation: Building on the 2000 finding that insulin independence could be achieved with islet transplantation coupled with a steroid-free immunosuppressive regimen, nine sites participating in the Immune Tolerance Network (ITN) successfully replicated the "Edmonton protocol" for islet transplantation. While most people in the study experienced a gradual loss of transplanted islet function over a period of years, even those individuals who retained only partial islet function and did not remain "insulin free" benefited greatly from improved post-transplant glycemic control. The study played a critical role in defining the challenges, obstacles, and feasibility of moving islet transplantation into the therapeutic arena and demonstrated that islet transplantation holds promise as a treatment for type 1 diabetes.

Launched Clinical Trials To Improve Islet Transplantation: The Clinical Islet Transplantation (CIT) Consortium has seven ongoing trials testing new strategies to improve islet transplantation. These trials are testing U.S. Food and Drug Administration (FDA)-approved and experimental agents to improve islet survival and insulin independence after transplantation and to prevent rejection of the transplanted tissue. In addition, new approaches for islet isolation are also being studied. The Collaborative Islet Transplant Registry (CITR) is collecting and disseminating data from the CIT Consortium and other islet transplant programs to expedite progress and promote safety in this research field.

Contributed to Unprecedented Islet Transplant: Research supported by the *Special Diabetes Program* laid the foundation for an unprecedented islet transplant to an American airman who was wounded while serving in Afghanistan. The airman's pancreas was damaged beyond repair by gunshot wounds, resulting in the need for removal of the entire pancreas. The pancreas was transported to researchers at the University of Miami who isolated and purified the islets and sent the purified islets back to Walter Reed Army Medical Center, where the cells were successfully infused into the patient's liver, freeing him from the insulin-requiring diabetes that would have ensued from loss of the pancreas. This advance was built on research supported by the *Special Diabetes Program* on islet isolation, purification, and transplantation.

Fostered "Bench to Bedside" Research Toward Goal of Cell Replacement Therapy: Translating key findings in the laboratory to clinical trials is critical to capitalizing on knowledge resulting from successful basic research, but can be difficult for scientists to do on their own. Programs supported by the *Special Diabetes Program* aim to facilitate this translation and have been successful. For example, researchers using mouse models demonstrated that an anti-inflammatory drug called lisofylline can protect newly transplanted islets from recurrent destruction by the immune system. Building on these results, the CIT Consortium is now testing the drug in humans using lisofylline manufactured through the T1D-RAID program, which helps scientists ready agents for testing in clinical trials. Likewise, the T1D-RAID program is generating a mixture of medicines, demonstrated by researchers in the Non-Human Primate Transplantation Tolerance Cooperative Study Group (NHPCSG) to promote long-term survival of islets after transplantation into non-human primates, for use in an ITN clinical trial to test this therapy in people with newly diagnosed type 1 diabetes.

Identification of Progenitor Cells in the Adult Pancreas that Form Insulin-producing Beta Cells: To gain further understanding about pancreatic progenitor cells, scientists surgically induced a specific type of wound to the adult mouse pancreas, which caused the number of beta cells to double. The scientists took advantage of this doubling in number to test for the presence of a well-established marker of embryonic pancreatic progenitor cells, called Ngn3, and observed that levels of Ngn3 not only increased in the pancreas in response to injury, but that Ngn3 played a role in increased beta cell numbers following the injury. By further examining the Ngn3-expressing cells within the injured mouse pancreas, the scientists demonstrated that these cells showed many of the same characteristics as embryonic progenitor cells, suggesting that the adult mouse pancreas contains progenitor cells that are able to regenerate beta cells. If, with further research, these embryonic-like progenitor cells are identified in the human pancreas, then this discovery may foster the development of therapies for both type 1 and type 2 diabetes.

Adult Pancreas Cells Reprogrammed to Insulin-producing Beta Cells: In order to promote the formation of new beta cells, scientists in the Beta Cell Biology Consortium (BCBC) are determining when and how certain pancreatic progenitor cells become "committed" to developing into specific pancreatic cell types and discovering flexibility in these cells. In one study, scientists made an exciting discovery that a type of adult cell in the mouse pancreas, called an exocrine cell, can be reprogrammed to become an insulin-producing beta cell. Using a genetically engineered virus and a combination of just three transcription factors, the researchers were able to reprogram some of the exocrine cells into beta cells. The newly formed beta cells produced enough insulin to decrease high blood glucose levels in diabetic mice. If the same type of approach can be developed to work safely and effectively in humans, this discovery could have a dramatic impact on the ability to increase beta cell mass in people with diabetes.

In another study, scientists uncovered plasticity in another pancreatic cell type—the alpha cell. Using genetic techniques in mice, the researchers increased the levels of a protein called Pax4, which is known to be involved in promoting cells to develop into a certain pancreatic cell type. They found that mice with high levels of Pax4 had oversized clusters of beta cells, which resulted from alpha-beta precursor cells and established alpha cells being induced to form beta cells. In addition, in a mouse model of diabetes, the high levels of Pax4 promoted generation of new beta cells and overcame the diabetic state. In a recent study, BCBC scientists observed spontaneous conversion in beta cell-depleted mice of alpha cells to insulin-producing cells. This discovery—that adult pancreatic cells have the potential to convert to beta cells—generates a fuller picture of pancreatic development and may pave the way toward new cell-based therapies for diabetes.

Mouse Model for Studying Beta Cell Regeneration: Scientists in the BCBC developed a mouse model useful for studying beta cell regeneration. When the genetically engineered mice are treated with a certain drug, a toxin is expressed in their beta cells. Expression of the toxin causes the beta cells to die, and the mice to develop diabetes.

Surprisingly, the researchers found that if they stopped the drug treatment after the mice developed diabetes, the animals recovered from the disease. The mice not only regained normal blood sugar levels, but also regenerated their beta cell mass. The scientists determined that the new beta cells came predominantly from preexisting beta cells, suggesting that beta cells have a significant capacity for regeneration. This research suggests that finding ways to promote regeneration of existing beta cells may be a therapeutic approach for treating diabetes. It also provides an important model system for testing the effect of therapeutic agents on beta cell regeneration.

Discovery of a New Indicator for Type 1 Diabetes Autoimmunity: To enhance understanding of the pathogenesis of type 1 diabetes and elucidate potential new therapeutic strategies, as well as to improve testing for autoimmunity, researchers in the BCBC sought to identify additional beta cell proteins that generate autoantibodies, factors that attack proteins within the body, rather than invading pathogens. By examining a set of proteins made exclusively or almost exclusively in beta cells, and testing with antibodies taken from people with new-onset diabetes, the scientists discovered that autoantibodies to a beta cell protein called ZnT8 are an excellent marker for type 1 diabetes autoimmunity. The scientists found that using ZnT8 autoantibodies can substantially improve prediction of diabetes when used in combination with the previously discovered autoantibodies commonly used to monitor for type 1 diabetes risk in research studies.

ISLET TRANSPLANTATION RESEARCH

Islet Transplantation Becomes a Reality: The field of islet transplantation was propelled forward by the success of a small clinical study in Edmonton, Canada. In 2000, seven consecutive patients achieved normal blood glucose levels following islet transplantation using a new protocol (referred to as the "Edmonton protocol"). This protocol did not use steroids to prevent rejection of the transplant; rather, a new combination of anti-rejection drugs was tested. Each patient received a large number of islets isolated from two to three donor pancreata as multiple transplants and infused into the recipient's liver. Progress in methods for isolating and storing islets from donor pancreata prior to transplantation also added to the success of this trial. However, the success of the transplants brought on new questions and challenges. While patients maintained normal blood glucose levels for a period after the transplant,

the islets tended to lose their insulin-producing function over time, prompting study of what caused this loss of function and how it could be halted. In addition, it remained to be demonstrated whether Edmonton's success could be replicated at other sites around the world in a standardized way. While the *Special Diabetes Program* did not support the original Edmonton trial, the *Program* has supported efforts to further progress in islet transplantation.

Replicating the Success at Edmonton in a Multicenter Trial: The ITN (see Goal II) took on the challenge to replicate the "Edmonton protocol" in a multicenter trial. ITN is an international consortium that receives support from the *Special Diabetes Program* and is led by NIAID in collaboration with NIDDK and JDRF. In the first multicenter trial of islet cell transplantation, from 2001-2006, nine sites in North America and Europe successfully replicated the "Edmonton protocol." One year after transplant, 44 percent of the participants (16 out of 36) achieved insulin independence with good glycemic control; 14 percent achieved insulin independence with a single donor islet function. By helping people with type 1 diabetes achieve better glycemic control and prevent episodes of hyper- or hypoglycemia and associated complications, the study was heralded a success. Importantly, even among patients who still required insulin injections, the survival of functioning transplanted islets led to an absence of severe hypoglycemic events due to hypoglycemia unawareness. As of January 2008, 21 participants had reached the 5-year evaluation after their final transplant—six were judged to be insulin-independent, and 15 were insulin-dependent. Although insulin independence declined over time in study participants, this important study confirmed and extended the demonstration that islet transplantation may be an alternative to whole organ transplantation, a major surgical procedure with significant risks. The results also highlight the continued need for research to develop safer, more tolerable, and longer-lasting anti-rejection therapies, as well as alternative engraftment sites and other approaches to enhance islet viability.

Research Challenges to Developing Islet Transplantation: While these results represent major clinical progress, several challenges remain before this technique can be implemented in a large-scale fashion. Researchers have now confirmed that many islet transplant recipients are able to maintain near normal blood glucose levels. They also have observed, however, that success of the transplantation process varies greatly and wanes over time, underscoring the need for more durable outcomes and further research. Moreover, patients are trading the need for insulin and

the dangers of hypoglycemia for the risks associated with drugs to prevent rejection. Thus, the procedure is only used in people with recurrent severe hypoglycemia or those who already require immunosuppression after kidney transplantation. The complexity of barriers associated with islet transplantation requires multiple avenues of research, many of which are supported by the *Special Diabetes Program*. Methods for acquisition and delivery of islets must be optimized, so that fewer donor organs are needed and islets are as healthy as possible prior to transplantation. An adequate supply of islets for all transplant patients must be created based on new understanding of how beta cells are formed and maintained. Better tolerated therapies to combat the body's tendency to destroy the transplanted islets need to be developed to avoid toxic side effects. Sometimes islets do not "take" and never produce insulin; efforts to identify the best graft site, and improve the survival and functionality of the transplanted islets are necessary. Finally, research to understand how to prevent the immune system destruction of transplanted islets and ideally to re-program the immune system so ongoing intervention is minimized will be critical to the success of this procedure.

Coordinating Studies To Advance Islet Transplantation: The CIT Consortium, an international network of 11 centers, was created to study and refine islet transplantation technology. The CIT Consortium is led jointly by NIDDK and NIAID and is supported by the *Special Diabetes Program*. As knowledge of islet cell biology and the processes associated with transplantation and immune rejection increase, and pre-clinical studies evaluating new approaches to immunomodulation in conjunction with islet transplantation in animal models progress, a means is needed by which to rigorously study these new approaches. Using a well-coordinated, collaborative approach, the CIT Consortium is conducting studies to find methods that have higher success rates and fewer risks. It also aims to validate standardized protocols for generation of islets of sufficient quality for FDA licensure as a biologic product. Since its inception, the CIT Consortium has developed and implemented a program of clinical and mechanistic studies to address the challenges in islet transplantation with or without an accompanying kidney transplant.

The CIT Consortium launched six single and multi-center trials, with associated immunologic, metabolic, and mechanistic studies, of islet transplantation in individuals with type 1 diabetes with severe hypoglycemic events despite intensive medical management. An additional trial, including Medicare beneficiaries as mandated by the Medicare Prescription Drug Improvement and Modernization Act of 2003 (Public Law 108-173), specifically consists of individuals with type 1 diabetes who have previously undergone kidney transplantation for diabetic nephropathy and are thus already receiving immunosuppressive therapy to prevent rejection of the donor kidney. These trials are testing FDA-approved and experimental agents to improve islet survival and insulin independence after transplantation and to prevent rejection of the transplanted tissue. In addition, new approaches are also being studied for islet isolation. These types of improvements can ultimately lead to more widespread use of this treatment strategy for individuals with type 1 diabetes.

Collecting Data on Islet Transplantation To Inform Future Research: To advance this field as rapidly as possible, scientists need access to information on every islet transplant that takes place, not just those in their local facility. Patients considering the procedure and their physicians also need information on success rates and risks. Therefore, the CITR, which is led by NIDDK and supported by the *Special Diabetes Program*, was created to collect data on islet transplantations for use by the entire research field and the public. It expedites progress and promotes safety in islet transplantation through collection, analysis, and communication of comprehensive and current data on all islet transplantations performed in North America. An annual report is widely disseminated throughout the islet transplant community, diabetes community, and general public with data on recipient and donor characteristics; pancreas procurement and islet processing; immunosuppressive medications; the function of the donated islets; lab results; and adverse events. Examples of progress made through CITR include reporting that 72 percent of islet transplant recipients achieved insulin independence at least once, and that 1 year after islet transplantation, individuals still requiring insulin injections had significant reduction in their insulin requirements. By collecting and analyzing these data, CITR is helping to define the overall risks and benefits of islet transplantation as a treatment option for people with type 1 diabetes, which is informing future research efforts.

Bridging Basic and Clinical Research To Propel Islet Transplantation: Integral to successful and effective clinical therapies are programs that bridge the discoveries made in basic research and studies to test these advances in animal models and clinical trials. The *Special Diabetes Program* has supported critical programs aimed to promote the translation of scientific advances to treatments. For example, improvement in the processing and handling of islets has been essential for increasing success and reducing the risks and costs associated with transplantation and extending the availability of islet transplant to a greater number of people with diabetes. Research to improve islet isolation techniques, islet quality, the shipping and storage of islets, and assays for characterizing viability of purified islets has been accelerated due to the efforts of the *Special Diabetes Program*-supported Islet Cell Resource Centers (ICRs) that made human islets available for research studies. A new program also supported by the *Special Diabetes Program*, the NIDDK-led Integrated Islet Distribution Program (IIDP), builds upon the experience obtained with the ICRs and provides human islets not suitable for islet transplantation to basic scientists as a critical resource to advance scientific discovery and translational medicine.

Investigating New Therapies in Transplantation in Large Animal Models: The NHPCSG was begun to move advances in transplantation toward human clinical trials. The NHPCSG, led by NIAID and supported, in part, by the *Special Diabetes Program*, is evaluating the safety and efficacy of novel therapies to induce immune tolerance in non-human primate models of islet, kidney, heart, and lung transplantation. In addition to establishing two species of non-human primate breeding colonies to derive specific pathogen-free animals and provide a shared resource of high-quality animals for these research studies, the NHPCSG has made several advances in islet transplantation. The NHPCSG was the first to demonstrate long-term and sustained beta cell function without continuous immunosuppressive therapy following islet transplantation in a drug-induced diabetic non-human primate model. In addition, studies of agents used to prolong transplanted islet cell survival in non-human primates have shown promise and have been moved into clinical trials, as described in this chapter.

Facilitating Success in "Bench to Bedside" Translation: The *Special Diabetes Program* vigorously supports "bench to bedside" research toward the goal of replacing insulin-producing beta cells. For example, researchers demonstrated that, in a mouse model of type 1 diabetes, treatment after islet transplantation with an anti-inflammatory drug, called lisofylline, protected the cells from recurrent destruction by the immune system. Building on these results, the CIT Consortium is now testing this drug in humans. The lisofylline being used in the trial was manufactured through the *Special Diabetes Program*-supported Type 1 Diabetes-Rapid Access to Intervention Development (T1D-RAID) program, which helps scientists ready agents for testing in clinical trials. In another example, researchers in the NHPCSG demonstrated long-term survival of islets after transplantation when the animals were given a novel mixture of factors that target the immune system. Based on these findings, the ITN approved a clinical trial to test this therapy in people with newly diagnosed type 1 diabetes, to determine if the agent can slow progression of the disease. The T1D-RAID program is undertaking production of the agent for these studies. These examples demonstrate how the *Special Diabetes Program* supports the discovery, manufacture, and testing of promising therapeutic agents, creating a robust pipeline of agents that have the potential to improve the health of people with type 1 diabetes.

DEVELOPING NOVEL STRATEGIES TO REPLACE ISLETS

Limitations in the islet supply create a major roadblock to developing islet transplantation as a cure because the number of donor pancreata does not meet the demand for islets nationwide. Therefore, a major focus has been placed on the development of new methods to stimulate human beta cell growth in the laboratory setting prior to transplantation. In addition, scientists have begun to explore methods to replace the insulin-producing beta cells in a person with type 1 diabetes without the need for donor pancreata and toxic anti-rejection drugs. Just a few decades ago, little was known about pancreatic development and whether it would be possible to recapitulate the process of normal beta cell development in the laboratory setting. It was understood that beta cells develop from a pool of precursors, or stem cells, but these were poorly defined and many of the factors critical to this process remained to be identified. However, the stage was set for significant advances in this field as scientists had increased their understanding of mechanisms that allowed individual cell types to develop, the events involved in development and regeneration of the pancreas, and the factors required for normal function and development of the beta cells.

A Team-based Approach to Studies of Beta Cell Biology: To accelerate research in the field of beta cell biology, a unique team-based and collaborative consortium was established—the BCBC. Led by NIDDK and supported in part by the *Special Diabetes Program*, the BCBC provides an infrastructure that is conducive to tackling critical issues that can revolutionize type 1 diabetes research and, ultimately, the treatment of people with type 1 diabetes. The BCBC is pursuing key challenges: (1) use cues from pancreatic development to directly differentiate beta cells from human stem/progenitor cells; (2) enhance functional beta cell mass; (3) reprogram progenitor or adult cells to beta cells; and (4) use patient-derived tissues and mouse models to generate and study human beta cells/islets in the context of a human autoimmune environment. Over

50 BCBC investigators and over 200 affiliates work collaboratively and regularly share data and information. In addition, research through the BCBC and the broader scientific community is accelerated by having BCBC core facilities that produce key laboratory reagents (*e.g.*, mouse models, antibodies, microarrays), which allow the scientists to spend more time performing experiments, rather than generating and preparing reagents. The team-based approach of the BCBC has been a success and has promoted major advances in the field by synergizing the skills and ingenuity of many creative scientists and minimizing duplication in research efforts. To date, the BCBC has made significant contributions to the field of beta cell biology, as described below and in the Feature "The Beta Cell Biology Consortium: An Experiment in Team Science" found later in this chapter.

Increased Understanding of Pancreatic Development Leads to Generation of Insulin-producing Cells: Today, in part due to advances from the BCBC, scientists understand a great deal more about the development of the pancreas. Many of the genes responsible for the establishment of different pancreatic lineages have been identified and much more is known about the integrated cascade of interactions that lead to the formation of the adult pancreas. Overall, these studies have led to a more detailed understanding of the factors that drive development of the pancreas and the islets. This knowledge has laid the foundation for the development of rational and informed strategies to successfully generate beta cells from human ES cells, and other stem/progenitor cell populations, such as iPS cells. Using a step-wise protocol to mimic how the pancreas forms during fetal development, scientists were able to direct human ES cells through stages resembling this process and obtain insulin-producing cells. Some of these human ES cell-derived insulin-producing cells have insulin content approaching that of adult beta cells. However, unlike the adult beta cells they need to replace, the cells are not very responsive to glucose. Although these cells do not yet display regulated insulin secretion, nor is the process to produce them highly efficient, this major achievement provides proof-of-principle that it is possible to replicate, in the laboratory, the steps leading to the production of insulin-producing cells—a significant leap forward toward the goal of developing beta cell replacement therapies to cure type 1 diabetes or severe type 2 diabetes.

New Knowledge Spurs Novel Strategies for Cell-based Therapies: The knowledge gained by studying basic pancreas development has also spawned studies of reprogramming, cell plasticity, and pancreatic beta cell regeneration. Scientists are studying the potential of many different non-insulin producing pancreatic cell types to be reprogrammed to insulin-producing cells. Research from the BCBC performed in diabetic mice has shown that introducing expression of just three genes is sufficient to reprogram non-insulin-producing adult pancreatic cells (and potentially other cell types) into beta cell-like insulin-producing cells. The reprogrammed cells lowered blood glucose in diabetic animals and represent important progress toward harnessing regenerative medicine to treat diabetes. This ability to reprogram other pancreatic cell types could be used in the laboratory to generate insulin-producing cells for islet transplants and/or could be used in the clinical setting to coax non-insulin-producing pancreatic cell types to insulin-producing cells within a patient. As a result of research supported by the *Special Diabetes Program*, both of these approaches hold significant potential to improve glycemic control in patients with type 1 diabetes.

Additional research is necessary, though, to develop the potential of these approaches into safe and effective cellular therapies.

Advances in Beta Cell Regeneration: In addition to studies to generate insulin-producing cells from other cell types, scientists are investigating the potential of beta cells to replicate and regenerate the beta cell mass. In people with type 1 diabetes, beta cell depletion is often not absolute, and scattered insulin-producing cells may often be observed even after many years of disease. Similarly, animal studies of how changes in beta cell mass are regulated during pregnancy to meet increased insulin demands have rendered new insights that the beta cell mass is dynamically regulated and beta cells can regenerate. One of the difficulties in studying beta cell regeneration has been the lack of a robust, animal system that would allow the controlled destruction of beta cells and study of subsequent cell proliferation in the adult pancreas. However, a mouse model developed by BCBC scientists now permits the study of the dynamics of beta cell regeneration from a diabetic state. Insights from the study of this new mouse model will aid in the evaluation of beta cell regeneration as a potential treatment for type 1 diabetes. Also, recent successes by BCBC investigators will allow scientists, for the first time, to study the regenerative capacity of human islets *in vivo*. The successful BCBC has advanced the field of pancreas development and beta cell biology, and will continue to propel this field toward the ultimate goal of curing type 1 diabetes.

SUMMARY

This chapter highlights some of the significant research progress that has been made possible by the *Special Diabetes Program* toward the goal of developing cell replacement therapy. Without support from the *Special Diabetes Program*, it would not have been possible to establish large, collaborative networks, such as the BCBC, at an unprecedented scale. As new insights and opportunities emerge from the basic research of the BCBC and from animal studies of the NHPCSG, the CIT Consortium is poised to test new strategies for islet transplantation in people with type 1 diabetes.

Additionally, discoveries from the BCBC have illuminated the potential of other approaches to regenerate the beta cells that are destroyed in people with type 1 diabetes. Progress has already been achieved, and additional progress is expected in the future as islet transplantation is improved and new cell-based therapies are identified and tested in the people who could benefit from them.

RESEARCH CONSORTIA AND NETWORKS RELATED TO THE DEVELOPMENT OF CELL REPLACEMENT THERAPY

Evaluation of research consortia and networks supported by the *Special Diabetes Program* and related to Goal III is found in Appendix C. Highlights of these are summarized below.

Beta Cell Biology Consortium (BCBC): The BCBC is an international consortium of over 50 principal investigators and over 200 affiliates. The BCBC brings a team-based approach to studies of pancreas and beta cell biology and development, as well as the generation of new research tools, reagents, and technologies that are vital for developing new cellular therapies in diabetes. The BCBC's Antibody Core has generated and/or validated more than 110 antibodies and distributed more than 700 orders since its inception. The BCBC's Mouse ES Cell Core has generated over 50 new lines of genetically altered mice or mouse embryonic stem cell lines. The BCBC has made numerous scientific discoveries reported in over 290 publications, including progress in understanding the steps necessary to turn stem/progenitor cells into insulin-producing cells, and generated many research resources, including a mouse model in which to study beta cell regeneration.

Clinical Islet Transplantation (CIT) Consortium: The CIT Consortium is conducting studies to improve the safety and long-term success of methods for islet transplantation in people with type 1 diabetes. The CIT Consortium has seven ongoing trials, with associated immunologic, metabolic, and mechanistic studies, testing new strategies for islet transplantation, including a congressionally-mandated clinical trial of islet transplantation in Medicare recipients.

Collaborative Islet Transplantation Registry (CITR): The CITR expedites progress and promotes safety in islet transplantation through the collection, analysis, and communication of comprehensive and current data on all islet transplants performed in North America. The CITR has prepared six widely disseminated annual reports to define the overall risk and benefits of islet transplantation as a treatment option for people with type 1 diabetes. Information on characteristics of donors, recipients, islets, treatments, and outcomes allows comprehensive analysis of over 200 factors that may influence results of the procedure. CITR has reported that 72 percent of islet-alone recipients achieved insulin independence at least once and that, one year after islet infusion, individuals requiring insulin injections had a significant reduction in their insulin requirements. CITR's current North American database includes information on 339 allogenic islet recipients, 658 allogenic infusion procedures, 722 donor pancreata, and 213 autograft recipients and their islets, from 28 centers that have performed islet transplantation since 1999.

Islet Cell Resource Centers (ICRs)/ Integrated Islet Distribution Program (IIDP): Formerly the ICRs provided a valuable resource by distributing islets to the scientific community for basic research studies and for clinical transplantation. They provided more than 92 million islet equivalents for transplantation and distributed more than 201 million islet equivalents to more than 270 investigators for research. In addition, the ICRs made progress to improve isolation techniques, islet quality, the shipping and storage of islets, and assays for characterizing purified islets. Now CIT supports production of islets for transplantation research protocols, and the need for human islets for fundamental research is met through the IIDP, a new program to process and distribute human islets. The IIDP builds on the experience of the ICRs for notification of islet availability to investigators and for optimized shipping conditions to ensure that precious human islets not needed for transplantation are efficiently distributed to approved researchers studying human beta cell biology to develop new approaches to therapy for all forms of diabetes.

Non-Human Primate Transplantation Tolerance Cooperative Study Group (NHPCSG): The NHPCSG is a multi-institution Consortium collaboratively developing and evaluating the safety and efficacy of novel therapies to induce immune tolerance in non-human primate models of islet, kidney, heart, and lung transplantation. The NHPCSG has made many scientific contributions, including significantly enhancing the utility of the non-human primate as a model of human transplantation. One agent with promising results from NHPCSG studies is now in trials conducted by the CIT Consortium and ITN; a second agent has been approved for an ITN clinical trial upon completion of pre-clinical studies. These studies are being coordinated with the T1D-RAID program which is also undertaking production of the agent for these studies.

Feature:
The Beta Cell Biology Consortium—
An Experiment in Team Science

The Beta Cell Biology Consortium (BCBC), created by NIDDK and supported in part by the *Special Statutory Funding Program for Type 1 Diabetes Research* (*Special Diabetes Program*), brings team science to the acquisition of new knowledge and production of new resources necessary to develop novel cell-based therapies for insulin delivery. Cell-based therapies could increase the mass of insulin-producing beta cells in a person with type 1 diabetes, either by inducing new beta cell growth in the pancreas or by transplanting new beta cells or islets. Therefore, the BCBC has been guided by three main goals: (1) understanding how endogenous beta cells are made through the study of pancreatic development, with the hope of making pancreatic cells in the laboratory for transplantation; (2) exploring the potential of animal and/or human stem cells as a source of making pancreatic islets; and (3) determining the basic mechanisms underlying beta cell regeneration in the adult as a basis for producing new cellular therapies for diabetes.

DEVELOPING THE TEAM

In 1999, the congressionally-established Diabetes Research Working Group recommended that NIH increase research on beta cell biology and development. This recommendation, in conjunction with the inception of the *Special Diabetes Program*, provided the opportunity to ignite research in this field with a new approach. Rather than solely supporting individual investigators pursuing projects independently, NIDDK launched an experiment in team science which would be continually propelled by a translatable clinical goal. In 2001, the BCBC (the first funding cycle of which is referred to as BCBC 1.0) was launched with the announcement of six collaborative agreement awards. As with other NIH grants, these awards were time limited, meaning that the investigators would be required to "recompete" to continue to participate in the BCBC. In 2005, the second round of BCBC investigators received their awards and the BCBC 2.0 was launched. In this round, 10 collaborative agreement awards were funded. As expected, the groups of investigators funded in the first and second rounds were similar, but not identical. The third round of the BCBC (BCBC 3.0) was launched in summer 2010 with the funding of 16 collaborative agreement awards. These awards bring nearly 50 multidisciplinary principal investigators and over 200 affiliates into the BCBC team. BCBC members are at different stages in their careers and are located at multiple institutions around the world.

A STUDY IN TEAM SCIENCE

Team science is not a concept unique to the BCBC; the past decades have been witness to a number of large-scale team science efforts. Some have been considered successes, while others have been less successful. This bloom of team science efforts may reflect the complexity of human disease and the urgency of developing therapies and strategies to combat increasing prevalences of diseases; solving complex problems may benefit from an integration of perspectives and disciplines. The rationale for team science is simple in concept. Collaboration can be a powerful driver for innovation and progress, and a team approach can both stimulate and facilitate the rapid development and translation of new discoveries. Meaningful advances can require the skills, often interdisciplinary, and ingenuity of many people. Synergies can be obtained and duplication can be minimized with coordinated efforts. Early results from the emerging field of the science of team science suggest that teams are, in general, more scientifically productive than individuals.[1]

Barriers and Challenges to Team Science: Team science, however, is not without significant barriers and challenges that impact its success. In the effort to establish and conduct the BCBC, many of these barriers and challenges have come to light and these examples are likely applicable to other team science efforts. For example, in the current institutional system, scientists are rewarded for their individual accomplishments, which often can be easily determined. Contributions to a team effort are difficult to measure and therefore may not be as valued. Understandably then, investigators have their own interests, scientific and professional, that must be considered when working in a team. These individual interests can lead to competition among members of a team. For the BCBC, managing rapidly evolving priorities—individual and otherwise—that were sometimes in conflict was a key challenge. Similar to investigators, institutions have their own priorities, and these may not align with the priorities of the team. Institutional regulations can sometimes make it difficult to transfer funds. Therefore getting research money to where it is needed is not trivial and can be a barrier to team science. For the BCBC, an additional challenge is integration of the large quantity of data being generated; highly functional informatics was, and still is to some extent, a challenge. Finally, with any team effort, individual personalities and abilities are an important factor in the success of the team. Studies in team science

indicate that individuals who value collaboration, a culture of sharing, and openness to diverse disciplinary perspectives are well-suited for team efforts.[2]

Lessons Learned—Build Trust: The BCBC, therefore, is an ongoing experiment in team science; NIDDK has closely monitored the group's challenges and successes and provided enhancements to the program where possible to overcome obstacles. As the BCBC matured, the Consortium identified themes that mirror those resulting from studies of team science. These themes led to the generation of "lessons learned" by the BCBC. Many of these lessons were realized during the early years and were used to guide the BCBC 2.0. They continue to be important themes for the BCBC and team science in general. First, the BCBC found that building trust among members of the team is essential, but also takes time. Studies of team science suggest that building and sustaining trust is critical to the success of a team, especially when the team is not in close physical proximity.[3] As the Consortium evolved and appreciated the importance of building trust, participants were particularly oriented to team goals, which enabled them to accept differences more readily and led to an environment of openness. This environment was one of the factors that increased and maintained trust within the BCBC.

This lesson was implemented from the beginning of BCBC 2.0. In August 2005, a kickoff meeting established the importance of trust and set a tone of high expectations among members. This provided an opportunity for members to meet in person and generate familiarity. Interactions among members were stimulated at this meeting, allowing new collaborations to be built and contacts to be made. Again, studies of team science echo more broadly what the BCBC has observed. Initial face-to-face contact seems to increase the level of trust among team members, facilitate the formation of team atmosphere and operating procedures, and aid the establishment of group identity. Face-to-face contact early in the formation of a team has been suggested to be a prerequisite for successful remote collaboration.[4] The BCBC kickoff meeting also provided an opportunity for participatory, team goal setting. Priorities were discussed and defined at the meeting. Studies note that group goal setting generates structure, connection, and shared goals and builds feelings of trust and inclusiveness.[5] A kickoff meeting for BCBC 3.0 is scheduled for October 3-5, 2010 and will focus on key aspects of how the BCBC will operate, including instruction of new functionalities for information exchange via the Web site, an enhanced Sharing Policy, and general discussion of timelines and deliverables. In addition, the leaders of all collaborative agreement awards will introduce their research plans to the group at large, and strategic discussions to identify new scientific opportunities that could become trans-BCBC projects will take place.

Lesson Learned—Have Frequent Communication: Another piece to building trust and a successful team is frequent communication. In general, it has been reported that teams with high levels of trust initiate communication more often to request clarification, to garner consensus, or to provide timely and substantive feedback.[6] Teams like the BCBC are now exploring how social networking can increase communication among team members and add value to team science. In addition to an initial meeting, retreats have also been shown to promote communication, reduce friction, and stimulate integration.[7] The BCBC holds semi-annual meetings: a planning meeting for investigators in the fall and a scientific retreat for all participants in the spring. These meetings provide another opportunity for investigators to interact in person, form contacts, discuss pressing issues, and establish new collaborations. Monthly teleconferences of the Executive Committee and newly established Workgroups enable attentive oversight; these discussions are crucial to exchange information and build consensus in order to quickly and effectively resolve operational issues.

Lesson Learned—Promote Open Sharing of Scientific Information: Another key to the BCBC and its success is that open sharing of information stimulates progress within the team and with the broader scientific community. Greater emphasis was placed on the timely sharing of unpublished information as the Consortium developed. To this end, the BCBC Web site is a vital resource that provides a forum for sharing research information throughout the BCBC. Data sharing is critical to the success of the BCBC, however significant issues to protect the confidentiality of unpublished results and to avoid conflict of interest issues generated a barrier to this activity. To ensure confidentiality and promote the sharing of preliminary research information and reagents, access to resource information on the BCBC Web site was restructured to enable a high degree of access control. This assures that BCBC investigators can access all information that they have privileges to see, while maintaining confidentiality of unpublished results and avoiding conflict of interest issues. Again, studies in team science indicate that "cyber-infrastructure" is essential to the success of distance collaboration.[8] Many reagents are described on and publicly accessible via the BCBC Web site. To enable this, the BCBC established a sharing policy in which all BCBC investigators agreed to the timely sharing of data and reagents. Sanctions are possible for individuals who do not comply, and new reagents must be distributed to academic investigators without regard to the requestor's identity or experimental plans. This promotes overall progress in the beta cell biology field. To date, the BCBC Web site has received over 65,000 unique visits from 152 countries, demonstrating its utility.

Lesson Learned—Need for Organization and Leadership: An important difference between the first and second funding cycles of the BCBC is the increase in organization as time progressed. It took time to build the resource cores, assemble the coordinating center, establish the cyber-infrastructure, and stimulate fruitful collaborations. Patience and time are required for establishing a productive team. The importance of thoughtful planning and goal-oriented results cannot be underestimated and require good leadership to achieve. Leadership in the BCBC does not rest on one person, ensuring that no single person is dominant and underscoring that every member has an important role and contributes to the goals of the BCBC. The BCBC found, however, that it was helpful to define these roles and monitor them to assist progress. For example, several committees with clearly defined responsibilities and which include BCBC investigators, scientists outside the BCBC, and NIDDK staff, are involved in guiding the Consortium. Communication and cooperation between BCBC scientists and NIDDK staff have been essential to establishing leadership in the BCBC and have led to a stimulating and collegial environment.

Lesson Learned—Employ Flexible Funding Mechanisms: The ability to distribute support in versatile and creative ways has helped to ensure rapid progress in the development and translation of new discoveries.

The BCBC utilizes Collaborative Bridging Projects (CBPs) which were created to support collaboration between various BCBC members and between the BCBC and other scientists; Pilot and Feasibility Projects (P&Fs) which attract new talent to beta cell biology; and the Seeding Collaborative Research Program that permits investigators outside the BCBC to collect preliminary data and form collaborative research teams prior to applying for full-scale funding during the BCBC re-competition. The CBP program, which supports projects that bridge two or more teams, has stimulated many productive interactions among investigators including higher impact and potentially riskier projects by providing the "glue" to bring BCBC investigators together in ways that are scientifically productive. These programs also bring non-BCBC investigators with relevant skills and talents into the Consortium. Many investigators who were brought into the BCBC through these programs went on to compete successfully to join subsequent funding cycles of the Consortium. These programs have allowed the BCBC to remain flexible, open, and responsive to new scientific developments and brought new skills and knowledge into the BCBC.

A Highly-Collaborative and Productive Team

The two completed funding cycles enable an evaluation of the Consortium's progress as the lessons learned were implemented and the program evolved. By comparing outcomes from the first and second cycles, it is possible to ascertain whether collaboration and productivity have been enhanced. Scientific interactions by BCBC investigators, as demonstrated in Figure 3, are tracked by the BCBC Coordinating Center and have increased as the Consortium matured. For 2001-2005 there was an average of 1-1.2 collaborations per investigator, while in 2005-2009 there was an average of 3 collaborations

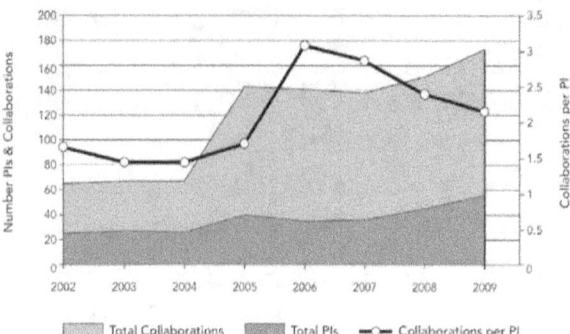

Figure 3: Collaborations in the BCBC
Total collaborations by the Consortium, as well as the number of collaborations per investigator, increased as the Consortium matured.
Graph courtesy of Dr. Jean-Phillipe Cartailler, Vanderbilt University.

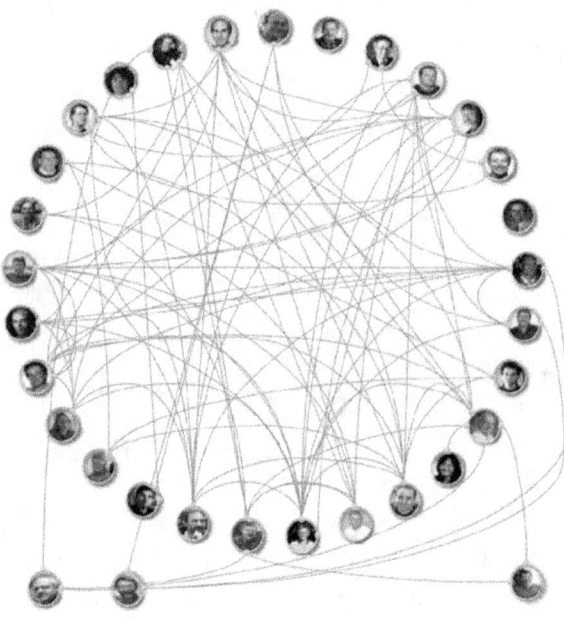

Figure 4: Scientific Interactions by BCBC Investigators
Scientific interactions by BCBC investigators. Collaborations are illustrated by a line between investigators. Collaborations have been stimulated by cooperative agreement awards (grey lines) or by the Collaborative Bridging Projects (blue lines). Many BCBC investigators participate in multiple collaborations.
Image courtesy of Dr. Jean-Phillipe Cartailler, Vanderbilt University.

per investigator, suggesting that efforts by the BCBC to enhance collaboration were successful. These collaborations, illustrated in Figure 4, were complicated with dynamic interactions and multiple ties for the majority of investigators. Enhancements to the BCBC, guided by the lessons learned, have likely contributed to the increased collaborations.

Generation of Publications and Resources: In science, one measure of productivity is publications, as these are a manner in which results of studies are transmitted to the scientific community. Over the past 8 years, the BCBC has published more than 290 articles, as determined by the BCBC Coordinating Center's query of PubMed for BCBC investigators. Over 200 of these publications occurred in BCBC 2.0, suggesting that improvements implemented as the Consortium progressed, in part, led to increased productivity.

Another goal of the BCBC, and measure of the Consortium's productivity, is the generation of tangible resources. The BCBC is responsible for collaboratively generating necessary reagents, such as mouse strains, antibodies, assays, protocols, datasets, and other technologies that are beyond the scope of any single research effort and that would facilitate research on the development of novel cellular therapies for diabetes (see Figure 5). In addition to resource generation, the BCBC lists resources, of which more than 70 percent are publically available, on its Web site (www.betacell.org). These resources are distributed to BCBC and non-BCBC investigators. As illustrated in Figure 5, generation of resources accelerated as the Consortium progressed: fewer than 100 resources had been produced by 2005 while over 400 have now been produced. These new tools, strategies, and reagents will have lasting value in beta cell biology research. In addition, these reagents

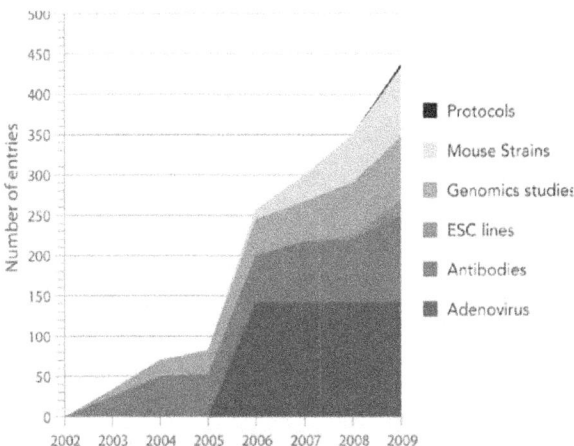

Figure 5: Expansion of BCBC Reagent Resources
Types and numbers of formal BCBC resources collected and made available by the Web site are illustrated.
Graph courtesy of Dr. Jean-Phillipe Cartailler, Vanderbilt University.

are being more broadly used for research by the scientific community, for example in pancreatic cancer research.

Achievements of the BCBC: As a result of the BCBC's efforts, new scientific insights have emerged and efforts toward cell-based therapies are progressing. Significant new knowledge has been gained of the genes involved in and events that occur during development that lead to the formation of pancreatic beta cells. This knowledge is being used in the development of strategies to generate beta cells from embryonic stem cells[9] and/or other stem/ progenitor cell populations, such as induced pluripotent stem cells, and may pave the way for new cell-based therapies for type 1 diabetes. Specific highlights of BCBC accomplishments include:

- Scientists in the BCBC identified progenitor cells in the adult mouse pancreas that form insulin-producing beta cells.

- Results from BCBC studies provided insight about the regenerative potential, or virtual lack thereof, of beta cells.

- BCBC investigators have also made significant strides toward being able to make beta cells from other cell types. For example, they reprogrammed adult mouse exocrine cells into beta cells and demonstrated spontaneous conversion of adult alpha cells into insulin-producing cells in beta cell-depleted mice.

- In addition to producing scientific knowledge that advances progress toward specific goals of the BCBC, such as the ability to coax cells along a pathway to make beta cells, the BCBC has also generated advances toward other goals. For example, researchers in the BCBC discovered that autoantibodies to a specific beta cell protein are an excellent marker for type 1 diabetes autoimmunity. They found that these autoantibodies can substantially improve prediction of diabetes when used in combination with other previously discovered autoantibodies commonly used to monitor for type 1 diabetes autoimmunity in research studies.

THE NEXT PHASE OF THE BCBC

The ever evolving nature of science and of team science provides new and continuing challenges for the BCBC. Transparency and sharing of data and results prior to publication are critical to accelerating progress and conducting team science. These features, however, must be balanced with the confidentiality of this information. As achievement in science is measured by publications and by being the first to report new information, BCBC investigators need to be able to pursue their results and publish their studies without risk of their results reaching a competitor. The BCBC also continues to balance its two efforts: resource generation and scientific performance. Both are critical to advancing progress in beta cell biology and to the success of the BCBC, and both interests require resources that are limited—time and funding. As the BCBC enters its second decade, the Consortium is reviewing its overall goals in order to assure that it continues to stimulate progress in this important field. By maintaining a fresh approach and responding to cutting edge discoveries and technologies, the BCBC aims to continue its success and enhance progress. This flexibility and responsiveness to the changing nature of science, technology, and the team itself will allow the BCBC to remain timely and composed of the top scientists in the field. As the science of team science and evaluation of scientific progress further develop, the BCBC will have more tools to realistically assess progress and impact and enhance the Consortium further.

In response to the needs of and feedback from members of the BCBC, as well as external evaluation committees, the BCBC continues to evolve. As BCBC 3.0 begins, the focus will be enhanced toward more translational outcomes. Results from BCBC investigators and the field have enabled this evolution and paved the path toward these outcomes. Therefore, the time is right for the BCBC to capitalize on this knowledge and take advantage of recent developments in cell reprogramming, induced pluripotent stem cell technology, and mouse models with greater fidelity to human disease. The BCBC will focus on the issues that stand in the way of developing cell-based and regenerative therapies, and will increase studies of the human islet to assist translation of this new knowledge to therapies.

Summary

The BCBC has been a highly collaborative, productive, and successful consortium, and is now being used as a model for other team science efforts at NIH. Implementation of program enhancements, guided by the lessons learned from the BCBC, promoted increased collaboration and productivity as the Consortium matured. This group has demonstrated that the challenges of team science can be mitigated with planning, patience, time, flexibility, and leadership. Critically, investigators pursue their personal scientific interests with collaborations in line with the goals of BCBC, providing a balance between personal interests and independence, and team needs. The team-based approach and activities of the BCBC maximize the scientific productivity of participating scientists and accelerate progress toward the development of effective cell-based therapies for type 1 diabetes. As a result of BCBC research, these therapies are one step closer to becoming a reality for patients with the disease.

Notes:
[1] Wuchty S, Jones BF, and Uzzi B: The Increasing Dominance of Teams in Production of Knowledge. Science 316: 1036-1039, 2007.
[2-8] Stokols D, Misra S, Moser RP, et al: The Ecology of Team Science. Am J Prev Med 35: S96-S115, 2008.
[9] The NIH supports research using human embryonic stem cells within the NIH Guidelines for Human Stem Cell Research.

Feature:
Investigator Comments on the Value of the Beta Cell Biology Consortium (BCBC) Team-science Approach

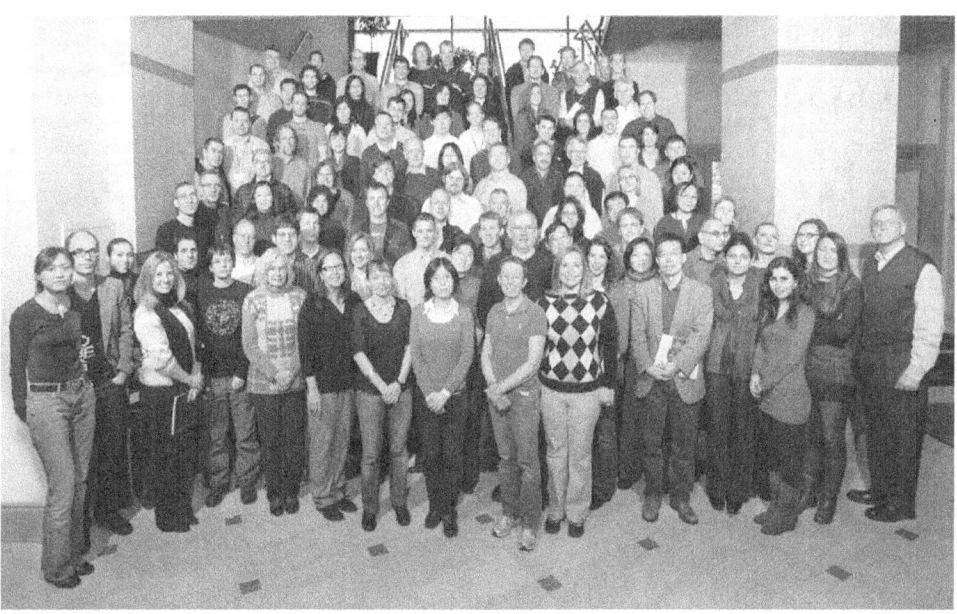

BCBC scientists at the 2010 BCBC Investigator Retreat; Bethesda, MD.
Photo courtesy of Dr. Mark Magnuson, Vanderbilt University.

"The team-based approach of the BCBC has benefited our research in two ways. First, it has enabled us to gain the expertise of diverse individuals working together to understand previously unappreciated signaling pathways that promote the development of the pancreatic beta cell. Second, by sharing our discoveries within the larger group of the Consortium, prior to publication, it allows certain findings to be confirmed more rapidly by others and new twists to be revealed as early as possible."

—*Ken Zaret, Ph.D., University of Pennsylvania*

"The team-based approach of the BCBC has transformed how I do research. We are now able to bring our knowledge and skills to bear on projects that were impossible for us to do before. By bringing leading scientists together, and then providing support for collaborative research, the BCBC accelerates the pace of discovery necessary for the development of novel, new therapies for both type 1 and type 2 diabetes."

—*Mark Magnuson, M.D., Vanderbilt University*

"The BCBC is, to me, the best example of how to partner a truly scientifically excited and expert NIH staff with a large cluster of first-tier research labs, working globally and in an integrated, rapid fashion. An interactive and flexible leadership group has generated an incredibly trusting and enabling infrastructure not only to innervate BCBC member labs, but also to reach out, via completely novel concepts and tools, to help tons of other basic and translational researchers who are tackling diabetes. A focused and milestone-oriented approach within the BCBC has shaved years off the time involved in drawing up a precise molecular-genetic blueprint for the production of our body's normal insulin-secreting beta cells. Personally, I am proud of my membership in the BCBC."

—Christopher Wright, D.Phil., Vanderbilt University

"Having the BCBC, and having different people develop and share reagents and technologies, has moved the [beta cell biology] field so much faster. The way that the BCBC as a whole has advanced the field is much more than the sum of the parts. As part of the BCBC, I have been able to probe deeper into the questions that I wanted to ask and to do the research in a much shorter time span. The BCBC has also allowed my lab to branch out into new areas. Having access to unique reagents through the BCBC has allowed us to ask questions that we simply would not have been able to ask otherwise."

—Maike Sander, M.D., University of California, San Diego

The BCBC is an international Consortium of investigators using a team-science approach to studies of pancreas and beta cell biology and development toward a cell-based therapy for type 1 diabetes. BCBC researchers from around the world work collaboratively and are encouraged to share data and information on a regular basis. For more information about the BCBC, please see "The Beta Cell Biology Consortium: An Experiment in Team Science" feature in this chapter and Appendix C.

Patient Profile

Charlotte Cunningham

With Type 1 Diabetes,
"Time is of the Essence"

Late in the summer of 2005, Lilo Cunningham noticed that her then 10 year-old daughter, Charlotte, was beginning to drink copious amounts of water. This seemed unusual to Lilo because Charlotte was not fond of drinking water. "But no matter where we went, she was always looking for a water fountain," says Lilo. Lilo also noticed that Charlotte was using the bathroom more frequently.

Lilo recognized these changes in Charlotte's behavior as potential symptoms of diabetes. As two of Lilo's sisters have sons with the type 1 form of the disease, Lilo decided not to take a chance. Within days of her observations, Lilo made an appointment with Charlotte's pediatrician and, sure enough, learned that Charlotte's blood sugar level was 680—about seven times above normal.

Charlotte was diagnosed with type 1 diabetes—previously known as juvenile diabetes—a devastating illness that often strikes in infancy, childhood, or young adulthood.

The diagnosis was frightening, but Lilo was able to turn to her sisters for advice. In addition to offering many practical suggestions for dealing with diabetes on a day-to-day basis, one of Lilo's sisters, who is very active in the Juvenile Diabetes Research Foundation International (JDRF), informed her that several diabetes research trials

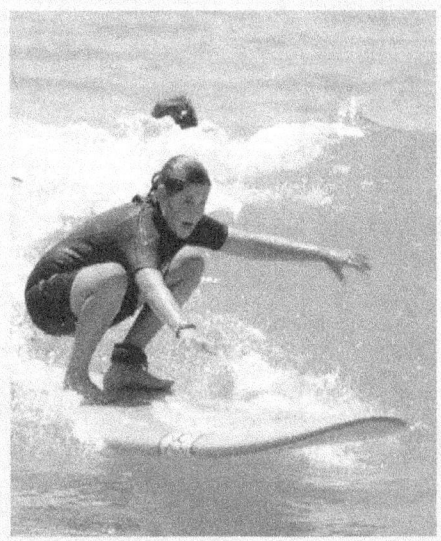

Charlotte Cunningham

were under way. She suggested that the Cunninghams might want to investigate these trials for Charlotte.

Because the Cunninghams were informed of several clinical trials shortly after Charlotte's diagnosis, she was eligible to participate in a clinical trial specifically designed for newly diagnosed patients. The therapy being tested in this trial may slow down the progression of the disease, which could reap long-term benefits for patients and make it easier for them to control their blood sugar levels.

Controlling blood sugar levels is critical. The NIDDK's landmark Diabetes Control and Complications Trial (DCCT) demonstrated that intensive blood sugar control offers remarkable long-term benefits when it comes to preventing or delaying complications frequently associated with type 1 diabetes, including eye, nerve, kidney, and cardiovascular disease.

At the time this profile was written, Charlotte was 13 years old and 3½ years post-diagnosis, and showed no signs of complications from diabetes. "Time is of the essence," says Lilo, "the more we can slow the progression of this disease and keep Charlotte healthy, the better chance she has of leading a longer, healthier life."

"The longer we can slow the progression of this disease and keep Charlotte healthy, the better chance she has of leading a longer, healthier life."

About the Study

Type 1 diabetes occurs when a person's immune system mounts a misguided attack and destroys the insulin-producing beta cells found in the pancreas. Insulin is critical for the body to absorb glucose from the blood and to use it for energy. Those with type 1 diabetes need daily administration of externally supplied insulin, either by injection or with a pump, and must monitor their blood sugar levels vigilantly. Researchers have discovered, however, that many individuals diagnosed with type 1 diabetes still make detectable amounts of insulin, even many years after they are diagnosed. The DCCT also showed that people with type 1 diabetes who still made some of their own insulin had fewer long-term disease complications, as well as reduced incidents of dangerously low blood sugar (hypoglycemia) from administration of too much insulin. These observations suggest that preserving patients' remaining beta cell function, so that they still produce some of their own insulin, could have dramatic, long-term health benefits.

The trial in which Charlotte is participating is trying to do just that. A previous NIDDK-supported clinical trial indicated that an antibody, called hOKT3gamma1(Ala-ala)

or "anti-CD3", halted the destruction of insulin-producing beta cells in a small number of newly diagnosed patients. Anti-CD3 alters the signal that triggers the disease-causing immune cells to attack the insulin-secreting cells. Charlotte is participating in a trial where researchers are determining if an additional treatment of anti-CD3 will provide further benefit, beyond that of the single treatment. This trial is being conducted by the Immune Tolerance Network, which is led by the National Institute of Allergy and Infectious Diseases, in collaboration with the NIDDK's Type 1 Diabetes TrialNet. Both networks also receive funding from the *Special Statutory Funding Program for Type 1 Diabetes Research*. Because one of the requirements for participation in this particular trial was that patients enroll within 8 weeks of their diagnosis, the Cunninghams are very grateful that a family member counseled them to act quickly after Charlotte's diagnosis.

"We were fortunate that Charlotte was diagnosed so early and was able to participate in this trial," says Lilo. "As a result, she's perhaps making more insulin than the average person in the early stages of diabetes and is doing very well."

The trial requires Charlotte to be infused daily over a 14-day period with the anti-CD3 antibody. Each daily infusion takes between 15 to 30 minutes, and is administered into Charlotte's upper arm. Charlotte received this 14-day set of infusions two times; the second treatment followed 19 months after the first. Charlotte returned to the trial site every 3 months in between the treatments and for 12 months following the second treatment. These visits were to monitor her response to the treatment and included a physical examination, a blood test, and a test to measure her insulin response. Except for a rash between her fingers, which lasted only 1 day, Charlotte has experienced no side effects from the treatment.

When asked about her overall experience in the trial study, Charlotte responded, "It was very cool." Not the typical response one would expect from an adolescent, but Charlotte has handled her diabetes extremely well from the beginning.

"We had an incredibly positive experience with Charlotte's study. We were exposed to so many people who know so much about this disease—we learned so much!"

Lilo & Charlotte's Message:
Don't hesitate. Act quickly.
When it comes to diabetes, Lilo and Charlotte's message to others is clear and simple: At the first sign of symptoms, do not hesitate; act quickly.

"If you have any suspicions or notice anything wrong with your child, go for a blood test [at your pediatrician's office] and follow up immediately," says Lilo. "If this study succeeds in allowing Charlotte to retain the ability to produce some of her own insulin, even for a little while longer than she might have otherwise, it will help to delay, reduce, and possibly even prevent the secondary complications that often accompany type 1 diabetes." "And make sure you check your blood sugar level regularly," adds Charlotte.

Lilo has not observed symptoms in other family members, but that does not mean she was going to take chances. The Cunninghams enrolled their two other children, Charlotte's 16 year-old brother and 19 year-old sister, in a study as well—the TrialNet Natural History Study.

This study is screening relatives of people with type 1 diabetes to determine what level of risk these family members have for developing the disease. These studies are being conducted to learn more about the causes and indicators of risk for the development of type 1 diabetes. So far neither one of Charlotte's siblings appears to be at increased risk. "But if either of them should show signs of the disease, I would enroll them in a clinical trial in a heartbeat," Lilo says. "We had an incredibly positive experience with Charlotte's study. We were exposed to so many people who know so much about this disease— we learned so much!" When asked her thoughts on participating in the trial, Charlotte proudly says "I'm an example of how diabetes research is helping people."

"Having diabetes hasn't really affected me much when I'm doing sports...my coaches are very understanding and let me do what I need to do to take care of myself."

About Charlotte
Since February 2008, Charlotte's need for injected insulin has increased dramatically. According to Lilo, it is hard to say exactly what is going on. "Charlotte is in the midst of puberty, which could mean her body is requiring more insulin because of hormonal changes," she says. Nineteen months after her first treatment, Charlotte received her second and final 14-day infusion as part of the trial. The good news is that, even though Charlotte needs more external insulin, tests performed in July 2010 (nearly 5 years after her initial diagnosis) indicate that she is still producing a clinically significant amount of insulin. Because her need for external insulin has increased, Charlotte started using an insulin pump, a portable device that injects insulin at programmed intervals.

If anything, Charlotte's life has become more active, rather than less, since being diagnosed with diabetes. Prior to her diagnosis, Charlotte played tennis and basketball. Now she has added surf boarding, lacrosse, and softball to her repertoire of physical activities. "Having diabetes hasn't really affected me much when I'm doing sports," she says. "I need to make sure my blood sugar count is okay both before and while I'm playing, but my coaches are very understanding and let me do what I need to do to take care of myself."

In the meantime, at the time this story was written, Charlotte was preparing to go to summer camp with 70 of her peers, all of whom have diabetes. She has been to the camp twice before and says she likes it a lot. "We meet with meal planners and check our blood sugar regularly, but mostly it's a regular, fun camp," Charlotte explained. Like any 13-year-old, Charlotte simply wants to lead as active and normal a life as possible.

EMERGING RESEARCH OPPORTUNITIES RESULTING FROM THE *SPECIAL DIABETES PROGRAM*

The *Special Statutory Funding Program for Type 1 Diabetes Research* has fueled the emergence of a wide range of research opportunities. These opportunities were identified in a strategic planning process as being critically important for overcoming current barriers and achieving progress in diabetes research. Key questions and research opportunities relevant to type 1 diabetes, including those related to the development of cell-based replacement therapy, are outlined in Appendix F.

GOAL IV

PREVENT OR REDUCE HYPOGLYCEMIA

Hypoglycemia is the major obstacle to achieving the tight glucose control that has been proven to reduce the deadly complications of type 1 diabetes. To overcome this obstacle, the *Special Statutory Funding Program for Type 1 Diabetes Research* has supported multifaceted efforts ranging from fundamental research to understand how the body recognizes and defends against hypoglycemia and how diabetes impairs this defense, to applied research in partnership with industry to develop technology for continuous glucose monitoring and automated insulin delivery; and has established a clinical network to test the latest technology that can stabilize glucose levels and prevent or reduce hypoglycemia in children with diabetes. In addition to the significant research progress described in this chapter, information on the program evaluation related to Goal IV can be found in Appendix A (Allocation of Funds), Appendix B (Assessment), and Appendix C (Evaluation of Major Research Consortia, Networks, and Resources).

While the results of NIDDK's landmark Diabetes Control and Complications Trial (DCCT) and its follow-up effort, the Epidemiology of Diabetes Interventions and Complications (EDIC) demonstrated that intensive control of blood glucose (sugar) levels can have long-lasting effects toward reducing the onset and progression of diabetes complications involving the kidneys, eyes, nerves, and heart, obstacles remain for many people with type 1 diabetes to achieving tight blood glucose control. Although finger pricks provide "snap shots" of a person's blood glucose levels, they are painful and do not provide data about "trends" that indicate whether blood glucose levels are increasing or decreasing. Even if patients test as much as a dozen times a day to help adjust insulin, they will spend prolonged periods each day outside the target glucose levels. Moreover, excessive treatment with insulin relative to food intake and physical activity can cause blood glucose levels to fall dangerously below a minimal threshold required to fuel the body's activities, particularly brain function. The immediate effects of abnormally low blood glucose (hypoglycemia) can be severe, including changes in cardiovascular and central nervous system function, cognitive impairment, increased risk for unintentional injury, coma, and death. Thus, in addition to the need for better tools to help people with type 1 diabetes achieve and sustain tight blood glucose control, the potential for hypoglycemic episodes has limited the use of intensive insulin therapy protocols. Research to develop and test new disease management technologies and to understand how to predict and prevent episodes of hypoglycemia is critical to helping people with type 1 diabetes prevent the deadly complications that can accompany the disease.

The *Special Statutory Funding Program for Type 1 Diabetes Research* (*Special Diabetes Program* or *Program*) has played an important role in the generation of new tools to improve patients' ability to control their blood glucose levels. As described in greater detail in this chapter, the *Program* supported the development of recently approved continuous glucose monitors (CGMs), which reveal the dynamic changes in blood glucose levels by assessing glucose levels hundreds of times per day and displaying trends. The *Program* filled an industry gap by first testing CGMs in children, a population that could benefit greatly from this technology, and supports research to "close the loop" by linking glucose monitoring to insulin delivery—what is often referred to as an "artificial pancreas." Additionally, the *Program* has supported research initiatives to better understand the causes of hypoglycemia and how to prevent this serious, life-threatening condition. Due to support from the *Program*, new technologies and research results have revolutionized the way that patients manage their disease, improved the outlook for people with type 1 diabetes, and accelerated the pace of research to close the loop.

HIGHLIGHTS OF RECENT RESEARCH ADVANCES RELATED TO GOAL IV

Approval of New Glucose Monitoring Technologies: In 2006, the U.S. Food and Drug Administration (FDA) approved a continuous glucose monitoring device displaying results on an insulin pump for use in people over age 18. Additional CGMs developed by other manufacturers with NIH support have recently been approved for use in both adults and children. This major technological advance represents the culmination of years of effort by the U.S. Department of Health and Human Services (HHS) and the *Program* in bringing together and funding collaborations of clinicians, engineers, and basic biologists from industry and academia. The new CGMs have been shown to improve control of glucose levels and reduce hypoglycemia and are a major milestone in the future development of an artificial pancreas.

Tested CGMs in Children: The Diabetes Research in Children Network (DirecNet) filled an industry gap by first testing the safety and efficacy of continuous glucose monitoring technology in children. DirecNet has carried out independent and scientifically rigorous studies to determine the true benefit of new monitoring technologies. Without the initial information from DirecNet, it could have been many years before the manufacturers of these devices conducted studies in the pediatric population. The DirecNet group is well positioned to assess new devices for their accuracy, as well as their clinical usefulness in the home environment.

Practical Steps To Avoid Nocturnal Hypoglycemia: DirecNet has examined factors that contribute to nocturnal hypoglycemia in children. Using the new CGMs, investigators found that exercising in the late afternoon caused a delayed nighttime drop in glucose levels and nearly doubled the risk for nocturnal hypoglycemia relative to exercise-free days. Additional DirecNet studies have shown that the risk of hypoglycemia can be markedly reduced in insulin pump-treated patients by suspending the basal insulin infusion during exercise. Exercise is important for these children, particularly in keeping blood glucose from rising too high, and these findings point to the importance of adjusting patients' diabetes regimen on active days.

Recurrent Episodes of Low Blood Glucose Do Not Impact Long-term Cognitive Function: The landmark DCCT found that tight blood glucose control—while reducing complications—increased the risk of severe hypoglycemia three-fold. There was fear that in addition to its dangerous short-term effects, hypoglycemia might also lead to a long-term loss of cognitive ability. Twelve years after the conclusion of the DCCT, researchers in its follow-up study, EDIC, reported the absence of a link between multiple severe hypoglycemia reactions and impaired cognitive function in people with type 1 diabetes in the study.

CONTINUOUS GLUCOSE MONITORS CHANGE MANAGEMENT OF TYPE 1 DIABETES

The results of DCCT/EDIC showed that good blood glucose control is a key factor in lowering the risk of many of the devastating long-term complications of diabetes, including blindness, kidney failure, and cardiovascular disease. For children and adults with type 1 diabetes, this has led to the use of intensified insulin therapy. However, the wide-spread application of this approach has been limited by a lack of technologies that would enable people with diabetes to easily and appropriately adjust delivery of insulin in response to minute-to-minute changes in circulating glucose. By the late 1990s, several daily measurements of glucose in the blood had proven useful, but did not provide patients with information about what happened in between readings and it was difficult to ascertain the highs, lows, and trends throughout the day and night. Scientists were actively pursuing new approaches to assess glucose continuously that were both safe and accurate (for more information about the development of CGMs, please see the accompanying Story of Discovery in this chapter). Research supported by NIH and industry led to FDA approval of the first CGM in 1999. While this device was a large step forward, measurements obtained from this CGM were not as accurate and could only be assessed retrospectively, not in real time.

Improving CGMs: Support from NIH and the *Program* accelerated the pace of research on glucose sensing technologies through research solicitations and investigator-initiated projects. This research culminated in FDA approval in 2006 of a continuous glucose monitoring device displaying results on an insulin pump for use in people over age 18. Additional CGMs developed by other manufacturers with NIH support have recently been approved for use in both adults and children. Currently, CGMs used in combination with finger sticks are FDA-approved. This major technological advance represents the culmination of years of effort by HHS and the *Program* in bringing together and funding collaborations of clinicians, engineers, and basic biologists from industry and academia to develop both the technology underlying the glucose sensors and the algorithms used to assist insulin delivery decisions. The new continuous glucose monitoring devices are a major milestone in the future development of an artificial pancreas. These CGMs combine a continuous glucose sensor with a unit displaying glucose levels. The sensors are inserted under the skin for up to 3 to 7 days and transmit readings of glucose levels in tissue fluid—an approximation of blood glucose levels—every 1 to 5 minutes to a receiver carried by the individual, whether the patient is awake or asleep, and trigger an alarm if levels become too high or too low. CGMs have the potential to dramatically improve patients' ability to control glucose levels, which is key for minimizing or preventing complications. They can also improve quality of life by reducing the need for frequent monitoring and alleviating the fears that children and their parents have of nocturnal hypoglycemia.

Testing CGMs in a Target Population: A critical component to any new technology is evaluating how well it will work in the people who use it. Therefore, the NICHD-led and *Program*-supported Diabetes Research in Children Network (DirecNet) took on the task of filling an industry gap by testing new continuous glucose monitoring technology in children. Because no regimen of insulin replacement in type 1 diabetes will be able to completely eliminate the risk of severe hypoglycemia in the absence of feedback control of insulin delivery based on real-time changes in blood glucose levels, DirecNet critically evaluated whether the recent advances in glucose sensor technology could be utilized to improve metabolic control and reduce the frequency of hypoglycemia without having adverse effects on health and psychosocial well-being in children and adolescents with type 1 diabetes. DirecNet developed a template inpatient protocol to test the accuracy of CGM devices and newer home glucose monitors in comparison with reference glucose determinations made at a central laboratory. Initial studies illustrated the limitations in accuracy of the first-generation CGM devices, especially for blood glucose values in the hypoglycemic range. In contrast, certain glucose meters were very accurate over the full range of glucose values. The results of these DirecNet studies have had a major impact on the analysis of CGM performance and indicated that reliability and ease of patient use are critically important factors in the clinical efficacy of CGM devices. DirecNet is continuing to study the efficacy, tolerability, safety, and effect on quality of life of CGMs in children 4 to less than 10 years of age with type 1 diabetes and has launched a pilot study to test this technology in children less than 4 years of age.

DirecNet accomplishments also include the development, modification, testing, and validation of several psychosocial and other outcome measures for use in future clinical trials. Subsequent JDRF- and industry-supported studies demonstrating improved glucose control with CGMs built upon the initial DirecNet studies. Scientists have begun to answer important clinical questions about the added value of CGM in people newly diagnosed with type 1 diabetes. Studies are also beginning in select people who have type 2 diabetes, such as those particularly prone to glucose fluctuations

due to the disabling diabetes complication gastroparesis. Not only are such trials key to identifying the population with the potential for maximum benefit from this technology, but these studies will lay the groundwork for trials to accelerate the development and evaluation of artificial pancreas technologies. DirecNet and TrialNet investigators (see Goal II) are currently collaborating on a clinical trial evaluating whether early and intensive blood glucose control can protect patients' remaining insulin-producing beta cells from the toxic effects of high blood glucose. The trial participants are placed on a closed-loop system, linking blood glucose monitoring via CGMs and insulin delivery via an insulin pump, to intensively manage their blood glucose levels shortly after disease onset. This trial will determine if near normalization of glucose levels at onset can protect beta cells from injury caused by high glucose levels and slow disease progression. For more information on the trial, see the Investigator Profile of Dr. Bruce Buckingham later in this chapter.

Research To Help Patients Use New Technologies: To optimize the potential impact of new technologies such as CGMs, research is needed that considers clinical and behavioral factors that may enhance or constrain their sustained use. There is an implicit assumption that more information will lead to better patient managed glucose control. But for patients and providers to make optimal use of the vast amounts of information these tools provide, additional knowledge, skill, and motivation is required. Individuals need to be able and willing to make the appropriate regimen course corrections on an ongoing basis and be savvy enough about their glucose trends to avoid over-correction with insulin. The user interface requirements will also be different across the lifespan. For example, the way a technology is used may require different behavioral approaches when it is employed in different age groups, such as young children, adolescents, and adults. Research is key to support the broad adoption of CGMs as a daily self-management tool and to identify the most effective ways to incorporate these technologies into clinical care. Behavioral research funded by the *Program* is seeking to improve outcomes of people with type 1 diabetes. Although this research is still in progress, it is expected that results will be used to enhance the usability of new technology and help patients in their decision-making regarding diabetes management. This research will identify ways to assist patients to effectively use new technologies to benefit their health and quality of life.

New Knowledge Toward Prevention of Hypoglycemia

Although CGMs enable people with type 1 diabetes to adjust their insulin doses to avoid extreme high and low glucose levels, this approach cannot replicate the exquisitely precise and dynamic regulation of insulin levels achieved by insulin-producing beta cells. Thus, despite a person's best efforts, glucose levels can rise excessively (hyperglycemia)—particularly after meals—and at other times can fall dangerously low (hypoglycemia), causing unconsciousness, seizures, and even death. Normally, a drop in blood glucose triggers the body's warning system to release stress hormones, including adrenaline, and to stimulate a part of the nervous system that raises glucose and results in symptoms such as shaking and sweating. However, in individuals who experience repeated episodes of hypoglycemia, these counterregulatory mechanisms are impaired so the typical signs and symptoms disappear. These affected individuals do not recognize, and therefore, cannot correct for, the low blood glucose—a

syndrome known as hypoglycemia unawareness. A vicious cycle is initiated as each hypoglycemic event makes it more likely that these compensatory signals will fail in the future, leading to another unrecognized hypoglycemic event. People with type 1 diabetes, especially children, are particularly vulnerable to hypoglycemia unawareness while they are asleep. Therefore "nocturnal hypoglycemia" is a primary concern and the source of many anxious nights for parents of children with type 1 diabetes who stay awake to check on the well-being of their children throughout each night.

Understandably, the fear of severe hypoglycemia represents the single greatest barrier to full implementation of the recommendations of the DCCT/EDIC. Therefore, in parallel to the development of better technologies to assist people with type 1 diabetes in managing the disease, it is critical to conduct research to understand the molecular mechanisms of hypoglycemia towards improvement of prevention strategies. Through DirecNet and other research, the *Special Diabetes Program* has supported a variety of efforts to improve understanding of hypoglycemia. While much still remains to be learned about this condition, studies supported by the *Program* have advanced progress in this field.

Practical Suggestions To Prevent Hypoglycemia: Data using continuous glucose monitoring have shown that low glucose levels are even more common than previously thought, but are often undetected; low levels sometimes go back up before the morning blood glucose check. DirecNet has examined factors that contribute to nocturnal hypoglycemia in children. Using the new continuous glucose sensors, investigators found that exercise in the late afternoon caused a delayed nighttime drop in glucose levels and increased the risk for nocturnal hypoglycemia relative to exercise-free days. Exercise is important for these children, particularly in keeping blood glucose from rising too high, and these findings point to the importance of adjusting patients' diabetes regimen on active days. A DirecNet follow-up study showed that the risk of hypoglycemia can be markedly reduced in patients treated with insulin pumps by suspending the basal insulin infusion during exercise. In addition, this work generated the practical suggestion of increased bedtime snacks on days when children with diabetes are particularly physically active even if the bedtime glucose measurement is not low. DirecNet further showed that both low-fat and high-fat bedtime snacks provide similar protection against nocturnal hypoglycemia. *Program*-supported efforts by DirecNet are yielding practical suggestions for children with diabetes and their caregivers to maintain healthy blood glucose levels more safely and effectively by managing diet and exercise.

Brain Function Not Permanently Damaged by Hypoglycemia: The landmark DCCT found that intensive glucose control—while reducing complications—increased the risk of severe hypoglycemia three-fold. There was fear that in addition to its dangerous short-term effects—confusion, irrational behavior, convulsions, and unconsciousness—hypoglycemia might also lead to a long-term loss of cognitive ability. Twelve years after the conclusion of the DCCT, researchers reported results of a study in which DCCT participants were evaluated using the same neuropsychological tests administered during the DCCT trial. The tests analyzed problem solving, learning, immediate memory, delayed recall, spatial information, attention, psychomotor efficiency, and motor speed. The tests revealed no link between multiple severe hypoglycemic reactions and impaired cognitive function in people with type 1 diabetes in the study. The results demonstrate that while acute episodes

of hypoglycemia can impair thinking and can even be life-threatening, people with type 1 diabetes do not have to worry that such episodes will damage their mental abilities and impair their long-term abilities to perceive, reason, and remember. However, investigation regarding this issue is ongoing to assess more subtle effects, and NIH is supporting imaging studies to elucidate whether brain structure is affected by recurrent hypoglycemia and to determine any possible correlation between recurrent hypoglycemia and cognitive capability.

Understanding Why Hypoglycemia Is Not Prevented in People with Type 1 Diabetes: Counterregulatory hormones, like glucagon, adrenaline, noreprinephrine, cortisol, and growth hormone, oppose the action of insulin by raising the level of glucose in blood in multiple ways. In healthy individuals, counterregulatory hormones act as a principal defense against hypoglycemia; levels of these hormones rise as glucose levels fall, thus promoting processes to raise the levels of glucose in the blood. It is not understood why this mechanism appears to fail in people with type 1 diabetes. In people with the disease, dangerous episodes of hypoglycemia reflect the failure of the body to trigger normal warning systems (like adrenaline and glucagon) that wake the patient and increase blood glucose in response to hypoglycemia. Progress in understanding these systems in people with type 1 diabetes has been made both by DirecNet and other research efforts through the support of the *Program*. For example, a DirecNet study demonstrated that young children (3-8 years of age) and adolescents (12-18 years of age) with well-controlled type 1 diabetes have impaired counterregulatory hormone responses to hypoglycemia. The results of this study showed that, regardless of age, these well-controlled pediatric patients failed to release the counterregulatory hormone epinephrine until blood glucose concentrations approach values that indicate a shortage of glucose in the brain.

To further understand why exercise increased the risk for nocturnal hypoglycemia, DirecNet investigators examined the levels of counterregulatory hormones on inactive and active (exercise) days. Through hourly measurement of hormone levels on nights following days of exercise or inactivity, this study demonstrated that counterregulatory hormone responses to spontaneous nocturnal hypoglycemia are blunted throughout the nighttime period with or without antecedent exercise. Similar DirecNet studies indicated that levels of adiponectin (a protein that is directly related to insulin sensitivity and is released from fat) are stable from day-to-day and are not affected by exercise or metabolic control. Moreover, higher levels of adiponectin appear to be associated with a decrease in hypoglycemia risk. Additional efforts will be necessary to understand this relationship and whether it can be utilized to prevent hypoglycemia.

Studies of the pancreatic alpha cell are also providing insights into why protective counterregulatory hormones fail to work in people with type 1 diabetes. The pancreatic islets are composed of several cell types. The counterpart to the insulin-producing beta cell is the glucagon-producing alpha cell. Just as insulin injections control high blood glucose, glucagon injections can be used in an emergency to raise glucose levels that may fall dangerously low after insulin therapy. Glucagon is the major counterregulatory hormone that causes glucose to be released by the liver into the blood stream. Researchers have long recognized that people with type 1 diabetes do not secrete glucagon in response to hypoglycemia, despite their ability to secrete glucagon under other circumstances. Findings from research supported by the *Program* suggest

that a decrease in intra-islet insulin is necessary for glucagon secretion, explaining why the protective glucagon response is impaired in type 1 diabetes. The inflammatory process seen in type 1 diabetes may affect nervous system regulation of the islets contributing to the deficient glucagon response, as reported recently in animal models by investigators supported by the *Program*. By discovering the mechanisms involved in the body's reaction to hypoglycemia, scientists may be able to develop therapies that break the vicious cycle of recurrent hypoglycemia.

CLOSING THE LOOP: DEVELOPMENT OF AN ARTIFICIAL PANCREAS

An artificial pancreas based on mechanical devices requires, at a minimum, three basic components: a continuous blood glucose sensor, an insulin delivery system, and a way to link the two in a loop. Such a system would automatically turn the measurement of blood glucose levels into a practical, precise, and "real-time" insulin-dosing system. Importantly, artificial pancreas technology could help people safely achieve the tight blood glucose control associated with preventing or delaying life-threatening disease complications. Thus, this technology has high potential to have a positive impact on patients' health and quality of life, alleviate an enormous amount of patient burden, and improve long-term health outcomes. There are numerous research opportunities to promote the development of the artificial pancreas. These include the development of more accurate and robust glucose sensing devices; improved methods of insulin delivery and faster acting insulin; and the development of improved computer algorithms that appropriately translate glucose measurements into changes in the delivery of insulin, including its interruption—*i.e.*, methods that can "close the loop" between glucose measurements and insulin delivery.

A key aspect of closing the loop between glucose sensing and insulin delivery in a mechanical artificial pancreas is the development of "instruction sets" for computers, called algorithms. In the case of the artificial pancreas, these computer programs are needed to interpret continuous glucose sensor data and instruct the insulin pump to dose the proper amount of insulin. Two primary algorithm approaches have been generated and are under investigation. The further development of these algorithms is essential for the rapid implementation of closed-loop glucose control. Another advance propelling progress toward an artificial pancreas is the development of in silico (computer-based) models as a resource for pre-clinical testing. In 2008, FDA accepted the use of an in silico model of diabetes as a pre-clinical testing tool for closed-loop research. This and other optimized simulators will facilitate the development of new control algorithms by enabling researchers to test and refine artificial pancreas algorithms quickly; it will allow for computer-based algorithm comparisons; and it may eliminate or minimize the need for animal testing, allowing investigators to focus instead on in-hospital human clinical trials, which may save time and money. This may also lead to a more expedited and better defined process of receiving regulatory approval for human trials of closed-loop systems. As the simulator is equipped with a wide array of tools for precise fine-tuning, it should help bring promising algorithms closer to perfection in a shorter time frame. Other studies are also pushing this field forward. Recently a study of 19 youth with type 1 diabetes suggested that closed-loop

systems could reduce the risk of nocturnal hypoglycemia. Tests of a bi-hormonal closed-loop artificial pancreas, one that delivers both insulin and glucagon, are also reporting promising results. Together these important advances are bringing the field closer to the development of an artificial pancreas.

To further accelerate the development of an artificial pancreas, there is close coordination among NIH, JDRF, and FDA. The NIH and JDRF fund research in this area, and FDA advises researchers as they develop new technologies needed to make the artificial pancreas a reality and assists them as they design studies to evaluate safety and effectiveness. In July 2008, NIH, in collaboration with FDA and JDRF, organized a workshop to discuss current advances and remaining challenges toward the development of an artificial pancreas. This workshop concluded that a mechanical artificial pancreas system has enormous potential benefit for a substantial proportion of people with diabetes. However, important technological obstacles impede long-term use of these devices and new and promising technologies are needed toward the development of an artificial pancreas. Therefore, NIH re-solicited cutting edge research conducted by small businesses leading to the development of innovative technologies toward an artificial pancreas and several Program-supported grants were awarded. The clinical testing of currently available closed-loop platforms and the development of innovative algorithms by academic investigators are also supported by the Program. While the results of this research remain to be determined, it is anticipated that this research will significantly contribute to making the artificial pancreas a reality for people with type 1 diabetes.

Summary

During the past 3 decades, in part due to support from the *Program*, a variety of technological advances have been introduced that have significantly improved the ability of people with diabetes and their physicians to treat diabetes with insulin, including home glucose monitoring devices that allow periodic measurements of blood glucose levels; improved insulin formulations; portable insulin pumps that provide continuous insulin delivery in a more controlled manner; and, most recently, early-phase CGMs that rely on inserting glucose sensors under the skin. The *Program*-supported DirecNet has filled an industry gap by testing these CGMs in children and has used these devices in studies that have produced practical suggestions to reduce the risk of nocturnal hypoglycemia. Research on counterregulatory hormones has provided new information about how hypoglycemia is normally prevented and what goes awry in people with type 1 diabetes. This knowledge could lead to the development of new strategies to prevent hypoglycemia. Finally, the pace of research to close the loop is more rapid due to support from the *Program*. Research efforts and advances in this Goal have improved diabetes care today and offer considerable potential for the creation of an artificial mechanical pancreas for the treatment of diabetes in the future.

RESEARCH CONSORTIUM RELATED TO THE PREVENTION OR REDUCTION OF HYPOGLYCEMIA

Details of the DirecNet evaluation are found in Appendix C. Highlights are summarized below.

Diabetes Research in Children Network (DirecNet): DirecNet is a multicenter clinical research network investigating the use of technology advances in the management of type 1 diabetes in children and adolescents. DirecNet filled an industry gap by testing new continuous glucose monitoring technology in children and has utilized six different brands of CGMs in its completion of nine different protocols. DirecNet has also yielded practical suggestions for people with diabetes and their caregivers to maintain healthy blood glucose levels more safely and effectively by managing diet and exercise.

Story of Discovery:
New Technology for Managing Type 1 Diabetes—Continuous Glucose Monitors

Sometimes, what you don't know can hurt you. For people with type 1 diabetes, undetected high or low blood glucose levels can have severe health consequences—including heart disease, blindness, and coma. With advanced technology, however, patients now have the opportunity to monitor their blood glucose (sugar) levels continuously, rather than just a few times a day. Developed with support from the *Special Statutory Funding Program for Type 1 Diabetes Research* (*Special Diabetes Program* or *Program*), NIH, industry, and others, these new, wearable continuous glucose monitors (CGMs) sound an alarm when glucose levels soar or plunge to dangerous levels—especially important during sleep. They also generate important data, in real time, on trends as they fluctuate throughout the day and night. With this new wealth of knowledge, people with type 1 diabetes may greatly improve their daily disease management by better adjusting the timing and dosages of insulin, and by eating or taking other action to raise low blood glucose. The monitors also have potential to help some other populations—such as people with type 2 diabetes—control their blood glucose levels. Finally, the realization of continuous glucose monitoring technology is a key step toward developing a mechanical replacement for insulin-producing pancreatic beta cells.

Decades ago, reliable and practical methods for glucose monitoring were not available, yet control of glucose levels in the body is crucial. In healthy people, insulin from pancreatic beta cells directs cells throughout the body to absorb glucose from the blood for use as energy. Without beta cells, however, people with type 1 diabetes face daily the arduous tasks of glucose monitoring, insulin administration, rigorous meal planning, and other efforts to control blood glucose. Without sufficient insulin, cells are deprived of energy, and, over time, high blood glucose levels greatly increase risks for heart disease, blindness, kidney failure, nerve damage, and other severe complications. Administering too much insulin, however, can lead to dangerously low glucose levels, or hypoglycemia, which can result in coma or death if untreated, and is especially feared during sleep. Thus, researchers have long sought to develop improved glucose-monitoring methods.

For years, people with type 1 diabetes could only check their glucose levels by testing urine, a method that was not very accurate or useful. In the 1960s, scientists invented the first meter to measure glucose in the blood. By the 1980s, blood glucose meters were widely used, and, with further improvements, remain so today. However, the need for tools for more frequent monitoring of blood glucose continued to drive research toward developing this technology. The availability of improved glucose-monitoring devices in the early 1980s was critical to enabling scientists to test the importance of blood glucose control to the prevention of the devastating complications of diabetes.

The Importance of Intensive Blood Glucose Control
The tremendous health benefits of intensive blood glucose control were demonstrated in the early 1990s by a landmark, NIH-supported clinical trial, the Diabetes Control and Complications Trial (DCCT). This trial showed that intensive control greatly reduced development of diabetic eye disease, kidney disease,

and nerve damage in people with type 1 diabetes, and an ongoing follow-up study demonstrated reduced risk for heart disease and stroke. The intensive control regimen is difficult, however, because it requires multiple painful finger sticks each day to draw blood for testing and frequent insulin administration. The DCCT also revealed that intensive control to avoid high blood glucose levels and future complications had a serious trade-off: an increased immediate risk for hypoglycemia. With the difficulties of intensive glucose control and the threat of hypoglycemia, people with type 1 diabetes still rarely achieve recommended glucose levels. The DCCT thus also underscored the critical importance of research to improve methods for blood glucose control.

Despite the impressive results obtained using glucose meters, these devices are far from optimal. By way of analogy, patients can see a few "snapshots" of their glucose levels per day with glucose meters, but miss what happens in between; with CGMs, patients would see an entire movie that captured glucose highs, lows, and trends throughout the day and night. Thus, scientists were actively investigating another route to assess glucose that would be both safe and practical for continuous monitoring—the interstitial fluid in tissues under the skin. A key research question was whether glucose levels measured by a sensor in the interstitial fluid would reflect glucose levels in the blood. The answer was "yes," as shown in studies in animals and humans, by several research groups supported by NIH and industry. A continuous monitor was first approved by the U.S. Food and Drug Administration (FDA) in 1999. The glucose values obtained from this device were not as accurate as direct blood glucose measures, and could only be assessed retrospectively, not in real time. But the continuous monitor could amass hundreds of glucose readings per day for subsequent analysis by health care providers and patients.

Producing a "Real-time" Continuous Glucose Monitor

The NIH and the *Special Diabetes Program* have accelerated the pace of research on glucose sensing technologies through research solicitations and investigator-initiated projects. Over the last decade, these efforts have led investigators in academia and industry to explore a variety of approaches to continuous glucose monitoring, including devices to measure glucose in body fluid extracted from skin, in eye fluid using a contact lens as a sensor, noninvasively with optical sensing of glucose in the blood, and with minimally invasive sensors inserted into the skin. Researchers have also been exploring the benefits and drawbacks of sensors designed for external use versus more permanent, fully implantable devices. Studies have also focused on validating and optimizing the different technologies.

This research culminated in FDA approval in 2006 of new CGMs for people with diabetes. These devices represented a significant improvement over the first devices approved by FDA. NIH support was instrumental in technology development for the new devices. The new monitors employ a slender sensor that can detect the biochemical reaction of glucose with an enzyme (glucose oxidase) present on the sensor tip. Inserted under the skin, these minimally-invasive sensors provide glucose readings in "real time," every few minutes; display trend data so patients know whether their glucose levels are rising or falling—and how quickly; and sound alarms when levels are too high or low—including at night, during sleep. Before taking action to adjust high or low glucose, patients still need to confirm readings from these new monitors with a traditional finger stick and blood glucose meter. However, the burden of care can be significantly reduced and further improvements in these devices can be expected with additional research and development.

The Potential of Continuous Glucose Monitors To Improve Outcomes

An ongoing and critical area of NIH-funded research is the evaluation of these monitors for use in children. New insights about the use of continuous glucose monitoring technologies have been gained from the Diabetes Research in Children Network (DirecNet) which is led by NICHD and supported by the *Program*. DirecNet is investigating the use of technological advances in the management of type 1 diabetes in children and adolescents and has carried out several independent and scientifically rigorous studies to determine the true benefit of continuous glucose monitoring technologies, including their accuracy and efficacy.

Clinical studies supported by the Juvenile Diabetes Research Foundation International have now shown significant benefits of CGM use by people with diabetes. To determine whether CGM can aid people who are already receiving intensive insulin therapy, researchers conducted a 26-week, randomized multi-center clinical trial in which one group of volunteers used CGMs, while a control group performed home monitoring with a blood glucose meter. The primary outcome, improved glucose control, as measured by hemoglobin A1c (HbA1c), was mainly achieved in people who were older than 25 years. HbA1c is a component of blood that is a good surrogate measure of long-term blood glucose control and, as such, reflects risk of diabetic complications. In children, benefit was seen specifically in those who used CGMs near-daily, underscoring the need to identify barriers to

CGM use in children and adolescents. Hypoglycemia did not increase, even in participants who improved blood glucose control. These encouraging results were reinforced by a second randomized, multi-center clinical trial. This study found that using CGM devices enables people who are already achieving excellent glucose control to spend more time per day in the target blood glucose range, while spending less time per day with glucose values in the potentially dangerous hypoglycemic range. A recent industry-supported study found that use of an insulin pump paired with a CGM, enabling users to adjust insulin doses based on glucose sensor values, resulted in much greater improvement in blood glucose control than the standard injection regimen. Most significantly, more people achieved recommended HbA1c targets with sensor/pump technology than with injection therapy, with no increase in hypoglycemia. It was especially encouraging that children had many fewer hypoglycemia episodes with the sensor/pump strategy than were seen, for example, in the DCCT. These trials have shown that CGMs, when used near-daily, not only help people with type 1 diabetes get into control—which can have a significant positive impact on lowering the risk of complications—but also enables them to stay in control without increasing the near-term risk of hypoglycemia.

In addition to facilitating self-monitoring of glucose levels by individuals, scientists are using CGMs to answer important research questions. Already an important lesson learned from the use of glucose sensor technology is the realization that blood glucose actually varies to a much greater extent during the course of the day than was previously thought, even in presumed "well-controlled" individuals. Further studies about the impact of this "glycemic variability"—both low- and high glucose—and not simply average glucose levels will provide important information on the development or progression of diabetes complications. CGMs also provide, for the first time, the opportunity to measure glycemic variability and undetected hypoglycemic events during insulin treatment in people with type 2 diabetes. Additionally, CGMs could be extremely beneficial in the management of individuals with gastroparesis, a slow emptying of food from the stomach caused by nerve damage from diabetic hyperglycemia. People with gastroparesis have great difficulty controlling glucose levels because meal absorption is variable. CGMs could be used to modify insulin delivery to prevent early hypoglycemia following a meal and delayed hyperglycemia. This technology has enormous potential to aid many different patient populations and extend its benefit beyond people with type 1 diabetes.

Today, the combined number of people who use CGMs is estimated to have reached several thousand and is still growing. There are still a number of caveats and limitations to current devices, however. For example, the sensor signals are not entirely specific for glucose and are adversely affected by a combination of factors, such as the body's wound healing and foreign body response, inactivation of the enzyme, and biochemical interference. As a result of these limitations, the sensors must be frequently recalibrated by the user based on finger stick glucose assays, and have not been approved by FDA as the primary standard for glucose measurement. Also, current glucose sensors cannot be fully relied upon for early hypoglycemia detection or warning. While CGMs have significantly benefitted many people with type 1 diabetes, research opportunities remain to improve these devices. Many of these emerging opportunities are described in Appendix F. Further research to overcome limitations to current devices, improve their usability, and expand their utility will be essential to capitalize on the progress to date and lead to the development of an artificial pancreas.

Pushing Continuous Glucose Monitoring Toward the Development of an Artificial Pancreas

An artificial pancreas—which would automate insulin delivery in response to the body's needs—requires, at a minimum, three basic components: a continuous blood glucose sensor, an insulin delivery system, and a way to link the two in a loop. Such a system would automatically turn the measurement of blood glucose levels into a practical, precise, and "real-time" insulin-dosing system for patients. Importantly, a key feature of one of the approved continuous glucose monitors is that it has been "paired" with an insulin pump through a wireless transmitter and transmits its data to the pump, making it easier for the patient to adjust the insulin dose. Although not an artificial pancreas since patients still must be actively involved in determining their insulin doses, this first pairing of a continuous monitor and pump has major implications. It represents the first step in joining glucose monitoring and insulin delivery systems using the most advanced current technology. To help "close the loop," the *Program* has awarded grants to small business and academic investigators to develop and test innovative technologies—like improved glucose sensors and more physiological algorithms—that may advance progress toward an artificial pancreas. Even before an artificial pancreas is developed, patients can improve their health now, with the unprecedented knowledge gained from continuous glucose monitors.

Investigator Profile

Bruce Buckingham, M.D.

Testing Closed-Loop Technology To Preserve Insulin Production in Children Newly Diagnosed with Type 1 Diabetes

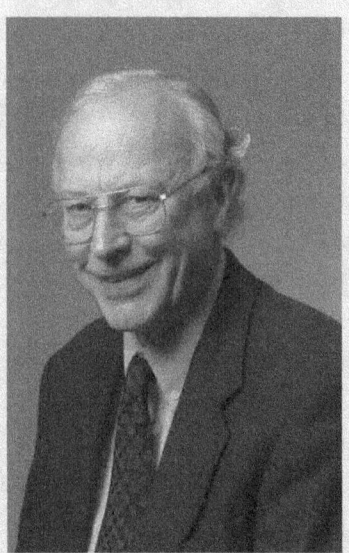

Bruce Buckingham, M.D.

Bruce Buckingham, M.D., is a Professor in the Department of Pediatrics at Stanford University and a renowned diabetes researcher. He participates in the Diabetes Research in Children Network (DirecNet) and Type 1 Diabetes TrialNet, which are led by NICHD and NIDDK, respectively, and are supported by the Special Statutory Funding Program for Type 1 Diabetes Research. Dr. Buckingham is the Principal Investigator of a clinical trial jointly conducted by DirecNet and TrialNet that is testing intensive glucose control at type 1 diabetes onset using a closed-loop system. This profile describes his experiences in the trial and his research testing new glucose monitoring technologies on a wide-range of patients.

A Clinical Trial in Newly Diagnosed Type 1 Diabetes Patients

Dr. Buckingham is leading a new clinical trial that, he says, "Is moving several fields forward."

He is testing whether early and intensive blood glucose control using a closed-loop artificial pancreas system can protect patients' remaining insulin-producing beta cells from the toxic effects of high blood glucose. "There are some earlier studies showing that, if the blood glucose is maintained fairly close to normal from disease onset, you have better and more prolonged insulin secretion, a prolonged 'honeymoon' phase," explains Dr. Buckingham. The "honeymoon" is the period of time shortly after diagnosis when patients still make significant amounts of their own insulin. Previous research has shown that preserving insulin production can have dramatic, long-term health benefits, which is why researchers are trying to intervene early in the disease.

"We enroll children within the first week of diabetes onset and put them on a closed-loop artificial pancreas. In this system, there is a subcutaneous sensor measuring glucose levels every minute and this information is sent to an algorithm which determines how much insulin they need," says Dr. Buckingham. The system then automatically delivers insulin to the patient. "When the blood glucose is going up, it delivers more insulin, when the blood glucose is going down, it decreases insulin delivery. By doing this over several days we can bring their blood glucose levels very close to the normal range," explains Dr. Buckingham.

After the children are treated for 3-4 days on the closed-loop system in the hospital, the intensive treatment continues at home for the next 2 years. "We send them home on a sensor-augmented pump, which is an insulin pump paired with a continuous glucose sensor," says Dr. Buckingham. This technology does not automatically deliver insulin based on glucose levels, but "It allows patients to see the fluctuations in their glucose, which are often not seen with routine blood glucose monitoring," explains Dr. Buckingham. Routine blood glucose monitoring involves a finger stick that measures blood glucose at a single point in time, but the continuous glucose sensor measures glucose levels every few minutes, giving the patients a more complete picture of how their levels are changing throughout the day and night. It also sounds an alarm if glucose levels are above or below glucose targets. "We thought that if they could see all their glucose levels, they could correct any elevations and continue to maintain their glucose values close to normal," notes Dr. Buckingham.

The trial is comparing outcomes (e.g., insulin production) in these "intensively treated" children to outcomes in children who, from disease onset, use routine blood glucose monitoring to manage their diabetes. Both groups will be followed for 2 years to determine if early, intensive treatment promotes and prolongs the "honeymoon" phase. "The concept is that if someone is exposed to high glucose, those sugars may be toxic to the remaining islet cells," explains Dr. Buckingham. In addition, "The immune attack [underlying type 1 diabetes] may be more aggressive/effective when the islets are in a high glucose environment," he says. Therefore, the hope is that keeping blood glucose levels close to normal for the duration of the 2 year trial will protect the islet cells from the toxic effects of high glucose, allowing them to continue to make insulin and this, in turn, makes it easier for them to maintain better glucose levels (a virtual circle).

The Benefits to Participants

The children in this clinical trial are doing very well, says Dr. Buckingham. "It's been very exciting, and for the kids who have entered a honeymoon, their blood glucose levels are almost a flat line throughout the day," which refers to the fact that the patients are not experiencing the high and low blood glucose excursions typical of type 1 diabetes.

It also turns out that the intensive treatment that these children receive doesn't just refer to their blood glucose levels, but also refers to the personal treatment they receive from the dedicated clinical research team. Because the closed-loop system is an experimental therapy, the U.S. Food and Drug Administration requires that, "A pediatric endocrinologist or someone trained in diabetes is at the patient's bedside 24 hours a day during their inpatient stay," explains Dr. Buckingham.

This dedication has not been overlooked by the children and their families—Dr. Buckingham has received a lot of positive feedback from them. He says that, because the children have just been diagnosed with diabetes, they and their parents are understandably a little overwhelmed. "We then provide them intensive education about how to use an insulin pump and how to use continuous glucose monitoring. They get a lot of one-on-one teaching. When they leave, I think they feel much more comfortable and in charge of their diabetes."

He also says that the patients and their parents appreciate using the new technology when they leave the hospital. "Having the glucose values all the time has been very helpful to them. It's nice to know that there is going to be an alarm at night to wake you if your blood glucose is low. They have been very appreciative and have done very well," explains Dr. Buckingham. In fact, the kids are doing so well that, "They have very few alarms because the majority of their blood glucose levels are in the normal range," he happily remarks.

The Benefits of Collaboration

The clinical trial is a collaboration between DirecNet, which has expertise in studying continuous glucose monitoring technologies, and TrialNet, which has expertise in recruiting and studying people with newly diagnosed type 1 diabetes. "It takes the expertise of both coordinating centers to really make this happen," notes Dr. Buckingham.

The strength of the DirecNet coordinating center is in collecting and analyzing large amounts of data from monitors and pumps. "When you think about it," Dr. Buckingham explains, "most of these monitors are measuring glucose levels every minute or every 5 minutes each day. With 5 minute measurements, that is 288 time points of data per day. Since the patients are also using an insulin pump, there is also data on insulin boluses and basal infusion rates that need to be integrated with the glucose data. This is a huge amount of data over 2 years. The DirecNet coordinating center has developed excellent methods of obtaining uploads from these devices, putting the data in a database, and verifying and validating the data as it arrives."

"On the other hand," continues Dr. Buckingham, "the trial is looking at the onset of diabetes and trying to prolong the honeymoon phase, which is one of the goals of TrialNet. TrialNet is also interested in how the treatment may affect the immune attack on islet cells, so we are collecting samples through TrialNet to look at immunologic markers to see if there are differences between the treatment and control groups to begin to see how the immune system was affected." Thus, the trial is utilizing the expertise of both networks and also saving resources by building on existing infrastructures.

Moving Several Fields Forward

"I think this is a big study in terms of the technical state-of-the-art," Dr. Buckingham explains, "in that the closed-loop studies are still pretty new. The sensor-augmented pump technology has been around a little while but it's still relatively new and using it in new-onset patients is also new."

Thus, this trial is moving several fields forward. First, it is advancing knowledge about closed-loop systems, which can provide insights regarding how to improve the technology to ultimately reach the goal of developing an artificial pancreas that can be used by patients outside of a hospital setting. Second, the trial is testing intensive therapy shortly after disease onset using the new technologies. If effective, it paves the way for people to use new technologies upon diagnosis to not only help manage their diabetes, but also to improve their health outcomes. "These studies could not have been done without NIH funding or without support of the *Special Diabetes Program*," says Dr. Buckingham.

Using New Technologies To Help a Wide-range of Patients

In the clinical trial described above, Dr. Buckingham is testing new technologies in children and youth who have just been diagnosed with type 1 diabetes. In other research, he is testing the technologies in a very different population—adults with type 1 or type 2 diabetes who have a disease-associated complication called gastroparesis. This complication is caused by nerve damage which may result from high blood glucose levels, and causes delayed emptying of food from the stomach. Thus, it is difficult for people with gastroparesis to predict when the sugar from food will enter their blood and when their body will need insulin. "It's hard for people with gastroparesis to administer insulin and keep their blood glucose in good control without having significant episodes of hyperglycemia and hypoglycemia," explains Dr. Buckingham, "so these patients have a really difficult time with their diabetes. We're going to utilize—for the first time in a clinical trial—continuous glucose monitoring and an insulin infusion pump therapy for these patients." By allowing patients to see their glucose values in real time, as well as having alarms to signal a low glucose, "It can hopefully help them keep their glucose values more in a normal range which could even potentially improve

their gastroparesis," Dr. Buckingham predicts. Thus, the new technologies have high potential for helping a wide-range of patients, from newly diagnosed children to people with late-stage disease complications.

Looking to the Future

With support from the *Special Diabetes Program*, Dr. Buckingham is conducting state-of-the-art research that can have a major impact on the health and quality of life of people with type 1 diabetes. Not only do new glucose monitoring and insulin-delivery technologies have the potential to make it easier for patients to manage their disease, but they may also improve health outcomes. Dr. Buckingham's dedication to testing the new technologies in a wide-range of patients can help this potential come to fruition.

Patient Profile

Gina Ferrari

Participating in a Clinical Trial Testing a Closed-Loop System To Slow Progression of Type 1 Diabetes

How a Life Can Change in an Instant

"I was eating more than I ever had before, but I kept losing weight," notes Gina Ferrari. It happened at the end of Gina's junior year in high school, just before her ballet showcase and final exams. A simple blood test at the doctor's office changed her life in an instant with a diagnosis she never saw coming—type 1 diabetes.

Gina had no family history of diabetes, so she was surprised and overwhelmed upon receiving the news that she had the disease. She remembers that while she was still processing her diagnosis, she was also a bit relieved. "I was just grateful to know what was wrong with me," says Gina. "I was convinced that, together with my family, I could beat this." Gina was fortunate to be referred through a family friend to Dr. Bruce Buckingham at Stanford University. During her first appointment with Dr. Buckingham, she learned about type 1 diabetes. Because of the daily need to monitor her diet and physical activity, and also closely monitor her blood glucose (sugar) levels and administer insulin, she quickly realized that type 1 diabetes was going to be a formidable opponent.

During that first appointment, Gina also learned about a clinical trial that Dr. Buckingham was leading to test the benefits of early and intensive blood glucose control in people with newly diagnosed type 1 diabetes. Gina's

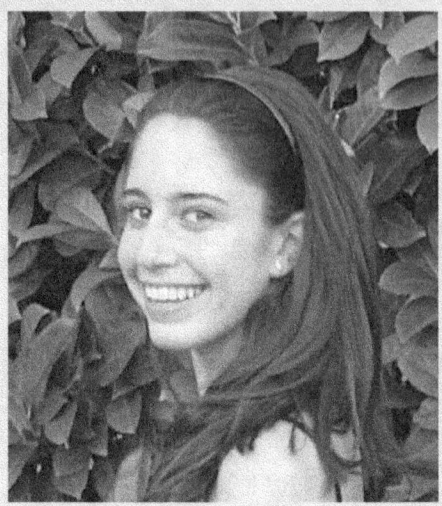

Gina Ferrari

dad Tom remembers, "Dr. Buckingham wanted us to know everything about diabetes and the trial up front. We went from having no information at all to a tidal wave of information in 1 day."

Joining the study required a commitment of 4 days in the hospital within 1 week of Gina's diagnosis. After the hospital stay, she would be sent home with an insulin pump and a continuous glucose monitor to use as part of the trial for the next 2 years. During that time, she would have doctor's appointments every 3 months. After 2 years, if her body is still producing insulin, Gina may continue to participate in the trial for another 2 years. "I was scared to commit so much so soon to a disease I knew so little about," Gina recalls. But she did not have much time to make her decision; participants must be enrolled in the trial within 1 week of their diagnosis. Her parents wanted Gina to participate, but they knew that it had to be her decision. "As hard as it was at the time, Tom and I didn't pressure her and allowed her to process all of the information we were given and arrive at her own decision," says her mom Lori. "Needless to say, we were relieved when she told us she wanted to sign up." The day after Gina learned about the trial she decided to participate.

"I am convinced that Gina is doing so well because of her participation in the trial," says Lori.

Participation in the Trial: Being Part of Something Special

The trial, which is supported by the *Special Statutory Funding Program for Type 1 Diabetes Research*, is a collaboration between the NIDDK-led Type 1 Diabetes TrialNet and the NICHD-led DirecNet to test whether intensive blood glucose control upon diagnosis can prolong a person's ability to produce insulin. Previous research demonstrated that preserving this ability can have positive, long-term health benefits in delaying the devastating complications of the disease. This trial employs a "closed-loop" system—a continuous glucose monitor linked to an insulin pump. In this system, a subcutaneous glucose sensor measures blood glucose levels every minute, and that information is transmitted to a computer that calculates how much insulin the pump should deliver. The insulin is delivered automatically based on the blood glucose readings.

The goals of this intensive management using a closed-loop system are to enable the research team to bring the participant's blood glucose levels close to normal range within the first week of diagnosis and hopefully to preserve the ability of the pancreas to produce some of its own insulin. Because the closed-loop system is experimental and not approved for home use, participants must remain in the hospital while using the system and be closely monitored by the research team,

which is why Gina was in the hospital for the first 4 days of the trial.

The first morning in the hospital was all about education. "We received a phenomenal amount of information and received one-on-one training by experts in the field," Lori remembers. "As the team was training Gina, Tom and I were learning, too." "We saw quickly that Gina was capable of managing her diabetes with the new technology and this was very comforting to us," notes Tom. "She took charge from the very beginning, and I think that helped to give her a sense of control over an overwhelming diagnosis." Gina remembers, "I spent the first 4 days of my summer in the hospital getting my blood sugar levels under control and learning everything I needed to know about the most advanced ways to manage my diabetes."

Gina was the second person to enroll in the study, and the excitement of the entire research team was evident to her and her family from the first day. "I love Dr. Buckingham. He was so excited about the trial. He would stay in the hospital with me all night and constantly check on me," remembers Gina. She recalls that Dr. Buckingham explained how eating different foods would affect her blood glucose levels. He also showed her how to use the continuous glucose monitor to watch how her blood glucose levels were rising and falling. "I knew that he was really busy, but he made me feel like I was his only patient," says Gina. "The whole team was excited about the trial. We really felt like we were part of something special, something much bigger than Gina's diabetes," says Tom. Gina remembers her hospital stay during the first part of the trial as a very positive experience. "My friends were able to come and stay with me in the hospital and as I was learning I was also teaching them about diabetes. I remember feeling more confident each day that I was in control of my diabetes," says Gina.

Gina received much more than knowledge about how to use the advanced technology to manage her type 1 diabetes. During her time in the hospital, the research team and Dr. Buckingham helped Gina to understand and believe that she could continue to live her life the way she wanted after leaving the hospital. "I think that after managing my diabetes, the most important thing that Dr. Buckingham and his team taught me was that I can continue to do what I want to do," says Gina. "Things become more complicated with diabetes and require more planning, but I left the hospital believing that diabetes doesn't have to slow me down."

"I remember feeling more confident each day that I was in control of my diabetes," says Gina.

Gina admits that she was a little scared when it was time to leave the hospital and go home. "I knew that I was prepared, and my parents and I stayed in close contact with Dr. Buckingham and his team. That helped a lot and was very comforting to all of us," remembers Gina. She was sent home with an insulin pump paired with a continuous glucose monitor to manage her type 1 diabetes. Unlike the closed-loop system that automatically delivered insulin, the new system required Gina to administer her own insulin. However, the hope is that the technology will help Gina achieve good control of her diabetes and preserve her ability to produce her own insulin. To help with this transition from hospital to home, Gina would get frequent calls from Dr. Buckingham and his team to check on her. "Even when he was traveling outside of the country he would call us. It was an incredible source of comfort for us all," says Lori.

Before type 1 diabetes, Gina's day would consist of waking up, going to school, dancing, more dancing, and then doing homework before bed. Now her days are back to that routine, but with the added responsibility and complexity of testing her blood glucose levels 8-10 times a day. All of this information—the amounts of insulin that Gina administers, her blood glucose readings—is uploaded from Gina's insulin pump and continuous glucose monitor and sent to Dr. Buckingham and his research team so they can monitor and analyze the data.

Finding the Silver Lining

At the time this profile was written, Gina had been participating in the trial for 15 months. The family reports that her doctors say that she is doing extremely well and continues to produce some of her own insulin. Her hemoglobin A1C, a measure reflective of blood glucose control over the preceding 2-3 months, is in the normal, "nondiabetic" range. "I am convinced that Gina is doing so well because of her participation in the trial," says Lori.

Gina was getting ready to leave for college at the time this article was written. She was excited about starting this new chapter in her life. "I try to not let diabetes define me, but my life is different now. Not only do I carry my insulin pump, glucose meter, medical bracelet, glucose tablets, syringes, and glucagon with me wherever I go," notes Gina, "but I carry the responsibility of managing a potentially lethal disease, one where a small mistake on my part could put me in the hospital and a big mistake could lead to death."

Living with type 1 diabetes and being part of the clinical trial have given Gina a new outlook on life. She worked hard the summer after her diagnosis to regain her strength and to get back to dancing. "Now I am back to where I was before diabetes," Gina says. "Going through this experience and having diabetes has made me really appreciate what I am able to do. I am not nervous before my dance performances like I used to be. Now, I am just grateful that I can perform." Her proud mother adds, "I am constantly amazed by Gina's positive attitude throughout this experience. She has found the silver lining in what could have been a devastating diagnosis."

EMERGING RESEARCH OPPORTUNITIES RESULTING FROM THE *SPECIAL DIABETES PROGRAM*

The *Special Statutory Funding Program for Type 1 Diabetes Research* has fueled the emergence of a wide range of research opportunities. These opportunities were identified in a strategic planning process as being critically important for overcoming current barriers and achieving progress in diabetes research. Key questions and research opportunities relevant to type 1 diabetes, including those related to the prevention or reversal of hypoglycemia, are outlined in Appendix F.

GOAL V

PREVENT OR REDUCE THE COMPLICATIONS OF TYPE 1 DIABETES

Persistent elevation of blood glucose (sugar) levels, despite insulin therapy, slowly damages the body's organs and can lead to life-threatening diabetes complications. Until the prevention or cure of type 1 diabetes is possible, the *Special Statutory Funding Program for Type 1 Diabetes Research* is vigorously supporting research toward preventing and treating the complications of the disease. In addition to the significant research progress described in this chapter, information on the program evaluation related to Goal V can be found in Appendix A (Allocation of Funds), Appendix B (Assessment), and Appendix C (Evaluation of Major Research Consortia, Networks, and Resources).

Insulin therapy enables survival for people with type 1 diabetes, by signaling their cells to take up needed glucose from the blood. One might expect this circumvention of the need for pancreatic insulin to allow people with the disease to live as long as people who do not have diabetes. Unfortunately, type 1 diabetes, like type 2 diabetes, is associated with an array of common complications that can be costly, debilitating, and deadly, and can shorten life. Diabetes ravages nearly every part of the body, including the heart, eyes, kidneys, nerves, lower limbs, mouth, and digestive and urologic systems. In the United States, diabetes is the leading cause of vision loss in working age adults, nontraumatic lower limb amputations, and kidney failure.[24] Heart disease risk is increased up to 10-fold in people with type 1 diabetes compared to the general age-matched population.[25] Type 1 diabetes is estimated to shorten the average life span by 15 years.[26] Until the prevention or cure of type 1 diabetes is possible, therefore, intensified research toward preventing and treating the complications of the disease is critically important. The *Special Statutory Funding Program for Type 1 Diabetes Research* (*Special Diabetes Program* or *Program*) has enabled significant progress toward combating diabetes complications.

[24] Centers for Disease Control and Prevention. National diabetes fact sheet: national estimates and general information on diabetes and prediabetes in the United States, 2011. Atlanta, GA: U.S. Department of Health and Human Services, Centers for Disease Control and Prevention, 2011.

[25] Krolewski AS, Kosinski EJ, Warram JH, et al: Magnitude and determinants of coronary artery disease in juvenile-onset, insulin-dependent diabetes mellitus. Am J Cardiol 59: 750-755, 1987; Dorman JS, Laporte RE, Kuller LH, et al: The Pittsburgh insulin-dependent diabetes mellitus (IDDM) morbidity and mortality study: mortality results. Diabetes 33: 271-276, 1984.

[26] Portuese E and Orchard T: Mortality in Insulin-Dependent Diabetes. In Diabetes in America (pp. 221-232). Bethesda, MD: National Diabetes Data Group, NIH, 1995.

Graphic: Image of artery occluded by lipid buildup which contributes to cardiovascular disease—a devastating complication of type 1 diabetes. Image credit: National Heart, Lung, and Blood Institute, NIH.

HIGHLIGHTS OF RECENT RESEARCH ADVANCES RELATED TO GOAL V

Continued Benefits of Improved Blood Glucose Control: The Diabetes Control and Complications Trial (DCCT) showed that intensive control of blood glucose levels reduced the risk of damage to small blood vessels and nerves in people with type 1 diabetes. The follow-up study, the Epidemiology of Diabetes Interventions and Complications (EDIC), continues to demonstrate the long-term benefits of intensive therapy. Patients who had been intensively treated during the trial had fewer than half the number of cardiovascular disease events—heart attacks, strokes, or death due to cardiovascular disease—than those in the conventionally-treated group. These results showed for the first time that intensive control of blood glucose levels has long-term beneficial effects on cardiovascular disease risk in people with type 1 diabetes. These findings have revolutionized the management of type 1 diabetes and the fruits of this research are resulting in improved health outcomes for people with type 1 diabetes: DCCT/EDIC researchers recently demonstrated that intensive control of glucose beginning as soon as possible after diagnosis can greatly improve the long-term prognosis of type 1 diabetes.

Long-term Clinical Trials Revealed the Phenomenon of "Metabolic Memory" in People with Diabetes: The DCCT/EDIC studies have shown that participants who intensively managed their blood glucose during the trial have maintained a lower risk of complications for more than 15 years, even though after the trial ended their glucose control gradually became indistinguishable from that of the participants who had received standard glycemic control measures. This apparent long-term benefit of a relatively short period of intensive glucose control has been termed metabolic memory. These results underscore the importance of intensive glucose management from the earliest stages of diabetes and point to the need for research in epigenetics and other potential mechanisms contributing to metabolic memory.

The Repair and Regeneration Process Is Impaired in Diabetes: Many of the serious complications associated with diabetes—including chronic, non-healing foot ulcers and poor recovery from impaired blood supply to the heart, brain, and/or limbs—stem from inadequate growth of new blood vessels where and when they are needed. A critical component of normal vessel growth is a population of cells called circulating endothelial progenitor cells (EPCs). Several recent studies report that diabetes is associated with impairments in EPC number and function, as well as problems in other stem cell populations involved in wound healing. Trials are under way to test injection of a person's own EPCs to promote blood vessel growth in sites where it is needed. Recent studies on wound healing in response to restricted blood supply show that a protein called hypoxia-inducible factor (HIF)-1alpha is a critical regulator of new blood vessel formation. HIF-1alpha, and other molecules involved in the repair process, might serve as targets for therapeutic intervention to promote wound healing in people with diabetes.

Value of Ranibizumab in Treating Diabetic Macular Edema: Diabetes has multiple effects on the vasculature. A paucity of small blood vessels prevents wound healing leading to amputation, but in the eye, diabetes leads to excessive new blood vessel formation. A recent Diabetic Retinopathy Clinical Research Network (DRCR.net) comparative effectiveness research study found that a drug that blocks vascular endothelial growth factor (VEGF), ranibizumab (Lucentis®), in combination with laser therapy, was substantially better than laser therapy alone or laser therapy with a different drug, at treating diabetic macular edema, a swelling in the eye that often accompanies and aggravates diabetic retinopathy. Nearly half of the patients receiving ranibizumab showed a substantial improvement in vision, compared to 28 percent receiving only laser treatments. This class of drugs could become the new standard of care for diabetic macular edema.

Development of a Mouse Model of Diabetic Nephropathy: Recent studies have implicated dysfunctional endothelial nitric-oxide synthase (eNOS) as a common pathogenic pathway in diabetic vascular complications. Researchers in the Animal Models of Diabetic Complications Consortium (AMDCC) have shown that eNOS deficiency in a widely used mouse model of type 2 diabetes causes profound glomerular changes with increased proteinuria, marked thickening of the glomerular basement membrane, mesangial expansion, prominent nodular sclerosis and an impressive reduction in glomerular filtration rate—all critical features of human diabetic nephropathy that had been missing from previous mouse models. Similar phenotypic changes were observed in a mouse model of type 1 diabetes. This is the first mouse model to exhibit all of the classic pathologic lesions of diabetic nephropathy observed in humans. The finding that endothelial eNOS loss produces a phenotype similar to diabetic nephropathy suggests that therapies targeted toward preservation of endothelial function may be useful in preventing or attenuating this complication in humans.

IMPORTANCE OF INTENSIVE BLOOD GLUCOSE CONTROL IN PREVENTING COMPLICATIONS

The NIDDK's landmark DCCT provided dramatic evidence that type 1 diabetes-related "microvascular" complications of the kidneys, eyes, and nerves can be prevented or greatly delayed through intensive control of blood glucose levels. The DCCT results also served to establish that these complications arise from the long-term effects of chronically elevated blood glucose rather than, for example, from the absence of some putative protective compound made by pancreatic beta cells. The initial DCCT results, published in 1993, therefore laid the groundwork for subsequent efforts to prevent or reduce the complications of type 1 diabetes.

Continuing To Learn from DCCT Participants:
The scientific benefits of the DCCT continue today through a follow-on effort with DCCT participants called the Epidemiology of Diabetes Interventions and Complications (EDIC) study, which is led by NIDDK and supported in part by the *Special Diabetes Program*, and which continues to yield important, life-saving data. EDIC, and some of its numerous major findings to date, are described in greater detail below and in the Story of Discovery later in this chapter. In subsequent studies, EDIC found that intensive blood glucose control could also prevent the "macrovascular" (heart-related) complications that are the most common cause of death among people with diabetes. These findings

have revolutionized management of type 1 diabetes and translated into dramatic health benefits. DCCT/EDIC scientists and other researchers recently reported that intensive control of blood glucose levels as soon as possible after diagnosis can greatly improve the long-term outcomes for people with type 1 diabetes, and result in reduced rates of complications. Thus, the fruits of type 1 diabetes research are paying off with respect to critical improvements in care.

IMPROVING CARE THROUGH STANDARDIZED HEMOGLOBIN ASSAYS

The DCCT also established and validated hemoglobin A1c (HbA1c) as a key marker of blood glucose control. Because HbA1c is an excellent indicator of how well a person's blood glucose has been controlled over the course of recent weeks and months, it has become enormously important as a tool for assessing the efficacy of new interventions, as well as for helping doctors and patients adjust their therapeutic regimen to obtain the best possible results. The utility of the test is dependent upon accuracy and reliability in measures of HbA1c. Another initiative supported in part by the *Special Diabetes Program*, the National Glycohemoglobin Standardization Program (NGSP), works to ensure that commercial HbA1c tests are accurate, free from artifactual errors due to naturally occurring variations in hemoglobin structure, and standardized to the methods used in the DCCT. This effort, which is supported by CDC and NIDDK, is critical to people with all forms of diabetes treated in the United States, and means that an HbA1c test result from one lab can meaningfully be compared to one from another.

Standardization of HbA1c test results has facilitated the implementation of vital public health campaigns such

as the National Diabetes Education Program's "Know Your Number" and "Control Your Diabetes. For Life." campaigns, co-led by NIDDK and CDC, which emphasize the importance of HbA1c control to extend life and reduce complications. Standardized laboratory HbA1c tests have now also been proposed as an alternative to fasting blood glucose tests for the diagnosis of type 2 diabetes, to help identify some of the many undiagnosed people with diabetes and pre-diabetes who would benefit from life-saving treatments. This is only practical because of the improvements in HbA1c testing that have been brought about through the NGSP.

PREVENTING OR DELAYING DIABETIC VISION LOSS

Blindness is a debilitating complication of diabetes. Laser photocoagulation is an effective therapy to prevent progression of diabetic retinopathy to blindness, but the technique itself can lead to impaired vision. Thus, new therapeutic options are needed and are being tested in the DRCR.net. Led by NEI and supported in part by the *Special Diabetes Program*, DRCR.net is facilitating multicenter clinical research on diabetic retinopathy, diabetic macular edema, and other associated conditions, and has launched 15 studies. A recent DRCR.net comparative effectiveness research study found that a therapeutic called ranibizumab, in combination with laser therapy, was substantially better than laser therapy alone or laser therapy with a different drug, at treating diabetic macular edema, a swelling in the eye that often accompanies and aggravates diabetic retinopathy. Ranibizumab with laser therapy often resulted in substantial improvements in vision among patients, and could become the new standard of care for diabetic macular edema. Ranibizumab works by inhibiting VEGF, a protein which contributed to diabetic macular edema by promoting blood vessel growth in the eye. The *Special*

Diabetes Program has also supported key basic research on VEGF and other factors affecting blood vessel growth.

Understanding the Risk Factors for Diabetic Complications

While the DCCT established that chronic hyperglycemia is a major risk factor for kidney disease and other complications of type 1 diabetes, some people with relatively well controlled blood glucose still develop certain complications, and some with more poorly controlled blood glucose do not. Therefore, it is believed that other factors may influence the risk of developing complications.

Epidemiologic Studies Provide Insight: SEARCH for Diabetes in Youth (SEARCH) is a multicenter, epidemiologic study led by CDC and supported by NIDDK and the *Special Diabetes Program* (see Goal I). Data collected by SEARCH is enabling studies to delineate the risk factors for diabetes complications in a racially and ethnically diverse population of youth with diabetes. For example, SEARCH has demonstrated that youth with type 1 diabetes and suboptimal control of their blood glucose levels had abnormal lipid (fat) profiles—indicators of heart disease risk—even after a short duration of disease. High prevalence of cardiovascular disease risk factors, including obesity, dyslipidemia, and hypertension, has been documented in youth with type 1 diabetes, as well as youth with type 2 or hybrid diabetes. These studies point to the complexity of the metabolic factors involved in diabetes and the need for careful monitoring of glucose, lipid, and blood pressure levels for people of all ages with type 1 diabetes. For more information on the use of

SEARCH data to inform understanding of heart-related complications of diabetes, see the Investigator Profile of Dr. Dana Dabelea later in this chapter.

Large-scale Studies on the Genetics of Diabetes Complications: Predispositions to specific complications within families suggest that some of the additional risk may come from genetics, but at the outset of the *Special Diabetes Program* in 1998, little was known definitively about the genetics of diabetes complications. To investigate the genetic underpinnings of diabetes complications, NIDDK's Family Investigation of Nephropathy and Diabetes (FIND) Consortium, and the JDRF's Genetics of Kidneys in Diabetes Study (GoKinD), also supported in part by the *Special Diabetes Program*, have taken different, complementary approaches to identifying genetic factors that predispose people with diabetes to—or protect them from—developing diabetic nephropathy (kidney disease). Based on the evidence that diabetic kidney disease results from chronically elevated blood glucose levels in both of the major forms of diabetes, the FIND study collected genetic material from participants with either type 1 or type 2 diabetes. This approach may make it easier to detect factors that influence genetic susceptibility in minority patients. Using genome-wide scans of these samples, FIND researchers identified four regions where subtle variations correlated with an increased risk of diabetic kidney disease. These findings confirmed earlier studies and identified a new region of interest. In addition, support from the *Special Diabetes Program* is enabling efforts to look for genes affecting the likelihood of diabetic eye disease using FIND genetic samples, thereby increasing the value obtained from these samples. FIND represents the first large-scale study of the genetic determinants of retinopathy.

GoKinD, in contrast, is a collection of samples from people who have both type 1 diabetes and kidney disease, as well as control samples from people with type 1 diabetes and other similar characteristics, but without kidney disease. The resulting data from GoKinD and DCCT/EDIC have been used by numerous investigators in various analyses to identify genetic regions associated with a disease, or to replicate promising findings from other studies, or to refine analytic methods. For example, genome-wide association data from the GoKinD collection has led to the identification of genes/genetic regions association with diabetic nephropathy, including *FRMD3*, *CARS*, and *ELMO1*. In another example, the DCCT/EDIC research group confirmed and helped define versions of the angiotensin converting enzyme gene that affect the likelihood of developing diabetic nephropathy.

Maximizing the Value of Collected Data and Samples: In addition to the genes and genetic associations with diabetes complications that have been discovered and are still emerging from DCCT/EDIC, FIND, and GoKinD, each of these consortia also serves as a resource for future efforts: tissue, genetic samples, data, and analytic methods from each study are stored in a repository or database. The large and diverse sample and data collections—with families, cases, and controls—are widely-used resources for genetic study of susceptibility to diabetic complications. The availability of immortalized cell lines for each participant provides a renewable source of DNA, allowing future investigators to explore novel hypotheses or analytical approaches. Identification of genes associated with diabetes complications may not only greatly improve understanding of the disease process, but also provide important new targets for therapy.

ADVANCING THE STUDY OF DIABETIC COMPLICATIONS THROUGH ANIMAL MODELS

Animal models of human disease often provide vital clues into the molecular pathways of disease and represent a critical tool for helping translate basic discoveries about disease pathobiology into candidate therapeutics for testing in clinical trials. While there were several notable animal models of type 1 diabetes when the *Special Diabetes Program* began, there were no animal models that faithfully recapitulated the pathology of human diabetic complications. The AMDCC was therefore established to develop and characterize such models. The AMDCC, which is supported by NIDDK, NHLBI, and the *Special Diabetes Program*, has made important strides in producing animal models that mimic human diabetic nephropathy, cardiovascular disease, and neuropathy. These models are advancing understanding of why complications occur, and how they can better be treated and prevented. For example, mouse models created through the AMDCC much more closely match the clinical pathology of human diabetic kidney disease than previous models had, and are helping tease out the key molecular players that lead to kidney damage in diabetes. Other work has helped further understanding of the molecular events that increase risk of cardiovascular disease in people with diabetes. Additionally, AMDCC researchers found that the therapeutic rosiglitazone helped prevent nerve damage in a mouse model of diabetic neuropathy.

SUMMARY

People with diabetes are leading longer, healthier lives with a reduced likelihood and severity of complications due to strides in medical treatment that derive from research advances such as the findings of DCCT/EDIC, which were made possible in part through support from the *Special Diabetes Program*. To realize further progress, the *Program* also supports research on the underlying causes of diabetic complications, including research on the genetic factors that may predispose or protect patients from developing certain complications. Numerous genes have now been identified, which is opening up avenues for new prevention and treatment approaches. This knowledge can pave the way toward personalized therapies based on patients' genetic profiles. The *Special Diabetes Program* also supported research that identified an improved treatment approach for treating diabetic eye disease. By supporting a broad research portfolio on the complications of diabetes, the *Special Diabetes Program* has already enabled significant progress, with additional insights expected in the future as research builds on the progress made to date.

RESEARCH CONSORTIA AND NETWORKS RELATED TO PREVENTING OR REDUCING THE COMPLICATIONS OF TYPE 1 DIABETES

Evaluation of research consortia and networks supported by the *Special Diabetes Program* and related to Goal V is found in Appendix C. Highlights of these are summarized below.

Epidemiology of Diabetes Interventions and Complications (EDIC): EDIC is a prospective study of the clinical course and risk factors associated with the long-term complications of type 1 diabetes, in the cohort of 1,441 patients who participated in the landmark Diabetes Control and Complications Trial (DCCT). Completed in 1993, the DCCT revolutionized diabetes management by demonstrating the benefit of intensively controlling blood glucose levels with frequent monitoring and insulin injection for preventing or delaying the early complications of the disease. EDIC follows both the "conventional" and "intensive" treatment groups from DCCT, although all participants are now recommended to follow the intensive therapy guidelines.

Genetics of Diabetic Complications: Genetics of Kidneys in Diabetes Study (GoKinD) has facilitated investigator-driven research into the genetic basis of diabetic nephropathy by creating a resource of genetic samples from people who have both type 1 diabetes and renal disease and "control" patients who have type 1 diabetes but no renal disease. The Family Investigation of Nephropathy and Diabetes (FIND) Consortium carries out studies to elucidate the genetic susceptibility to kidney disease (nephropathy) in patients, especially those with diabetes, as well as genetic susceptibility to eye disease (retinopathy) in people with diabetes. Five to ten percent of the people in FIND have type 1 diabetes. A genetics component of the EDIC study is analyzing expanded data regarding the progression of complications in EDIC participants and their affected and non-affected family members to identify DNA sequence differences that influence susceptibility to diabetic complications.

Diabetic Retinopathy Clinical Research Network (DRCR.net): The DRCR.net is a collaborative, nationwide network of eye doctors and investigators conducting clinical research on diabetes-induced retinal disorders (diabetic retinopathy, diabetic macular edema, and associated conditions). The DRCR.net supports the identification, design, and implementation of multicenter clinical research initiatives, including standardization of multiple study procedures, utilization of novel technology, extensive integration of information technology, and the ability to leverage resources to evaluate promising new therapies that might otherwise not be tested. The Network has spearheaded 15 protocols. Because diabetic retinopathies are associated with both type 1 and type 2 diabetes, DRCR.net enrolls both type 1 and type 2 diabetes patients.

Animal Models of Diabetic Complications Consortium (AMDCC): The AMDCC is an interdisciplinary consortium designed to develop animal models that closely mimic the human complications of diabetes for the purpose of studying disease pathogenesis, prevention, and treatment. In addition to creating animal models, the AMDCC sets standards to validate each experimental animal model of diabetic complications for its similarity to the human disease; tests the role of candidate genes or chromosomal regions that emerge from genetic studies of human diabetic complications; and facilitates the sharing of animals, reagents, and expertise between members of the Consortium and the greater scientific community via its bioinformatics and data coordinating center. The AMDCC has developed about 40 animal models of type 1 diabetes that closely mimic various aspects of the human complications of diabetes.

Story of Discovery:
The DCCT/EDIC Research Group: Improving the Lives of People with Type 1 Diabetes

Diabetes slowly damages major organs in the body, such as the eyes, kidneys, and heart. Impressive research progress toward combating diabetes complications was achieved through a large clinical trial launched by NIDDK in 1983. The Diabetes Control and Complications Trial (DCCT) was a multicenter clinical trial in 1,441 people with type 1 diabetes. Completed in 1993, the trial compared the effects of intensive versus conventional treatment of blood glucose levels on the development of microvascular complications (those affecting the small blood vessels in the eyes, kidneys, and nerves). Participants in the intensive treatment group kept their blood glucose levels and hemoglobin A1c (HbA1c) levels (which reflect average blood glucose levels over a 2- to 3-month period) as close to normal as safely possible through a regimen that included frequent monitoring of blood glucose and at least three insulin injections per day or use of an insulin pump. Conventional treatment consisted of one or two insulin injections per day, with once-a-day urine or blood glucose testing. The two treatment groups achieved markedly different average HbA1c levels over the course of the trial, and strikingly different rates of microvascular complications. The DCCT proved conclusively that intensive therapy reduces the risk of microvascular complications, such as diabetic eye, kidney, and nerve disease, by 35 to 76 percent compared with what was then conventional treatment. This dramatic, positive result has had a profound impact on clinical practice for the management of type 1 diabetes: it led to the development of clinical guidelines by the American Diabetes Association and other groups; it spurred the creation of the National Diabetes Education Program to disseminate the findings to the public (www. ndep.nih.gov); and it stimulated multifaceted research efforts to develop tools and therapies that aid patients in achieving close control of blood glucose levels.

Long-term Benefits of Intensive Blood Glucose Control

Upon completion of the DCCT, participants who had received conventional treatment were taught the intensive treatment methods, and all were encouraged to use intensive treatment, although the intervention itself stopped. Nearly all who participated in the DCCT volunteered for the follow-on Epidemiology of Diabetes Interventions and Complications (EDIC) study, which began in 1994. EDIC was established to determine the long-term outcome of reducing exposure of the body's tissues and organs to high blood glucose levels.

In 2002 and 2003, EDIC investigators reported that the period of intensive glucose control during the DCCT continued to reduce risk for microvascular complications 7 to 8 years after the end of DCCT. These long-term benefits were observed despite nearly identical blood glucose control in the two treatment groups after completion of the DCCT. The phenomenon of long-lasting effects of a period of intensive or non-intensive glucose control has been termed "metabolic memory," and it suggests that implementing intensive glucose control as early in the course of type 1 diabetes as possible could help people avoid life-threatening complications. More recent results showing that new cases of retinopathy among participants who received the intensive treatment are beginning to approach the number of new cases in the control group, however, suggest that metabolic memory may wane over time.

While the DCCT proved that blood glucose control could prevent small vessel damage, the effect of glucose control on cardiovascular disease (CVD) was unknown. Through support in part by the *Special Statutory Funding Program for Type 1 Diabetes Research* (*Special Diabetes Program* or *Program*), scientists were able to address this critically important topic. In December 2005, the DCCT/EDIC research group reported that, during an average period of 17 years since their enrollment in the DCCT, people who had been intensively treated during the trial had fewer than half the number of CVD events—heart attacks, strokes, or death due to CVD—than those in the conventionally-treated group. These results showed for the first time that intensive control of blood glucose levels has long-term beneficial effects on CVD risk in people with type 1 diabetes. These findings are particularly significant because people with the disease face a 10-fold increased risk of CVD death compared to the general age-matched population.[27]

More than 17 years after the end of the DCCT, insights continue to emerge regarding the long-term benefits of intensive blood glucose control. In 2009, DCCT/EDIC researchers found that, after 30 years of diabetes, DCCT participants randomly assigned to intensive glucose control had about half the rate of eye damage compared to those assigned to conventional glucose control (21 percent versus 50 percent). They also had lower rates of kidney damage (9 percent versus 25 percent) and cardiovascular events (9 percent versus 14 percent) compared to those receiving conventional glucose control. These findings suggest that, with early intensive therapy to control blood glucose levels, the outlook for people with type 1 diabetes is better than ever.

Research To Understand and Combat Hypoglycemia

Even though the results of the DCCT/EDIC studies show that intensive therapy is beneficial for long-term prevention of complications, a severe limitation to the practice of intensive therapy is the potential for acute episodes of hypoglycemia, or low blood sugar. The immediate effects of hypoglycemia can be severe, including changes in cardiovascular and central nervous system function, cognitive impairment, increased risk for unintentional injury, coma, and death. Thus, researchers supported by the *Special Diabetes Program* are seeking new methods to keep blood glucose low, but not dangerously low, through improved blood glucose monitoring and insulin delivery, and through beta cell replacement therapy to potentially cure type 1 diabetes. Researchers supported by the *Program* have already been successful in contributing to the development of continuous glucose monitoring technology that has been approved by the U.S. Food and Drug Administration (FDA) (see Goal IV). Other research is ongoing to develop artificial pancreas technology, which represents an important current opportunity to help people with diabetes implement intensive blood glucose control.

Encouraging news about the long-term effects of hypoglycemia emerged from evaluation of EDIC participants 12 years after the conclusion of the DCCT. The study revealed no link between multiple severe hypoglycemic reactions and impaired cognitive function. This result means that people with type 1 diabetes do not have to worry that acute episodes of hypoglycemia will damage their mental abilities and impair their long-term abilities to perceive, reason, and remember.

---

[27] Krolewski AS, Kosinski EJ, Warram JH, et al: Magnitude and determinants of coronary artery disease in juvenile-onset, insulin-dependent diabetes mellitus. Am J Cardiol 59: 750-755, 1987; Dorman JS, Laporte RE, Kuller LH, et al: The Pittsburgh insulin-dependent diabetes mellitus (IDDM) morbidity and mortality study: mortality results. Diabetes 33: 271-276, 1984.

New Insights into the Genetics of Diabetes Complications

The DCCT and EDIC studies have also provided an enormous wealth of information on the genetics of diabetes complications and related questions. Genetic samples taken during the DCCT, for example, helped researchers to identify a region of the genome near the *SORCS1* gene that is associated with HbA1c levels. Other genetic regions were also found to be associated with HbA1c levels, and some of the regions were also associated with low blood glucose levels. These results could be used to identify people at risk for poor blood glucose control and aid in developing their personalized treatment plans. Genetic data from DCCT/EDIC have also proved useful in other ways, by providing control data for use in other studies, and therefore represent a significant scientific contribution that goes beyond the study of diabetes and its complications.

A Long-term Investment in Research Improves the Lives of People with Type 1 Diabetes

The DCCT and EDIC studies demonstrate how the long-term investment in research continues to have a profound impact on the health of patients. Almost 30 years after the beginning of the DCCT, researchers are still demonstrating significant findings that continue to improve the care of people with type 1 diabetes and also have implications for people with type 2 diabetes. Because the cohort of DCCT patients was too young for examination of cardiovascular complications when the study began, the long-term follow-up was necessary to assess the effect of intensive glucose control on this most life-threatening diabetic complication. Likewise, it is anticipated that the long-term research efforts that have been launched with support of the *Special Diabetes Program* will also result in dramatic and positive benefits for people with or at-risk for type 1 diabetes in the future.

Dana M. Dabelea, M.D., Ph.D.

SEARCH-ing for Diabetes in Youth and Studying the Natural History of Heart Disease

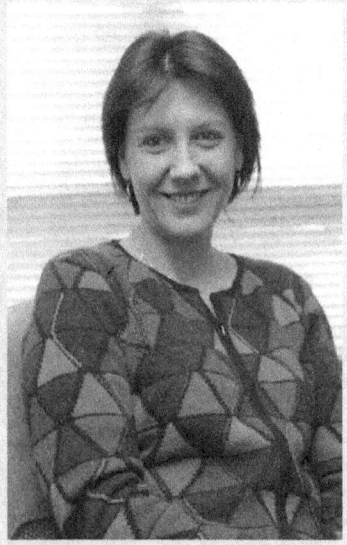

Dana M. Dabelea, M.D., Ph.D.

Dana M. Dabelea, M.D., Ph.D., is an Associate Professor in the Department of Epidemiology, School of Public Health, at the University of Colorado Denver. She is one of six principal investigators and serves as national vice-chair person for the SEARCH for Diabetes in Youth (SEARCH) study, which is led by CDC with support from NIDDK and the Special Statutory Funding Program for Type 1 Diabetes Research. SEARCH is identifying cases of diabetes in youth less than 20 years of age in six geographically dispersed populations in the United States, including Colorado. This profile describes some of SEARCH's remarkable progress and how Dr. Dabelea is capitalizing on the SEARCH infrastructure to study the natural history of heart disease in youth with type 1 diabetes.

"I have been doing diabetes research for nearly 20 years and was first attracted to diabetes research because of my clinical training as a diabetologist," says Dr. Dabelea. In particular, she is interested in pediatric diabetes. "I believe that diabetes research—and especially pediatric diabetes research—is very important because kids have a higher lifetime burden of diabetes than adults. By studying younger people with diabetes, we increase our chances of finding risk factors for the disease and for disease progression before it's too late and before chronic complications develop," she adds. This interest led her to participate in the SEARCH for Diabetes in Youth (SEARCH) study. She moved from Romania to Colorado specifically to work on SEARCH, demonstrating her personal commitment to participating in this important research study.

New Insights into Childhood Diabetes

While substantial increases in the incidence (number of new cases) of type 1 diabetes have been reported in Europe, reliable data on whether the rates of childhood diabetes in the United States are changing over time, or even how many children in the United States have diabetes, were lacking. To address this gap in knowledge, the SEARCH study was launched in 2000.

"SEARCH is unique," says Dr. Dabelea. "It is the only comprehensive population-based study of childhood diabetes by type in a population with a diverse racial background in the U.S. and, I dare to say, in the world. Some of the other registry studies in Europe are based on youth with type 1 diabetes of Caucasian origin. SEARCH is unique in that it includes various racial and ethnic backgrounds and both types of diabetes."

Dr. Dabelea notes that many new insights are emerging from SEARCH. For example, for the first time, SEARCH defined the prevalence (total number of cases) of childhood diabetes in the United States: 1 of every 523 youth had physician-diagnosed diabetes in 2001. SEARCH also determined the incidence of diabetes in American youth: annually, about 15,000 youth are diagnosed with type 1 diabetes and about 3,700 youth are diagnosed with type 2 diabetes. Thus, SEARCH is providing new insights not only on type 1 diabetes, but also on type 2 diabetes, which is an emerging health problem in youth driven by increasing rates of obesity. In fact, Dr. Dabelea explains that "With the epidemic of obesity and the younger age of onset in both type 1 and type 2 diabetes, the lines between the two major forms of diabetes are becoming blurred." In other words, although most children are accurately diagnosed with type 1 or type 2 diabetes, a subset of children may have clinical characteristics that overlap between the two major forms of diabetes, making it difficult for physicians to easily determine diabetes type. To address this issue, SEARCH is leading an effort to classify diabetes type in youth by developing clinical definitions and epidemiologic definitions of diabetes type, which is important not only for SEARCH research, but also for clinical purposes to ensure that all children are accurately diagnosed and given the proper treatment.

SEARCH is also shedding light on the complications of diabetes in youth, and, "The findings are not necessarily painting an optimistic story," says Dr. Dabelea. For example, SEARCH found that youth with diabetes have a high prevalence of risk factors for kidney disease and heart disease. Although these findings are troubling, Dr. Dabelea notes that they are important because they tell us that "Even at a young age, in a population with short duration of disease, we are seeing risk factors for chronic complications that will develop later. We must

start programs that address this increased risk and try to prevent the development of chronic complications." Dr. Dabelea is building on the observations from SEARCH to further study heart disease in type 1 diabetes.

Studying the Natural History of Heart Disease in Youth with Type 1 Diabetes

Heart disease risk is increased by up to 10-fold in people with type 1 diabetes compared to the general age-matched population—a statistic that underscores the importance of identifying and implementing strategies to prevent this life-threatening complication. Research from the NIDDK's landmark Diabetes Control and Complications Trial/Epidemiology of Diabetes Interventions and Complications study showed that early and intensive blood glucose control prevented or delayed future heart-related complications of type 1 diabetes. However, achieving good glucose control is difficult for many patients. "SEARCH has found that a high percentage of youth with diabetes, especially those of minority racial/ethnic backgrounds, have poor glycemic control," says Dr. Dabelea.

Furthermore, little is known about when the course of heart disease actually begins in people with type 1 diabetes. This knowledge is important to inform decisions about when additional therapy to prevent heart disease—such as treatment with statin medications that lower LDL (bad) cholesterol—should be started. For example, does the development of heart disease begin in childhood or adulthood? If it begins in childhood, should statin therapy be introduced at a young age? SEARCH data show that physicians rarely prescribe statin medications to their young patients with type 1 diabetes.

"Prevalence of statin use is very, very low in the SEARCH population," notes Dr. Dabelea. "It is possible that we may need to intervene earlier in life than in adulthood and at lower lipid and blood pressure levels to prevent chronic complications from developing." However, more research is needed to inform those types of recommendations.

Dr. Dabelea is capitalizing on the SEARCH infrastructure to conduct an ancillary study that can begin to address these important questions. "The study is enrolling a subset of SEARCH children, adolescents, and young adults with type 1 diabetes and non-diabetic controls from Colorado and Ohio and is comparing the prevalence of sub-clinical cardiovascular abnormalities in these two groups," explains Dr. Dabelea. "We are looking at carotid intimal-medial thickness (carotid IMT), which is a marker of atherosclerosis, and at arterial stiffness, which is a stiffening of both the large and small vessels that occurs early in the progression of heart disease. Such abnormalities can be detected early in life in teenagers and young adults before heart events even occur. That is why we are interested in studying this population that doesn't have heart disease, but who may have early signs of pre-clinical heart disease."

The first part of the study will examine whether there are any differences in carotid IMT and arterial stiffness between youth with type 1 diabetes and non-diabetic youth. "We suspect that we will find differences," Dr. Dabelea predicts, "and if there are differences, we will explore whether they could be explained by glycemic control, obesity, a family history of heart disease, or other factors." This study also has a longitudinal component, which will examine whether there is progression in arterial stiffness in youth with type 1 diabetes over

time. This research can contribute much needed knowledge about the natural history of heart disease in youth, which could inform recommendations about when preventive strategies, such as introducing statin therapy, should begin.

Capitalizing on the SEARCH Infrastructure
To conduct the ancillary study, Dr. Dabelea is collaborating with SEARCH colleagues in Ohio and also taking advantage of the existing SEARCH infrastructure. She cites numerous advantages to conducting her research as an ancillary study to SEARCH, rather than starting a new study. "The children and youth participating in a study like SEARCH are already attending baseline and follow-up visits and are committed to participating in the study," Dr. Dabelea explains. "When you tell them about the possibility of participating in an ancillary study, you have a very receptive population."

Another benefit is that Dr. Dabelea can utilize the existing SEARCH network system for the ancillary study. "The network system includes providers throughout the state of Colorado and at each of the other SEARCH sites, so when we want to start an ancillary study, it is easy to talk to providers and participants—you don't have to start that network from scratch," she says. Furthermore, Dr. Dabelea already has a wealth of SEARCH data that can be incorporated into the ancillary study. "We don't have to spend time and resources collecting those data *de novo*," she notes. Thus, Dr. Dabelea is able to build on the investment that has been made in SEARCH, with support from the *Special Diabetes Program*, to maximize research progress and address key questions related to the management of type 1 diabetes.

Looking to the Future

Dr. Dabelea believes that it is important to continue collecting data through SEARCH, to paint a better and broader picture of childhood diabetes in the United States. "SEARCH is unique," she explains, "and diabetes in youth is an important problem with many public health implications." Dr. Dabelea also has a vision for using SEARCH data to benefit children with diabetes. "SEARCH has increased our understanding of childhood diabetes and its complications. We hope that in the next several years, the knowledge provided by SEARCH will translate into better quality of care and better quality of life for children with type 1 diabetes, and maybe someday to successful prevention of the disease."

Patient Profiles

Robert Watts and Sallie Cartwright
Participating in a Landmark Clinical Trial that Improved Vision

Blindness is a debilitating complication of diabetes that has a profound impact on people's quality of life. To combat this complication, the *Special Statutory Funding Program for Type 1 Diabetes Research* supports clinical research to accelerate the development of new therapies and treatments for diabetic eye disease (retinopathy). One major research effort is the Diabetic Retinopathy Clinical Research Network (DRCR.net), which is led by NEI and supported in part by the *Special Diabetes Program*. The DRCR.net is a nationwide collaboration of eye doctors and scientists conducting research on diabetes-induced retinal disorders. Because diabetic retinopathy is a complication associated with both type 1 and type 2 diabetes, DRCR.net enrolls people with both forms of diabetes into its studies. In April 2010, the DRCR.net announced the results from its landmark comparative effectiveness clinical trial showing that a new therapy combining eye injections of the drug ranibizumab with laser treatment to the eye was more effective than the standard practice of laser treatment alone. This profile includes the personal stories of two people—one with type 1 diabetes and the other with type 2 diabetes—who achieved significant vision improvement in this clinical trial.

About the Trial
The goal of the DRCR.net trial was to translate recent discoveries about a molecule that affects blood vessel growth and permeability into potential new treatment approaches for diabetic retinopathy. Diabetic retinopathy is caused by changes in blood vessels in the retina, the part of the eye that detects light and produces signals that enable the brain to "see" images—thus functioning much like the sensor in a digital camera, or like camera film. One condition that can affect people with diabetic retinopathy is called diabetic macular edema. In this condition, blood vessels in the eye leak fluid in an area of the retina responsible for sharp central vision, causing swelling and blurring sight. Regular eye exams are important to help detect this and other diabetic eye problems early and protect vision. Diabetic retinopathy can be treated with laser surgery to the eye, significantly reducing the development of severe vision loss. However, laser treatment itself can lead to some diminution of vision. New approaches are thus highly desirable. A normal body protein called vascular endothelial growth factor, or VEGF, has emerged as a prime suspect in some of the blood vessel problems seen in diabetic retinopathy, including blood vessel "leakiness." Researchers decided to test whether administration of a drug (ranibizumab) that inhibits VEGF activity, in combination with laser treatment, could benefit people with diabetic retinopathy.

The DRCR.net trial included a total of 854 eyes of 691 participants. The reason that there are more eyes than people is because some people had only one eye treated, while others had both eyes treated. Each eye was randomly assigned to one of four treatment groups: sham injections (containing no medicine) plus prompt laser treatment; ranibizumab injections plus prompt laser treatment; ranibizumab plus deferred (for a short time) laser treatment; or injections of corticosteroid medication known as triamcinolone, plus prompt laser treatment. However, if a person was receiving treatment in both eyes, then one eye was treated with laser and sham injections and the other eye was treated with laser and a medicine (ranibizumab or triamcinolone).

For the first 12 weeks of the study, the participants received treatment based on their assigned group. After that time and for the remainder of the study, retreatment followed a detailed algorithm. In general, treatment was continued until a participant's vision or retinal thickness returned to normal, or until additional treatment did not improve vision or retinal swelling. Once retreatment was withheld, it typically was resumed if retinal thickness worsened at a subsequent visit.

The exciting results demonstrated that nearly 50 percent of eyes treated with ranibizumab and either prompt or deferred laser treatment showed a substantial visual improvement after 1 year, compared to 28 percent of eyes that received the standard laser treatment plus sham injections. In some instances, the combination treatment reversed a person's vision impairment, an advance that has greatly improved quality of life for those individuals. Many in the field refer to this finding as the most significant treatment advance in diabetic retinopathy in 25 years.

Robert Watts

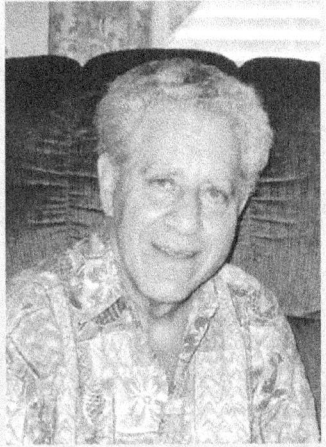

Robert Watts was diagnosed with type 1 diabetes at the age of 24, and he has been injecting himself with insulin for the past 46 years. Robert admits that he works hard at taking care of himself and monitoring his blood sugar levels. He tests his blood sugar levels seven or eight times each day, and he believes that it is because of this constant monitoring that he has not yet experienced many of the common complications from diabetes.

However, 10 years ago, Robert began to notice that his vision was declining. "The street signs became difficult to read when I was driving at night, and it became challenging to read the numbers at the bottom of my television screen during a sporting event," he recalls. "When I went to my eye doctor a little over 3 years ago, he told me that my vision was going to continue to deteriorate. He told me about a clinical trial that was testing a new course of therapy for people with my condition, and I wanted to learn more." Robert was fortunate that his doctor was participating in DRCR.net, and he was able to receive information about the trial quickly.

"It was an easy decision to enter the trial," says Robert. "I have four grandchildren, ages 14, 13, 9 and 6. I want to see them grow up. I love them more than anything, and that is why I try to take good care of myself." Robert also recognized the opportunity he had been given to help others with diabetes. "I knew that by participating in this trial, I would be helping the researchers gather more information about diabetic retinopathy that would help them develop new treatments for others," he says.

"My vision has improved big time," Robert says proudly.

Robert enrolled in the trial 3 years ago and, since the start of the trial, he has visited his doctor every month for an exam that lasts approximately 2 hours. Robert was one of the trial participants who received treatment in one eye only. He received ranibizumab injections in combination with laser treatment. During the time that Robert was receiving the treatment, he remembers that the procedure was not pleasant. "After my monthly exam, if the research team determined that I needed to receive the treatment, it would involve a needle in my eye," Robert notes. "It was not a procedure that I looked forward to. But there was a team of people in the doctor's office who took great care of me. That made it a lot easier." Robert attributes his positive experience in the trial to his doctor and his team. "I have lots of tests done at each visit," he says. "The team is very professional and works together. They are outstanding." Even his wife, a retired nurse, has commented on the care Robert has received. "My wife took me to each appointment and was always by my side. She is a retired nurse and has been so impressed with the quality of care I have been receiving as a participant in the trial."

"After about a year of receiving the treatment, my vision improved greatly," Robert remembers. "I keep going back to the doctor monthly for my exams, but I haven't had to have a treatment in about a year and a half. My vision has improved big time," Robert says proudly.

Sallie Cartwright

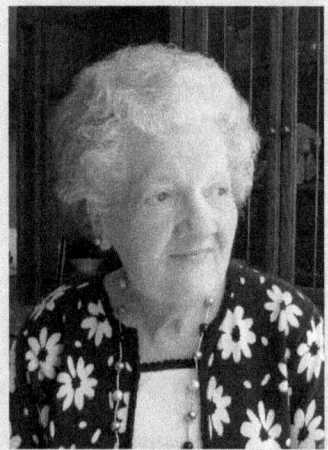

Shortly after Sallie Cartwright and her husband moved to Maryland 4 years ago, she noticed a problem with her vision. "I realized when I was driving that I couldn't see the road signs and my first thought was that I needed driving glasses," remembers Sallie. "Reading became increasingly difficult. I had trouble reading the phone book and my prescription bottles. But the hardest thing for me," she recalls, "was not being able to read music properly. I am a retired professional musician and sharing my musical skills still brings joy to me."

When Sallie went to the eye doctor, she received an unexpected diagnosis. After a thorough examination, the ophthalmologist told her that her right eye was worthless and her left eye was legally blind. He said that glasses would not help her and that she needed to go to a retina specialist as soon as possible. The vision problems she was experiencing were a complication of her type 2 diabetes.

Shortly after that visit, Sallie went to a retina specialist recommended by her ophthalmologist. During her first visit, she learned about a DRCR.net clinical trial that was testing a new therapy to treat diabetic retinopathy. She was told that she was eligible to participate in the trial and what would be involved if she chose to participate. Sallie remembers that the decision to enter the trial was not an easy one to make. "I have had severe allergies to food and medicines since I was a child, so the decision to participate was a difficult one," she recalls. "I had no idea how I was going to react to the medication I would be given. Over the years I had been rushed to the emergency room for adverse reactions to drugs and nearly lost my life several times." Sallie has been married to a research scientist for 45 years, so her knowledge of the importance of clinical research played a big role in her decision to participate. She says, "With the professionalism, caring, kindness, commitment and dedication to healing and research of the retina specialist to whom I was referred, I felt that it was my obligation to participate and possibly help others. I was willing to take a personal risk for the opportunity to help so many."

Sallie had both eyes treated as part of the trial. One eye was treated with ranibizumab injections plus laser, while the other eye was treated with sham injections plus laser. Happily for Sallie, her vision dramatically improved in both eyes since she enrolled in the trial— she now sees "20/20" and is back to reading music and playing the piano. She says, "Everyone is so excited when I have my vision tested and I am reading 20/20. The research team and support staff are like a big cheering squad for me. Throughout the trial, they have always been professional, caring, and incredibly dedicated. The quality of care I have received has been exceptional."

"For my eyes to go from worthless and legally blind to being able to see at 20/20 without glasses is incredible," says Sallie.

When asked about her experience in the trial, Sallie pauses and searches for the right words. Expressively she says, "My experience during this trial is hard to describe. For my eyes to go from worthless and legally blind to being able to see at 20/20 without glasses is incredible."

For more information on the DRCR.net, please visit: www.drcr.net

EMERGING RESEARCH OPPORTUNITIES RESULTING FROM THE *SPECIAL DIABETES PROGRAM*

The *Special Statutory Funding Program for Type 1 Diabetes Research* has fueled the emergence of a wide range of research opportunities. These opportunities were identified in a strategic planning process as being critically important for overcoming current barriers and achieving progress in diabetes research. Key questions and research opportunities relevant to type 1 diabetes, including those related to preventing and reversing diabetes complications, are outlined in Appendix F.

GOAL VI

ATTRACT NEW TALENT AND APPLY NEW TECHNOLOGIES TO RESEARCH ON TYPE 1 DIABETES

The *Special Statutory Funding Program for Type 1 Diabetes Research* has expanded the research opportunities in type 1 diabetes and its complications by harnessing cutting edge tools and technologies and attracting creative and skilled scientists with diverse background. This has resulted in significant scientific progress, which is described in this chapter and in other chapters throughout the report. Additional information on the program evaluation related to Goal VI can be found in Appendix A (Allocation of Funds), Appendix B (Assessment), and Appendix C (Evaluation of Major Research Consortia, Networks, and Resources).

Type 1 diabetes affects many organ systems and involves diverse areas of science. Thus, it is imperative to pursue a broad range of research to have the greatest impact on the health of people. Toward that end, it is important to recruit scientists with different areas of expertise and to promote collaboration to conduct research on type 1 diabetes. It is also imperative to capitalize on new and emerging technologies and fields of science to propel research progress. Research supported by the *Special Statutory Funding Program for Type 1 Diabetes Research* (*Special Diabetes Program* or *Program*) has led to major scientific advances by attracting new scientific talent with diverse backgrounds and applying new and emerging technologies to the study of this complex disease.

HIGHLIGHTS OF RECENT RESEARCH ADVANCES RELATED TO GOAL VI

Attracted New Talent to Research on Type 1 Diabetes: Evaluation of research supported by the *Special Diabetes Program* showed that approximately 38 percent of scientists who received R01, R21, or DP2 grants were new investigators, and that number is likely an underestimation. In addition, the *Program* supported a training and career development program for a cadre of pediatricians specializing in childhood diabetes. An evaluation of the K12 (Physician Scientist Award) component of this training program showed that 28 pediatric endocrinologists received training, and 27 of them (96 percent) remain in academic medicine. Thus, the *Special Diabetes Program* has attracted new researchers to the study of type 1 diabetes and has also trained a new generation of pediatric endocrinologists to conduct diabetes research.

Positron Emission Tomography (PET) Imaging Agents Target the Pancreatic Beta Cell: ^{11}C-DTBZ (^{11}C-dihydrotetrabenazine) is an imaging agent developed for PET imaging of the dopaminergic neurons of the brain. Its target, the Vesicular Monoamine Transporter 2 (VMAT2) protein, was identified in gene array screens of islet cells. The imaging agent binds specifically to beta and pancreatic polypeptide-producing cells of the islet and has been used to visualize these cells in the human pancreas in healthy people and in people with diabetes. Currently, researchers are working to modify the molecule in order to improve its imaging and binding characteristics to the point where it can be reliably used to monitor beta cell mass in people. Other research is ongoing to determine the

Graphic: Noninvasive in vivo magnetic resonance imaging (MRI) of transplanted human islets, designated by white arrows, in the livers of healthy mice. Islets were labeled with a magnetically "visible" contrast agent for imaging. Image credit: Dr. Anna Moore.

specific location and expression of its molecular target in the pancreas. Additional highly promising imaging agents are being developed that target markers enriched in the beta cell, such as the glucagon-like protein (GLP)-1 receptor. Development of the imaging agent ^{11}C-DTBZ has thus spurred noninvasive studies of beta cells.

Magnetic Resonance Imaging (MRI) Agents Hold Promise for Imaging Transplanted Islets: The current practice of transplanting islets into the livers of people with diabetes presents both challenges and opportunities for imaging. The liver takes up many of the molecular imaging agents in a non-specific way, and therefore tends to have a high background signal in most experiments. Considerable progress has been made by labeling either the islets themselves with iron-based contrast agents prior to transplantation, or by encapsulating the isolated islets in immunoprotective coatings that contain iron- or gadolinium-based contrast agents. Signals persist long after transplantation in rodent, porcine, and primate models, and correlate very well with islet survival. Human trials are under way using this approach.

Ability To Image Islet Inflammation *In Vivo*: The presence of islet autoantibodies, and perhaps metabolic changes as detected in the circulation, are the current standards to measure islet autoimmunity, but are an indirect measure. In preliminary experiments, the specific T cell populations that cause insulitis have been directly visualized using molecular imaging approaches, but the most promising and least invasive approach is to take advantage of the vasculature 'leakiness' that develops during inflammation. Large, iron-based MRI contrast agents tend to remain in the bloodstream except in sites of compromised vasculature, and a persistent signal in the pancreas due to islet inflammation has been successfully monitored in type 1 diabetes mouse models and in people recently diagnosed with type 1 diabetes.

ATTRACTING NEW TALENT TO TYPE 1 DIABETES RESEARCH

A major goal of the *Special Diabetes Program* is to attract new talent to the study of type 1 diabetes and its complications. Encouraging new researchers to study type 1 diabetes brings fresh talent to the field and promotes the careers of young scientists poised to make a difference in public health. From the *Program*'s inception in Fiscal Year (FY) 1998 through FY 2009, approximately 38 percent[28] of scientists who received R01, R21, or DP2 grants were new investigators, and this number is likely an underestimation. In addition to attracting new scientists, the *Special Diabetes Program* has also facilitated novel collaborations among scientists with diverse interests to study type 1 diabetes and its complications.

Type 1 Diabetes Pathfinder Awards: Through support from the *Special Diabetes Program*, the NIDDK employed a novel strategy to attract new scientists to type 1 diabetes research. Ten scientists who had not previously received an NIH grant successfully competed for Type 1 Diabetes Pathfinder Awards for highly innovative research studies. Some of the scientists supported by the Pathfinder Awards were new to type 1

---

[28] Data collected through the NIAID electronic Scientific Portfolio Assistant (e-SPA). More information on data and methodology related to new investigators is found in Appendix B.

diabetes research, demonstrating how this innovative strategy attracted scientists to apply their expertise to a new research field. Profiles of two scientists who received Type 1 Diabetes Pathfinder Awards are found later in this chapter.

Supporting the Next Generation of Scientists: Management of diabetes in children is particularly arduous and requires an exceptional level of effort from the children, their families, and their health care providers. These extraordinary clinical care demands make it challenging for pediatric endocrinologists involved in diabetes care to also pursue research careers. Furthermore, there is a long process of training and career development before a new independent investigator is ready to obtain grant support and lead a research laboratory. Through support from the *Special Diabetes Program*, a cadre of pediatricians specializing in childhood diabetes received such research training and career development. A recent evaluation of the K12 training program showed that 28 pediatric endocrinologists received training under the program, and 27 of them (96 percent) remain in academic science. Many of them have also successfully competed for independent funding to conduct research. As just one example of the success of this training program, one of the trainees, Dr. Stuart Weinzimer, attained a faculty position at Yale University and is making significant contributions to research on continuous glucose monitoring technology and the development of an artificial pancreas (see Dr. Weinzimer's Investigator Profile later in this chapter).

Promoting Research Collaborations: The *Special Diabetes Program* has promoted successful collaborations among scientists with diverse interests to combat type 1 diabetes. The *Special Diabetes Program*

has facilitated the creation of multiple research consortia to tackle specific challenges that will impact the health of people with type 1 diabetes. Collaboration has been a key component to the success of these efforts. For example, the Beta Cell Biology Consortium (BCBC; see Goal III) has brought together experts in diverse fields such as developmental biology, bioinformatics, animal model development, immunology, and other areas, to work collaboratively toward the goal of developing cell replacement therapy for type 1 diabetes. The BCBC has been extremely successful, has resulted in major scientific advances, and is now being used a model for other new collaborative research programs being established by NIH. In another example, researchers in DirecNet (experts in continuous glucose monitoring technology) and Type 1 Diabetes TrialNet (experts in clinical trials focused on type 1 diabetes prevention and early treatment) forged a collaboration to test whether a closed-loop system could preserve beta cell function in newly diagnosed patients. (For more information about the collaboration on this trial, please see the Investigator Profile of Dr. Bruce Buckingham in Goal IV.) Collaboration between these two groups of scientists was crucial to undertake this type of study and such coordination and collaboration continues to be essential as type 1 diabetes research evolves.

Pilot and Feasibility Projects: Pilot and Feasibility (P&F) projects have been used successfully to attract new talent to type 1 diabetes research. Several of the consortia supported by the *Special Diabetes Program*, such as the BCBC, the Animal Models of Diabetic Complications Consortium, and the Cooperative Study Group for Autoimmune Disease Prevention, support P&F projects to attract new talent. These programs give new researchers the opportunity to test novel hypotheses that have conceptual promise, established investigators a chance to explore a new application or direction for their research, or scientists not studying type 1 diabetes an opportunity to apply their talents to a completely new research field. Thus, this mechanism has provided a means to attract new talent to research on type 1 diabetes and its complications.

APPLYING NEW TECHNOLOGIES TO TYPE 1 DIABETES RESEARCH

The tools of biomedical research have changed rapidly due to the biotechnology revolution. Many methods that were used as recently as 10 or 20 years ago have been replaced by technologies that permit scientists to conduct research more efficiently and to ask and answer new research questions.

Capitalizing on New Genetics Tools and Technologies: Recent advances in the genetics of type 1 diabetes are a prime example of progress that has been achieved due to the development of new technologies. Technological developments in the 1980s sped up the ability to sequence genes, which in turn enabled NIH to launch the Human Genome Project in 1990. Completed in 2003, the Human Genome Project mapped all the genes in the human genome. The elucidation of the entire human genome made possible another effort, called the International HapMap Project, to develop a "haplotype" map of the human genome. The haplotype map, or "HapMap," is a tool that allows researchers to find genes and genetic variations that affect health and disease.

The new research tools that emerged from the Human Genome Project and the International HapMap Project laid the foundation for new "genome wide association studies" (GWAS) to identify even subtle genetic differences between people with specific illnesses and unaffected individuals. As recently as 2003, just three type 1 diabetes genes were known. Now, through GWAS and other genetics studies, scientists supported by the *Special Diabetes Program* and others have identified over 40 genes or genetic regions associated with type 1 diabetes. This remarkable progress demonstrates how researchers supported by the *Program* capitalized on new tools and technologies to make major strides in understanding the genetic underpinnings of type 1 diabetes. Researchers supported by the *Special Diabetes Program* are now building on these scientific discoveries to pinpoint the exact genes that influence type 1 diabetes susceptibility and to understand their role in health and disease. This knowledge can lead to the development of new prevention and treatment strategies, and possibly personalized therapies. For more information on the genetics of type 1 diabetes, please see Goal I.

Supporting Research in a New Era of "Omics" Technologies: Historically, scientists have looked at individual genes or proteins to understand how they influence disease. This has been a useful strategy and has led to revolutionary progress and new treatment approaches, but could be limiting—much like looking at one piece of a puzzle. The era of "omics" technologies is providing researchers an opportunity to understand how networks of cellular components work together to produce a state of health and to identify key players that go awry in disease. Toward that goal, researchers supported by the *Special Diabetes Program* are using "omics" technologies to generate a system-wide picture of all of the molecules in a cell and how they are affected by type 1 diabetes. This research includes determining the sequences and expression of all genes in a certain cellular context (genomics), mapping out all interactions of different proteins and how they are modulated in disease (proteomics), and following the path of all metabolic intermediates (metabolomics).

For example, scientists are using proteomics to elucidate beta cell function and to identify new proteins on the beta cell that may be targets of the immune system's attack. In addition, research supported by the *Special Diabetes Program* demonstrated that, in mice, the trillions of bacteria that live in the gut may protect against the immune system attack that causes type 1 diabetes. Thus, knowledge stemming from the NIH Human Microbiome Project, which is identifying and characterizing the microorganisms found in the body, can be utilized to explore this fascinating insight into type 1 diabetes. In fact, the samples that are being collected by TEDDY (see Goal I) could be analyzed with new technologies emerging from the Human Microbiome Project, to uncover potential environmental triggers of type 1 diabetes. Also, because celiac disease shares the same genetic risk factors as type 1 diabetes, TEDDY will also study the environmental triggers for celiac disease. Therefore, application of "omics" technologies to type 1 diabetes provides a chance to see the entire puzzle, facilitating a greater understanding of the disease process than ever before possible, which can lead to the identification of new targets or strategies for prevention and therapy.

Development of New Continuous Glucose Monitoring Technology and Research Toward an Artificial Pancreas: While there has been remarkable progress due to involvement of bioengineers in developing current continuous glucose monitoring technology, a next generation of sensors, algorithms, and insulin formulations are needed. Recent research supported by

the *Special Diabetes Program* is intended to build on earlier success and develop even more accurate devices. More information on continuous glucose monitoring and artificial pancreas technologies is found in Goal IV.

Applying New Technologies To Improve Detection of Diabetic Eye Disease: Scientists supported by the *Special Diabetes Program* are developing new tools and technologies that can be used for increasing patient access to eye exams for detecting diabetic retinopathy, a complication of diabetes that can lead to blindness. Many people with diabetes live in communities without ophthalmologists trained in examining the retina for signs of diabetic damage. New tools combined with telemedicine can address this problem and overcome a barrier to regular eye exams that can lead to prompt vision-sparing therapy. For example, researchers are seeking to develop a low-cost, handheld camera that is capable of assessing the human retina. This type of device could be used by non-eye specialists, such as primary care physicians, to acquire and transmit retinal images to a remote processing site for interpretation and diagnosis by retinal specialists. This technology could help improve detection of diabetic retinopathy because patients would not necessarily have to make a trip to an eye specialist for an exam. Early detection could lead to early treatment to prevent blindness.

Imaging the Pancreatic Beta Cell: Another research area that has been fostered by the *Special Diabetes Program* is imaging the pancreatic beta cell. The NIDDK, through support from the *Program*, spearheaded a series of targeted research solicitations and scientific workshops to accelerate research progress in this area. At the first workshop, in 1999, only a handful of scientists were in attendance. At the most recent workshop, in April 2009, a few hundred scientists and trainees were in attendance to discuss research progress and future directions. The overall intended goal of the research is to develop clinically useful imaging approaches for monitoring the mass, function, and inflammation of naturally occurring or transplanted beta cells in the body, in people with type 1 or type 2 diabetes, or people who are at risk for these diseases. Imaging the beta cell holds promise as a means to allow scientists to visualize the extent of pancreatic damage and, potentially, to see directly if a therapy is effective. This ability could lead to smaller, shorter, and less expensive clinical trials for both type 1 and type 2 diabetes. It could also allow physicians to see damage to the pancreas before onset of symptoms, thus possibly allowing for earlier intervention. Furthermore, imaging could help physicians monitor islets after transplantation, which could permit them to intervene when necessary to prevent the islets' destruction.

Applying Other New and Emerging Technologies to Research on Type 1 Diabetes: In addition to the examples given above, the *Special Diabetes Program* has supported research on a wide range of scientific areas using new and emerging technologies. For example, research supported by the *Special Diabetes Program* suggests that manipulating dendritic cells of the immune system is a promising strategy to prevent, delay, or reverse type 1 diabetes (see Goal II). Scientists are also using small interfering RNA (siRNA) technology to identify target genes that promote type 1 diabetes, and developing strategies for therapeutic application of siRNA to turn off genes of interest. Bioengineers are studying ways to protect transplanted islets for immune system attack, such as by encasing cells in a protective barrier.

SUMMARY

The diabetes research enterprise requires a diversely-trained, multidisciplinary, and interactive workforce to fully address the complexity of disease etiology and treatment. The *Special Diabetes Program* has augmented such a workforce to combat complex problems related to diabetes prevention, treatment, and cure. Scientists with expertise in areas not historically associated with type 1 diabetes, such as bioengineers, are now applying their talents to type 1 diabetes research. As scientists from diverse fields continue to study type 1 diabetes and its complications, additional progress will be achieved.

The highlights of scientific accomplishments described in this chapter showcase how the *Special Diabetes Program* is capitalizing on new and emerging technologies toward the goal of improving health and quality of life of people with type 1 diabetes. Research that was not possible at the inception of the *Program* is now possible because of these new technologies. New technologies applied to type 1 diabetes research have resulted in major scientific advances, such as the identification of numerous genes associated with the disease and its complications. In many cases, such as in the development of continuous glucose monitoring technology and imaging inflammation, the *Special Diabetes Program* supported the development of the new technologies themselves, which is having a far-reaching impact.

Investigator Profile

Stuart Weinzimer, M.D.

Nurturing Research Careers in Pediatric Endocrinology

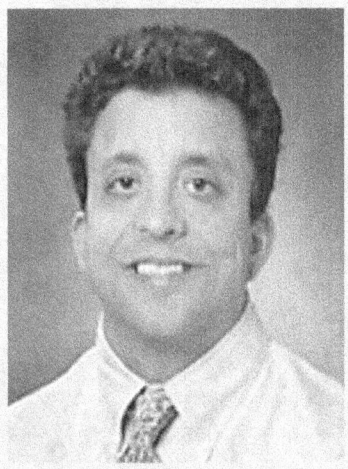

Stuart Weinzimer, M.D.

Stuart Weinzimer, M.D. is an Associate Professor in the Department of Pediatrics at the Yale University School of Medicine. He was a recipient of an NIH Clinical Scientist Career Development Program (K12) award, which was supported by the Special Statutory Funding Program for Type 1 Diabetes Research to cultivate clinical researchers in pediatric endocrinology. Now he is an independent investigator pursuing cutting-edge research on new technologies in diabetes management for children, including research toward the development of an artificial pancreas. This profile describes Dr. Weinzimer's research, the impact of the K12 award on his career, and the importance of fellowship awards to recruit pediatric endocrinologists to research.

A Marriage of Technologies: The Artificial Pancreas

"We need to improve the lives of people now," says Dr. Weinzimer passionately when describing the objective of his research. Toward this goal, his research focuses on the use of technology to improve diabetes care for children. This has included studies on technological advancements such as insulin pumps and continuous glucose monitors through the *Special Diabetes Program*-supported Diabetes Research in Children Network (DirecNet). Dr. Weinzimer is now working on a "marriage of those two technologies," an artificial pancreas that "closes the loop" between the insulin pump and continuous glucose monitors. "Closed loop is really nothing more than insulin delivery that's automated so that a person with diabetes or a caretaker doesn't have to manually do it," describes Dr. Weinzimer.

This technology has the potential to significantly improve the quality of life of people with type 1 diabetes by automatically measuring glucose levels in real time and administering the proper amount of insulin. By replicating what the body does naturally, it is hoped that the artificial pancreas will help people with type 1 diabetes achieve tighter control of their blood glucose levels, reduce risks of long-term complications from chronic hyperglycemia (high blood glucose), and eliminate dangerous episodes of hypoglycemia when blood glucose levels drop too low. Research from the landmark NIDDK-supported Diabetes Control and Complications Trial and the follow-on Epidemiology of Diabetes Interventions and Complications study has demonstrated that intensive control of blood glucose levels can have long-lasting effects toward reducing the onset and progression of diabetes complications involving the kidneys, eyes, nerves, and heart. "With closed loop technologies, it will be the first time we've ever been able to offer people a new tool for diabetes that's associated with less burden of care rather than more burden of care," explains Dr. Weinzimer.

"It's humbling," he says, describing what it is like to work with patients with type 1 diabetes. "I went into pediatric endocrinology because it was very logical and rational and all the metabolic pathways were beautiful and elegant. And the reason I went into diabetes is because it's completely irrational and makes no sense," he explains. In addition to his research, Dr. Weinzimer is the Medical Director of Yale's Type 1 Diabetes clinic, seeing children with diabetes every week. While that may seem like a lot to juggle, it's the right balance for Dr. Weinzimer. "I need to have different facets—where I'm seeing patients and working on research protocols and I can very easily pick up what I'm doing in my research and apply it to the clinic. It allows me a lot of variety, but [they are] similar enough where one informs the other." For example, after performing basic pharmacology studies looking at the rate of insulin absorption, he was able to immediately apply the results to how his patients were being treated with insulin pumps. Conducting type 1 diabetes research and seeing patients in the clinic is a perfect combination for him.

Enticing Pediatric Endocrinologists to Research

When Dr. Weinzimer started his training in pediatric endocrinology (diabetes is an endocrine disease), he worked in a laboratory studying the molecular determinants of growth and growth factors. Although he found the research interesting, he decided to pursue another facet of pediatric endocrinology—diabetes. "I always had a clinical interest in diabetes management,"

notes Dr. Weinzimer, "and I wanted a change in my career trajectory." He began speaking with clinical diabetes researchers, in search of a program that would be a good fit for his interests in diabetes research, and met with Dr. William Tamborlane, a renowned type 1 diabetes researcher at Yale University. Yale had received funding from NIH to recruit pediatric endocrinology fellows into research and had dedicated and committed senior investigators with the mentoring qualities for which Dr. Weinzimer was looking.

To enlarge the pool of pediatric endocrinologists conducting diabetes research, NIH, in partnership with the American Diabetes Association (ADA) and the Juvenile Diabetes Research Foundation International (JDRF) and with support from the *Special Diabetes Program*, awarded institution-wide research training and career development grants to seven medical centers with strong research programs in childhood diabetes. Dr. Weinzimer's award, the Clinical Scientist Career Development Program (K12) grant mechanism of the NIH, was designed to provide 2-3 years of support for junior clinical investigators. The funding supported up to five positions at each medical center; each center was free to decide how many of the five slots were to be reserved for pediatric endocrinology fellows or investigators who were transitioning from fellow to independent scientist.

"This kind of funding mechanism really made this whole thing possible," says Dr. Weinzimer, referring to his transition to a new field and advancement to an independent investigator. "He [Dr. Tamborlane] was able to bring me to Yale from my previous institution, without my own hard funding, and I was basically able to train in a whole new area. By having the K12 I was able to learn techniques, develop a whole new research expertise, and have the 'protected time' to do it." The award meant that Dr. Weinzimer could be trained in type 1 diabetes clinical research and conduct research, rather than having to spend the majority of his time in the clinic. He learned how to carry out clinical diabetes research studies in children and started studying how the body uses and responds to insulin delivered by an insulin pump.

Transition to an Independent Researcher

At the end of his fellowship, Dr. Weinzimer would transition from being a fellow to a faculty member, at which time he would be expected to find his own source of funding to support his research program. The K12 award allowed him to begin to develop his own research program as an independent investigator. "We were able to do some of our earliest closed loop studies under the K12 as well," Dr. Weinzimer notes. "That led very directly to both JDRF funding and my current R01 [an NIH Research Project Grant] funding." Dr. Weinzimer decided to continue his research at Yale where he is now an Associate Professor.

When asked if training awards like the K12 are a good mechanism to attract pediatric endocrinologists to diabetes, Dr. Weinzimer responds, "I will say that it's necessary, it's not just good. Pediatric endocrinology is a small field, and we have to be able to offer something to young investigators to help them either become interested or stay interested in pediatric diabetes research." Now as the fellowship director for Yale's pediatric endocrinology program, Dr. Weinzimer has an even broader perspective of the importance of awards like the K12: "It's really great for me to take a person who's interested in diabetes, be able to protect his or her time, and say 'Go off and do this, learn this' at a place such as Yale where we have the resources to do that. And I'll know at the end of the 3 to 4 years that we can develop an investigator who can go out and do great things. It's a tremendous investment and is incredibly important." Dr. Weinzimer himself fits this description well, as he continues to do great things through research and clinical practice to improve the lives of children with diabetes.

Pathfinder Investigator Profile

Deyu Fang, Ph.D.

Insight from Traditional Chinese Medicine Paves a Path to a Career in Type 1 Diabetes Research

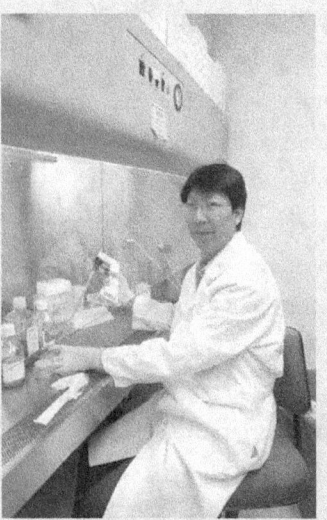

Deyu Fang, Ph.D.

Deyu Fang, Ph.D., is an Associate Professor of Pathology at Northwestern University. He is a recipient of the Type 1 Diabetes Pathfinder Award, which is supported by the Special Statutory Funding Program for Type 1 Diabetes Research and provides funding for new investigators pursuing innovative research on type 1 diabetes. Dr. Fang is conducting research to uncover how a specific protein ensures that potentially harmful cells of the immune system are kept inactive. This profile describes how he came to be involved in type 1 diabetes research, his research that is supported by the Pathfinder Award, and how this award has impacted his career as an independent investigator.

"The overall goal for my research," begins Dr. Fang, "is to understand how type 1 diabetes develops. Why does a person with type 1 diabetes have immune cells that attack insulin-producing cells, but other people do not?"

The question is simple in its presentation, but finding the answer is complicated. Normally the immune system protects from foreign invaders—bacteria or viruses—that have entered the body. To be effective, the immune system needs to be able to distinguish cells in the body (self) from foreign invaders (non-self). "Tolerance" is the normal process that prevents the immune system from attacking self. When the body produces an immune system cell that may pose a threat to it, the body can delete the cell or ensure it stays inactive. Autoimmune diseases like type 1 diabetes develop from a defect in tolerance. In people with type 1 diabetes, the defect results in the fact that the aberrant immune cells are not destroyed or inactivated, so they target and destroy the insulin-producing beta cells in the pancreas. How tolerance works, and why and how it is altered in people with type 1 diabetes, are critical research questions that innovative researchers like Dr. Fang are trying to answer.

Demonstrating a Role for SIRT1 in Tolerance

Dr. Fang is investigating the function of a specific protein—known as SIRT1—in tolerance. He became interested in the role of SIRT1 in the immune system from an observation he made while in medical school in China. Says Dr. Fang, "The Chinese herbal medicine *Hu Zhang* has been used to treat autoimmune disease, particularly lupus, for thousands of years and no one thought about why." When it was discovered that this particular herbal medicine contained a small molecule called resveratrol, Dr. Fang saw a connection. Resveratrol is being studied for potential metabolic benefits, including enhancing insulin signaling and protecting tissues from damage caused by reactive oxygen. Thus, Dr. Fang thought that the resveratrol in *Hu Zhang* might have protective effects in type 1 diabetes. He was prompted to study the role of SIRT1—a key enzyme which resveratrol is thought to influence—on tolerance, and hypothesized that "SIRT1 was likely to be a critical regulator for the immune response." If SIRT1 is important in the immune system, he thought that "dysregulated or misregulated SIRT1 function could be critically involved in the development of type 1 diabetes."

With funding from the Pathfinder Award, Dr. Fang and his colleagues have already made significant progress in testing this hypothesis. Results from his laboratory demonstrated that SIRT1 inhibits activation of T cells, a type of immune cell involved in autoimmunity, and is required for tolerance in mice. Mice genetically engineered to lack SIRT1 developed spontaneous autoimmunity in Dr. Fang's studies, suggesting that SIRT1 plays an important role in suppressing the autoimmune response.

With these exciting observations, Dr. Fang returned to his initial observation. If loss of SIRT1 can lead to the development of type 1 diabetes in mice, can treatment with resveratrol prevent the disease? In a pilot study, Dr. Fang and his colleagues tested the effects of resveratrol on mice that spontaneously develop type 1 diabetes. He summarized the result simply: "If we feed mice this small compound, then they won't develop diabetes." Dr. Fang is currently conducting a more-detailed study to conclusively demonstrate the preventative effects of resveratrol on type 1 diabetes in mice. If effective in mice, further studies would then be needed to determine if the compound is also effective in people.

Implications for Type 1 Diabetes and Beyond

Resveratrol has significant promise as a therapy for type 1 diabetes, but much remains to be understood about this compound and the role of SIRT1 in tolerance and autoimmunity. Dr. Fang will continue his research with the Pathfinder Award to address how SIRT1 regulates T cell activation and tolerance, and to determine the effects of resveratrol on type 1 diabetes development. Dr. Fang sees potential with this compound and aims to see his studies move beyond the laboratory bench: "My goal is to push this research toward a clinical trial."

Dr. Fang's research also has implications beyond type 1 diabetes. Because impaired tolerance is critical to the development of autoimmunity, his research may provide insights into other autoimmune diseases as well. "This Pathfinder Award allows us to figure out the common mechanism behind other types of autoimmune disease," explains Dr. Fang, "and whether we can find some small molecules to treat those diseases." Additionally, there is evidence to suggest that resveratrol may be effective in treating type 2 diabetes. With support from the Pathfinder Award, Dr. Fang has been able to establish collaborations with scientists studying type 2 diabetes to investigate the potential of resveratrol in treatment of both forms of the disease.

The Importance of the Pathfinder Award

Obtaining support through a Pathfinder Award has been critical in Dr. Fang's opinion. "Essentially, this award established my career and made this research project possible," he says. Before receiving the award, his laboratory studied rheumatoid arthritis, another type of autoimmune disease. The Pathfinder Award allowed

Dr. Fang to extend his research specifically to type 1 diabetes. In addition, the award has enabled him to recruit new graduate students to the laboratory and to type 1 diabetes research. "I think this award is extremely important, not only to develop a new generation of new investigators, but to develop the next generation. For example, because of this award, I was able to recruit several graduate students—very bright, smart, and highly motivated students—and train them to do research to combat type 1 diabetes," he says. Thus, like the potential of Dr. Fang's research to alter the treatment of type 1 diabetes and extend to other autoimmune diseases and perhaps even type 2 diabetes, the influence of the Pathfinder Award in Dr. Fang's laboratory will extend as well. As new graduate students are recruited to studying type 1 diabetes and trained to do research in this field because of Dr. Fang's Pathfinder Award, the impact of this award will continue long after its conclusion.

Pathfinder Investigator Profile

Bridget K. Wagner, Ph.D.

Bringing Small Molecules to a Career in Type 1 Diabetes Research

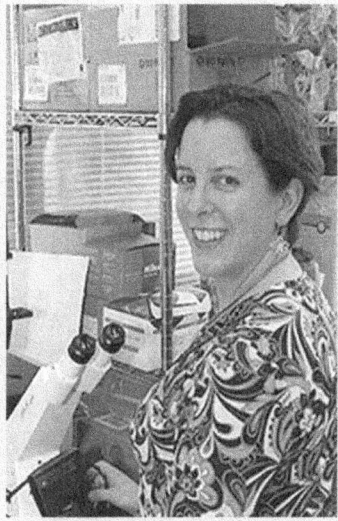

Bridget K. Wagner, Ph.D.
Photo credit: Maria Nemchuk, Broad Institute

Bridget K. Wagner, Ph.D., is a Group Leader in the Chemical Biology Program at the Broad Institute of MIT and Harvard. She is a recipient of the Type 1 Diabetes Pathfinder Award, which is supported by the Special Statutory Funding Program for Type 1 Diabetes Research and provides funding for new investigators pursuing innovative research on type 1 diabetes. With the Pathfinder Award, Dr. Wagner is pioneering the use of small molecules to affect the biology of type 1 diabetes. This profile describes Dr. Wagner's research and the impact of the Pathfinder Award on her career in type 1 diabetes research.

With a fiery enthusiasm for chemical biology and a burning spirit of discovery, Dr. Wagner is using the "spark of a grant," as she refers to the Type 1 Diabetes Pathfinder Award, "to ignite a career path towards type 1 diabetes research."

Finding Small Molecules To Affect Biological Processes

In line with the goals of the Pathfinder Award, Dr. Wagner is developing highly innovative new approaches to address problems in type 1 diabetes. "We are trying to bring small-molecule science to beta cell biology," Dr. Wagner says in explaining her overall goal of using small molecules to preserve the function of beta cells—the insulin-producing cells of the pancreas—during the course of development of type 1 diabetes.

Small molecules are, as their name implies, small—usually a few hundred or even a thousand times smaller in terms of mass than a typical protein molecule that carries out a biological function in a cell. Despite their diminutive size, small molecules are extremely important for studying and affecting the function of genes, cells, and biological pathways. Small molecules have proven valuable for treating diseases, and they often can be administered orally and can be less costly to produce than protein-based therapies. A key challenge, however, is to identify small molecules that can modulate a given biological process or disease state. To do this, researchers like Dr. Wagner are developing high-throughput screening approaches that can systematically test, or screen, tens or hundreds of thousands of small molecules to find one or a few compounds that produce the desired effect.

Novel Application to Beta Cell Biology

While there has been a lot of effort to understand type 1 diabetes using traditional aspects of basic biology, immunology, and animal models, Dr. Wagner points out that "there haven't been many efforts to systematically perturb beta cell biology with small molecules." Under the Pathfinder Award, Dr. Wagner is applying her expertise in chemical biology and high-throughput screening to find small molecules that affect beta cell function.

In one project, her team is screening libraries of small molecules to identify compounds that preserve beta cell viability. In type 1 diabetes, beta cells are attacked and destroyed by the immune system. Dr. Wagner and her research team can mimic this process in the lab by growing beta cells from rodents in culture and treating them with inflammatory molecules. "If you treat the cells with particular inflammatory molecules, you can induce them to start to die in a programmed way. We use this as a mimic of what goes on during type 1 diabetes when beta cells are attacked by the immune system," says Dr. Wagner. Her team converted this simple assay to a high-throughput format, and, she explains, "We are looking for compounds that in the presence of the inflammatory molecules can allow beta cells to survive."

Using this system, Dr. Wagner has screened some 400,000 compounds available through the Broad Institute and the NIH Molecular Libraries Program. In preliminary studies, Dr. Wagner already has found a few promising compounds. "These compounds are very good at preserving beta cell viability not only in our primary screen, but they also improve various aspects of beta cell function," Dr. Wagner exclaims.

Pushing Forward Promising Compounds

But the problem does not end at just finding compounds that seem to affect the cells. "We are pursuing these compounds very eagerly now to figure out what they do in cells," says Dr. Wagner. "This is one of the key challenges in screening. The challenge is always figuring out, now what? What do they do, how are they accomplishing what you are detecting in cells?" Answering these questions can provide fundamental insights to the cellular processes that lead to the development of type 1 diabetes.

With many of the cellular processes that lead to type 1 diabetes still unknown, Dr. Wagner is excited to think about the answers her research might uncover. "This is one of the things I like best about a screening project—that we don't know ahead of time what's going to happen," she says. "The Pathfinder Award program is unique in that it has really allowed me to do experiments towards discovery—it's hypothesis-generating as opposed to hypothesis-driven science." While recognizing the inherent risks of this approach, Dr. Wagner feels her research will pay off with discoveries that lead to the development of clinically relevant compounds and fundamental understanding of disease processes in type 1 diabetes.

"This is very mission-oriented research," Dr. Wagner says. "We are trying to find compounds that we can really push forward as leads." While she acknowledges the challenges in going from finding "something that is interesting in a mouse to something that can be given to a human," Dr. Wagner's goal is to move promising compounds forward to eventual clinical trials. "That is definitely something that would just be terrific to get to that point," she says.

A Career in Type 1 Diabetes Research

Dr. Wagner brings to type 1 diabetes research more than a decade of success in developing and applying high-throughput screening to address problems in biology. Although some of her earlier work focused on aspects of muscle biology, Dr. Wagner points out that "it was still in the spirit of metabolic disease" as she was trying to understand "how small molecules can be brought to bear on metabolic processes."

With her experience in chemical screening and the recent expansion of type 1 diabetes research in the Chemical Biology Program at the Broad Institute, the timing was perfect for Dr. Wagner to pursue the Pathfinder Award. "I had enough of a background in small-molecule science," she recalls, "and I was starting to get more of a background in beta cell biology to have some interesting ideas towards perturbing beta cells with compounds."

The Pathfinder Award allows Dr. Wagner to pursue these ideas with a "new level of independence," she says. "I have been able to build a small team of researchers towards my overall goal. That really helps the research progress at a much faster rate."

This progress is already being realized. Having identified some promising compounds that affect beta cell biology in preliminary screens, Dr. Wagner is making discoveries that are spurring new ideas for future directions. As her research supported by the Pathfinder Award continues to move forward, Dr. Wagner is optimistic about the opportunities that lie ahead. With the data and interesting leads her current work is generating, Dr. Wagner believes that her Pathfinder Award—her spark of a grant—is setting a foundation for her to build upon with ongoing research to impact type 1 diabetes.

EMERGING RESEARCH OPPORTUNITIES RESULTING FROM THE *SPECIAL DIABETES PROGRAM*

The *Special Statutory Funding Program for Type 1 Diabetes Research* has fueled the emergence of a wide range of research opportunities. These opportunities were identified in a strategic planning process as being critically important for overcoming current barriers and achieving progress in diabetes research. Key questions and research opportunities relevant to type 1 diabetes, including those related to new and emerging technologies and attracting new research talent, are outlined in Appendix F.

APPENDIX A

ALLOCATION OF THE *SPECIAL STATUTORY FUNDING PROGRAM FOR TYPE 1 DIABETES RESEARCH*

T he complete budget allocation of the *Special Statutory Funding Program for Type 1 Diabetes Research (Special Diabetes Program or Program)* from Fiscal Year (FY) 1998-2009 is provided in this Appendix. It is important to note that the six overarching Goals of type 1 diabetes research are interdependent. For example, "Attracting New Talent and Applying New Technologies" (Goal VI) is important for every area of type 1 diabetes research and thus relevant to all Goals. Furthermore, the scientific aims of many of the initiatives coincide with multiple Goals. However, to facilitate management of this *Program*, most initiatives have been assigned to a single, specific Goal.

BUDGET OF THE SPECIAL DIABETES PROGRAM

The expenditure of funds from the *Special Statutory Funding Program for Type 1 Diabetes Research* is detailed in Table A1. Budget figures for FY 1998 through 2009 represent actual spending levels. Some of the projects received additional support from non-governmental sources and/or from funds provided to

NIH or CDC through the regular appropriations process or from the American Recovery and Reinvestment Act of 2009. Scientific descriptions of each funded initiative are located in this Appendix, Appendix C, and the 2007 *"Evaluation Report"* on the *Special Diabetes Program* (www.T1Diabetes.nih.gov/evaluation).

Table A1: Detailed Budget by Goal of the Special Statutory Funding Program for Type 1 Diabetes Research

GOAL I: IDENTIFY THE GENETIC AND ENVIRONMENTAL CAUSES OF TYPE 1 DIABETES

	1998	1999	2000	2001	2002	2003	2004	2005	2006	2007	2008	2009
Type 1 Diabetes Genetics Consortium (T1DGC) (NIDDK, NIAID, NHGRI, JDRF, Diabetes UK)	0	0	0	1,536,000	5,047,330	8,958,898	13,000,000	17,541,724	13,444,975	5,031,275	244,320	0
Repository Services for T1DGC (NIDDK)	0	0	0	0	0	0	0	1,000,000	4,500,000	500,999	0	1,000,000
Fine Mapping and Function of Genes for Type 1 Diabetes (DP3) (RFA DK08-006) (NIDDK)*	0	0	0	0	0	0	0	0	0	0	0	23,261,208
13th International Histocompatibility Working Group (NIAID, NIDDK, NCI, NHGRI, JDRF)	0	0	0	3,000,000	1,000,000	0	0	0	0	0	0	0
SEARCH for Diabetes in Youth (SEARCH) (CDC, NIDDK)	0	0	0	4,200,000	3,000,000	3,000,000	4,000,000	2,000,000	2,262,000	2,262,000	2,188,843	3,024,000
The Environmental Determinants of Diabetes in the Young (TEDDY) (RFA DK02-029; RFA DK07-500) (NIDDK, NIAID, NICHD, NIEHS, CDC, JDRF, ADA)	0	0	0	0	5,000,000	7,568,300	17,500,000	24,542,679	17,500,000	50,913,817	15,745,948	27,326,779
Repository Services for TEDDY (NIDDK)	0	0	0	0	0	0	0	0	0	0	3,000,000	4,000,000
Type 1 Diabetes Mouse Resource (NIDDK)b	0	0	0	4,000,000	0	0	0	0	0	4,478,006	0	1,150,000
Bioinformatics Integration Support Contract (RFP AI-DAIT02-16) (NIAID)	0	0	0	0	1,000,000	0	0	0	0	0	0	0
Mammalian Gene Collection (NCI, NIDDK)	0	0	0	500,000	0	0	0	0	0	0	0	0
Sequence the NOD Mouse for Immune System Genes for Type 1 Diabetes (NIAID)	0	0	0	4,500,000	0	0	0	0	0	0	0	0
Biotechnology Resource Centers (RFA DK00-002) (NIDDK)	0	0	454,575	693,750	502,250	0	0	0	0	0	0	0
Functional Genomics of the Developing Endocrine Pancreas (RFA DK99-007) (NIDDK)	0	1,500,000	3,241,602	3,081,250	609,652	0	0	0	0	0	0	0
Public Health Pilot Programs in Newborn Screening (CDC)	246,718	301,544	548,261	804,826	0	0	0	0	0	0	0	0
Proficiency Testing for Laboratory Assays of Dried Blood Spots (CDC)	0	0	0	0	0	190,256	0	0	0	0	0	0
High-Throughput, High-Sensitivity Methods for Measuring Markers of Type 1 Diabetes (CDC)	246,718	268,648	219,305	219,305	219,305	0	0	0	0	0	0	0
Cadaveric Pancreata of Autoantibody Positive Individuals (NIDDK)	0	0	0	0	0	0	308,000	0	0	0	0	0
Total - Goal I:	493,436	2,070,192	4,463,743	22,535,131	16,378,537	19,717,454	34,808,000	45,084,403	37,706,975	63,186,097	21,179,111	59,761,987

GOAL II: PREVENT OR REVERSE TYPE 1 DIABETES

	1998	1999	2000	2001	2002	2003	2004	2005	2006	2007	2008	2009
Type 1 Diabetes TrialNet (RFA DK01-004; RFA DK08-011) (NIDDK, NIAID, NICHD, NCCAM, JDRF, ADA) and Immune Tolerance Network (RFP-AI-99-30) (NIAID, NIDDK, JDRF)	0	0	0	17,320,000	15,489,174	12,920,894	11,242,933	7,350,382	0	15,423,706	50,615,272	28,501,983
Repository Services: Diabetes Prevention Trial for Type 1 Diabetes (DPT-1) and Type 1 Diabetes TrialNet (NIDDK)	0	0	0	0	0	0	0	0	0	0	0	1,415,641
Recruitment for Clinical Research Studies (Matthews Media)	0	0	0	0	0	0	943,215	716,010	747,920	781,310	816,249	0
Type 1 Diabetes-Rapid Access to Intervention Development (T1D-RAID): Prevention Projects (NIDDK, NCI)	0	0	0	0	0	0	105,000	1,575,503	4,908,798	1,555,145	1,506,152	1,453,143
Type 1 Diabetes-Preclinical Testing Program: Preclinical Study of Efficacy in Animal Models of Type 1 Diabetes (RFP 05-05) (NIDDK)	0	0	0	0	0	0	0	0	2,000,000	0	767,501	1,047,335
Cooperative Study Group for Autoimmune Disease Prevention (RFA AI00-016; RFA AI05-026) (NIAID, NICHD, NIDDK, ORWH, JDRF)	0	0	0	2,154,000	2,318,796	2,336,681	2,354,595	2,392,355	2,521,427	2,936,864	2,888,196	1,802,740
Trial to Reduce IDDM in the Genetically-At-Risk (TRIGR) (NICHD, CIHR, EFSD, EU, JDRF, Mead Johnson, NDF)	0	0	0	2,000,000	500,000	500,000	3,000,000	1,799,998	2,200,000c	2,942,000	2,883,160	2,798,000
Diabetes Autoantibody Standardization Program (DASP) (CDC, IDS)	816,680	746,014	438,609	778,609	755,199	1,158,101	675,000	566,000	675,000	675,000	675,000	675,000
C-Peptide Standardization (CDC, NIDDK)	0	0	0	0	0	57,225	64,301	34,854	37,255	37,698	76,155	62,116
Data and Biosample Repository (RFP DK02-04) (NIDDK)	0	0	0	0	0	3,000,000	0	0	0	0	0	0
Gene Therapy Approaches for Diabetes and its Complications (RFA DK01-006) (NIDDK, NHLBI, NIAID)	0	0	0	993,000	1,112,600	0	0	0	0	0	0	0
Biomarkers of Autoimmunity in Type 1 Diabetes (R21) (RFA DK06-002) (NIDDK, NIAID, NICHD)	0	0	0	0	0	0	0	0	2,000,398	1,712,411	0	0
Innovative Grants on Immune Tolerance (RFA AI00-006) (NIAID, NIDDK)	0	0	0	2,443,000	1,658,523	1,658,523	982,665	741,765	0	0	0	0
Pilot Studies for New Therapies for Type 1 Diabetes and its Complications (RFA DK99-013) (NIDDK, NIAID)	0	1,146,742	1,170,524	0	0	0	0	0	0	0	0	0
Immunopathogenesis of Type 1 Diabetes (RFA DK98-010) (NIDDK, NIAID, NICHD)	4,086,215	4,124,050	3,806,447	0	0	0	0	0	0	0	0	0
Autoantibodies in Type 1 Diabetes (NIDCR)	0	100,000	200,344	200,000	100,000	0	0	0	0	0	0	0
DPT-1 Supplements (NIDDK, NIAID, NICHD, NCRR)	3,350,000	95,000	0	0	0	0	0	0	0	0	0	0
One Year Supplements to Ongoing Projects (NIDDK, NIAID, NCRR)	994,340	0	0	0	0	0	0	0	0	0	0	0
Total - Goal II:	9,247,235	6,211,806	5,615,924	25,888,609	21,934,292	21,631,424	19,367,709	15,176,867	15,090,798	26,064,134	60,227,685	37,755,958

GOAL III: DEVELOP CELL REPLACEMENT THERAPY

Program	1998	1999	2000	2001	2002	2003	2004	2005	2006	2007	2008	2009
Beta Cell Biology Consortium (RFA DK01-014; RFA DK04-018) (NIDDK)	0	0	0	7,250,000	7,589,779	6,790,240	6,126,956	8,891,656	16,614,540	11,870,578	2,377,157	12,981,013
Clinical Islet Transplantation Consortium (RFA DK04-005; RFA DK04-004) (NIDDK, NIAID)	0	0	0	0	0	0	24,569,188	14,977,134	15,480,664	5,503,579	6,474,452	9,878,298
Toward Imaging the Pancreatic Beta Cell in People (R01) (RFA DK06-003) (NIDDK, NIA, NIAID, NIBIB)	0	0	0	0	0	0	0	0	1,575,115	1,734,810	1,887,475	0
Beta Cell Regeneration for Diabetes Therapy (RFA DK05-007) (NIDDK)	0	0	0	0	0	0	0	0	777,245	743,070	0	0
Comprehensive Programs in Beta Cell Biology (RFA DK02-014) (NIDDK)	0	0	0	0	3,154,850	3,055,850	2,393,922	1,942,751	802,420	0	0	0
Non-Human Primate Transplantation Tolerance Cooperative Study Group (RFA AI01-006; RFA AI06-018) (NIAID, NIDDK)	0	0	0	518,000	1,822,876	1,772,003	4,979,323	4,156,398	4,036,852	3,508,815	4,602,277	4,999,786
Immune Tolerance Network - Islet Transplantation (RFP AI99-30) (NIAID, NIDDK, JDRF)	0	0	0	3,500,000	0	0	1,417,000	0	0	0	0	0
Immunobiology of Xenotransplantation Cooperative Research Program (RFA AI04-042) (NIAID, NIDDK)	0	0	0	0	0	0	0	1,929,129	1,909,234	1,594,071	1,467,868	0
NIDDK Intramural Program (NIDDK)	0	492,458	0	1,370,000	0	0	0	0	0	0	0	0
Islet Cell Resource Centers (RFA RR01-002) (NCRR, NIDDK)	0	0	0	5,000,000	1,999,998	5,000,000	5,000,000	5,000,000	5,000,000	4,854,996	4,757,896	0
Islet Cell Distribution Coordinating Center (NIH-NIDDK-08-099-SB) (NIDDK)	0	0	0	0	0	0	0	0	0	0	0	6,000,000
Collaborative Islet Transplant Registry (CITR) (RFP DK00-002) (NIDDK)	0	0	0	3,964,000	0	0	0	336,988	5,179,085	0	0	0
Pilot and Feasibility Program in Human Islet Biology (RFA DK03-021) (NIDDK)	0	0	0	0	0	0	2,010,158	3,830,341	1,764,903	0	0	0
Islet Encapsulation Research (NIDDK)	0	0	0	0	894,471	0	0	0	0	0	0	0
Gene Transfer Approaches to Enhance Islet Transplantation (RFA DK02-020) (NIDDK, NIAID)	0	0	0	0	1,744,423	1,727,771	0	0	0	0	0	0
Imaging Pancreatic Beta Cell Mass, Function, Engraftment, or Inflammation (RFA DK02-002) (NIDDK)	0	0	0	0	1,258,302	1,356,106	651,723	651,723	0	0	0	0
New Strategies for Treatment of Type 1 Diabetes (RFA DK00-001) (NIDDK)	0	0	1,135,749	1,107,681	882,200	0	0	0	0	0	0	0
Pilot Studies for New Therapies for Type 1 Diabetes and its Complications (RFA DK99-013) (NIDDK)	0	779,293	783,039	0	0	0	0	0	0	0	0	0
Cellular and Molecular Approaches to Achieving Euglycemia (RFA DK98-007) (NIDDK, NIAID, NICHD)	4,883,944	4,921,491	3,962,434	0	0	0	0	0	0	0	0	0
Beta Cell Proteomics (NIDDK, NHGRI)	0	0	0	2,495,000	0	0	0	0	0	0	0	0
Glucagon-like Peptide as a Differentiation Factor for Pancreatic Beta Cells (NIA)	94,379	99,995	0	0	0	0	0	0	60,000	0	0	0
Imaging Supplement to Diabetes Center (NIDDK, NIAID, NICHD)	0	0	0	0	0	0	0	0	0	0	0	0
One Year Supplements to Ongoing Projects (NIDDK, NIAID, NICHD)	1,401,654	0	0	0	0	0	0	0	0	0	0	0
Total - Goal III:	6,379,977	6,293,237	5,881,222	25,204,681	19,346,899	19,701,970	47,148,270	41,716,120	53,200,058	29,809,919	21,567,125	33,859,097

GOAL IV: PREVENT OR REDUCE HYPOGLYCEMIA IN TYPE 1 DIABETES

	1998	1999	2000	2001	2002	2003	2004	2005	2006	2007	2008	2009
Diabetes Research in Children Network (DirecNet) (RFA HD01-009; RFA HD06-020) (NICHD, NIDDK, NINDS)	0	0	0	2,000,000	3,148,071	1,886,158	2,500,000	2,499,994	1,401,789	2,023,663	1,983,191	2,000,001
Closed Loop Technologies: Clinical and Behavioral Approaches to Improve Type 1 Diabetes Outcomes (R01) (RFA DK08-012) (NIDDK, NICHD)	0	0	0	0	0	0	0	0	0	0	0	5,268,637
Closed Loop Technologies: Pilot and Exploratory Clinical and Behavioral Approaches to Improve Type 1 Diabetes Outcomes (R21) (RFA DK08-013) (NIDDK, NICHD)	0	0	0	0	0	0	0	0	0	0	0	192,500
Standardization Program To Improve the Measurement of Blood Glucose (CDC)	0	148,284	188,931	231,526	101,319	209,282	0	0	0	0	0	0
Hypoglycemia in Patients with Type 1 Diabetes (RFA DK03-017) (NIDDK, NINDS)	0	0	0	0	0	0	2,475,590	2,532,821	2,330,253	2,277,821	1,862,538	0
Effects of Hypoglycemia on Neuronal and Glial Cell Function (RFA NS02-008) (NINDS, NIDDK, JDRF)	0	0	0	0	1,454,310	1,438,495	646,480	645,090	0	0	0	0
Sensor Development and Validation (RFA EB02-002) (NIBIB, NIDDK)	0	0	0	0	2,091,949	2,073,237	1,405,465	641,154	0	0	0	0
Understanding Hypoglycemia Unawareness in Patients with Diabetes (RFA DK01-031) (NIDDK, NINDS, JDRF)	0	0	0	0	2,055,648	2,036,527	1,362,001	1,361,842	693,195	0	0	0
Pilot Studies for New Therapies for Type 1 Diabetes and its Complications (RFA DK99-013) (NIDDK)	0	141,408	130,216	0	0	0	0	0	0	0	0	0
Glucose Sensors in the Treatment of Diabetes (RFA DK98-008) (NIDDK, NCRR)	3,298,740	3,239,772	2,117,998	0	0	0	0	0	0	0	0	0
Developing New Tools for Detecting and Monitoring Low Blood Glucose (CDC)	0	142,548	142,548	142,548	142,548	0	0	0	0	0	0	0
Development of Surrogate Markers for Clinical Trials: Supplements (NIMH, NIDDK)	0	0	0	300,000	0	0	0	0	0	0	0	0
One Year Supplements to Ongoing Projects (NIDDK, NCRR)	172,000	0	0	0	0	0	0	0	0	0	0	0
Total - Goal IV:	3,470,740	3,672,012	2,579,693	2,674,074	8,993,845	7,643,699	8,389,536	7,680,901	4,425,237	4,301,484	3,845,729	7,461,138

GOAL V: PREVENT OR REDUCE THE COMPLICATIONS OF TYPE 1 DIABETES

	1998	1999	2000	2001	2002	2003	2004	2005	2006	2007	2008	2009
Genetics of Kidneys in Diabetes (GoKinD) Study (CDC, JDRF)	921,792	872,114	974,809	1,315,827	1,315,827	1,247,536	1,500,000	1,019,150	675,000	0	0	0
GoKinD: Repository Services	0	0	0	0	0	0	0	0	1,000,000	0	1,000,000	0
GoKinD: Genotyping Services	0	0	0	0	0	0	0	0	0	968,184	0	0
Epidemiology of Diabetes Interventions and Complications (EDIC): Genetics Study and Measurement of Cardiovascular Disease, Uropathy and Autonomic Neuropathy	1,000,000	0	0	7,000,000	3,807,082	290,000	0	2,021,077	5,637,353	0	0	0
EDIC: Repository Services	0	0	0	0	0	0	0	0	1,250,000	0	0	0
Type 1 Diabetes-Rapid Access to Intervention Development (T1D-RAID): Complications Projects (NIDDK, NCI)	0	0	0	0	0	0	75,000	344,728	527,972	0	0	0
Type 1 Diabetes-Preclinical Testing Program: Preclinical Study of Efficacy in Animal Models of Diabetes Complications (RFP 05-04) (NIDDK)	0	0	0	0	0	0	0	0	1,031,117	1,015,854	1,038,629	1,065,875
Family Investigation of Nephropathy and Diabetes (FIND) (NIDDK, NEI, NCMHD)	0	0	0	500,000	500,000	500,000	500,000	500,000	488,250	0	0	0
Diabetic Retinopathy Clinical Research Network (DRCR.net) (RFA EY01-001) (NEI)	0	0	0	0	2,000,000	2,000,000	2,000,000	1,000,000	1,000,000	1,000,000	1,000,000	1,000,000
Animal Models of Diabetic Complications Consortium (RFA DK01-009; RFA HL01-010; RFA DK 05-011; RFA DK05-012) (NIDDK, NHLBI, NINDS)[a]	0	0	0	3,982,000	4,135,862	4,055,585	4,252,287	4,296,778	3,689,907	3,136,299	3,136,256	3,203,807
High-Density Genotyping of Diabetes and Diabetic Complications Sample Collections (R01) (RFA DK06-005) (NIDDK, NHLBI, NIAID)	0	0	0	0	0	0	0	0	1,903,002	2,101,633	1,898,360	0
Genetics of Diabetes Complications–Genotyping (NIDDK)	0	0	0	0	0	0	0	0	2,996,821	0	0	0
Biomarker Development for Diabetic Complications (R21) (RFA DK06-004) (NIDDK, NHLBI, NEI)	0	0	0	0	0	0	0	0	0	1,689,153	1,530,798	260,680
Improving the Clinical Measurement of HbA1c (CDC)	768,092	520,848	487,537	466,649	384,903	534,825	600,000	600,000	750,000	750,000	600,000	600,000
Collaborative Studies on Angiogenesis and Diabetic Complications (RFA DK04-022) (NIDDK, NINDS, NHLBI, NEI)	0	0	0	0	0	0	0	1,736,225	1,673,307	1,337,602	1,310,868	0
Progression of Cardiovascular Disease in Type 1 Diabetes (RFA HL04-013) (NHLBI, NIDDK)	0	0	0	0	0	0	3,258,309	3,470,479	3,253,541	2,984,407	0	0
Feasibility Projects To Test Strategies for Preventing or Slowing the Progression of Diabetic Nephropathy (RFA DK02-025) (NIDDK)	0	0	0	0	1,325,273	1,190,190	0	0	0	0	0	0

GOAL V: PREVENT OR REDUCE THE COMPLICATIONS OF TYPE 1 DIABETES (cont'd)

	1998	1999	2000	2001	2002	2003	2004	2005	2006	2007	2008	2009
Surrogate Markers for Diabetic Microvascular Complications (RFA DK02-016) (NIDDK, NEI, NINDS)	0	0	0	0	3,427,339	3,468,856	2,731,380	2,031,157	0	0	0	0
Imaging Early Markers of Diabetic Microvascular Complications in Peripheral Tissue (RFA DK02-001) (NIDDK)	0	0	0	0	1,282,371	1,288,444	729,250	729,250	0	0	0	0
Oral Microbiology/Immunology of Type 1 Diabetes (RFA DE01-001) (NIDCR)	0	0	0	645,000	500,000	0	0	0	0	0	0	0
Neurobiology of Diabetic Complications (RFA NS00-002) (NINDS, NIDDK, JDRF)	0	0	907,406	895,971	610,916	442,485	712,852	0	0	0	0	0
Pilot Studies for New Therapies for Type 1 Diabetes and its Complications (RFA DK99-013) (NIDDK, NHLBI, NEI)	0	1,174,221	1,159,255	0	0	0	0	0	0	0	0	0
Neurological Complications of Diabetes (RFA NS99-005) (NINDS, NIDDK)	0	2,243,319	2,193,073	2,007,389	1,603,619	0	0	0	0	0	0	0
Pathogenesis and Therapy of Complications of Diabetes (RFA DK98-009) (NIDDK, NEI, NHLBI, NICHD, NINDS)	6,713,260	6,914,914	5,622,671	440,431	452,086	0	0	0	0	0	0	0
Development of Clinical Markers for Kidney Disease (NIDDK)	0	0	0	834,000	0	0	0	0	0	0	0	0
Advanced Glycation Endproducts (CDC)	0	0	0	280,710	57,567	0	0	0	0	0	0	0
Development of Surrogate Markers for Clinical Trials: Supplement (NIEHS, NIDDK)	0	0	0	318,000	0	0	0	0	0	0	0	0
Administrative Supplements for a Drug Screening Program for Diabetic Complications (NIDDK, NHLBI, NCI, NEI, NINDS)	0	0	0	0	0	0	0	0	1,072,536	339,299	0	0
Functional Genomics Approaches to Diabetic Complications - IHWG SNPs (NHGRI, NIDDK)	0	0	0	750,000	0	0	0	0	0	0	0	0
One Year Supplements to Ongoing Projects (NIDDK, NEI, NIDCR, NICHD, NHLBI)	936,150	0	0	0	0	0	0	0	0	0	0	0
Total - Goal V:	10,339,294	11,725,416	11,344,751	19,435,977	21,402,845	15,017,921	16,359,078	17,748,844	26,948,806	15,322,431	11,514,911	6,130,362

GOAL VI: ATTRACT NEW TALENT AND APPLY NEW TECHNOLOGIES TO RESEARCH ON TYPE 1 DIABETES

	1998	1999	2000	2001	2002	2003	2004	2005	2006	2007	2008	2009
Training Programs in Diabetes Research for Pediatric Endocrinologists (RFA DK02-024) (NIDDK, JDRF, ADA)	0	0	0	0	2,571,342	3,472,772	3,274,907	3,169,415	1,352,032	1,283,294	0	0
Innovative Partnerships in Type 1 Diabetes (RFA DK02-023) (NIDDK, NEI, NIAID)	0	0	0	0	5,778,702	5,620,843	4,337,638	4,258,939	0	0	0	0
Bench to Bedside Research on Type 1 Diabetes and its Complications (RFA DK02-022) (NIDDK, NIAID)	0	0	0	0	3,443,507	3,587,082	392,500	1,236,677	1,274,733	342,611	0	0
Bench to Bedside Research on Type 1 Diabetes and its Complications (RFA DK03-001) (NIDDK, NIAID, NEI, NHLBI)	0	0	0	0	0	3,449,975	3,415,870	1,629,440	956,405	1,008,408	0	0
Bench to Bedside Research on Type 1 Diabetes and its Complications (RFA DK03-019) (NIDDK, NIAID, NEI, NHLBI, NINDS, ODS)	0	0	0	0	0	0	4,376,639	4,184,253	1,650,918	1,396,776	1,011,645	0
Innovative Patient Outreach Programs and Ocular Screening Technologies to Improve Detection of Diabetic Retinopathy (SBIR [R43/R44]) (RFA EY09-001) (NEI)	0	0	0	0	0	0	0	0	0	0	0	1,796,756
Proteomics and Metabolomics in Type 1 Diabetes and its Complications (RFA DK03-024) (NIDDK, NIAID, NEI, NHLBI, NINDS, NICHD)	0	0	0	0	0	0	3,789,400	3,410,294	1,790,149	2,413,532	2,399,609	0
Small Business Innovation Research (SBIR) and Small Business Technology Transfer (STTR) RFA in Type 1 Diabetes and its Complications (RFA DK03-020) (NIDDK, NEI, NIAID, NHLBI, NINDS, NICHD, NINR) and SBIR: Measurement Tools for Altered Autonomic Function in Spinal Cord Injury and Diabetes (RFA HD04-018) (NICHD, NIDDK)	0	0	0	0	0	0	4,202,727	4,167,000	3,167,335	1,795,594	1,870,487	0
STTR to Develop New Therapeutics and Monitoring Technologies for Type 1 Diabetes and its Complications (STTR [R41/R42]) (RFA DK05-015) (NIDDK, NEI, NHLBI, NIAID, NICHD, NINDS)	0	0	0	0	0	0	0	0	552,665	447,000	447,000	447,000
SBIR to Develop New Therapeutics and Monitoring Technologies for Type 1 Diabetes and its Complications (SBIR [R43/R44]) (RFA DK05-016) (NIDDK, NEI, NHLBI, NIAID, NICHD, NINDS)	0	0	0	0	0	0	0	0	446,985	1,924,336	1,849,513	0
SBIR to Develop New Therapeutics and Monitoring Technologies for Type 1 Diabetes (T1D) Towards an Artificial Pancreas [R43/R44]) (RFA DK09-001) (NIDDK, NIBIB, NICHD)	0	0	0	0	0	0	0	0	0	0	0	1,923,244
Type 1 Diabetes Pathfinder (DP2) (RFA DK08-001) (NIDDK)*	0	0	0	0	0	0	0	0	0	0	23,499,500	0
Type 1 Diabetes Pilot and Feasibility Awards (awarded through Diabetes Centers)	0	0	0	0	0	0	0	0	634,000	0	0	0
Phased Innovation Partnerships (NIDDK)	0	0	0	4,049,000	0	0	0	0	0	0	0	0
Total - Goal VI:†	0	0	0	4,049,000	11,793,551	16,130,672	23,789,681	22,056,018	11,825,222	10,611,551	31,077,754	4,167,000
Conferences and Other Expenses	69,318	27,337	114,667	212,528	150,031	156,860	137,726	536,847	802,904	704,384	587,685	864,458
TOTAL	30,000,000	30,000,000	30,000,000	100,000,000	100,000,000	100,000,000	150,000,000	150,000,000	150,000,000	150,000,000	150,000,000	150,000,000

Footnotes for Table A1:

a   FY 2009 funds provide funding for FY 2009-2013.
b   A portion of the budget from FY 2007-2009 has supported AMDCC activities.
c   In addition to the $2.2 million shown in the table, an additional $1 million was subcontracted from TrialNet to TRIGR in FY 2006.
d   The total yearly budget for the AMDCC for FY 2006-2009 is $4.38 million, which includes funding that was awarded to the Type 1 Diabetes Mouse Resource (see Goal I) and used for AMDCC activities.
e   FY 2008 funds provide funding for FY 2008-2012.
f   In addition to solicitations focused exclusively on attracting new talent to type 1 diabetes research, Goal VI was addressed by solicitations for research projects that encouraged the participation of new investigators and the submission of applications for pilot and feasibility awards, as well as the development of new technology in the context of Goals I-V. These early efforts relative to Goal VI are thus embedded in other Goals during the FY 1998-2000 period of the *Program*. Starting in FY 2001, specific initiatives were also launched relative to Goal VI.

EXTRAMURAL RESEARCH GRANTS

Extramural NIH grants, cooperative agreements, contracts, and supplements, which were awarded through the *Special Statutory Funding Program for Type 1 Diabetes Research* between FY 1998-2009, are listed in Table A2. Some initiatives supported additional awards with regularly appropriated funds; some awards were supported by both the *Special Diabetes Program* and regularly appropriated funds. Abstracts describing research topics pursued through these grants are available through the NIH Research Portfolio Online Reporting Tools Expenditures and Results (RePORTER) Web site (http://projectreporter.nih.gov/reporter.cfm). Bibliometric analysis of publications resulting from these awards as of January 1, 2010, is found in Appendix B.

TABLE A2: Research Grants and Contracts Awarded with *Special Diabetes Program* Funds

	Year*	Project No.	Project Title
GOAL I: IDENTIFY THE GENETIC AND ENVIRONMENTAL CAUSES OF TYPE 1 DIABETES			
Type 1 Diabetes Genetics Consortium (T1DGC)			
Donald Bowden, Wake Forest University‡	2001	R01 DK056289	ID of Diabetes Genes on Human Chromosome 20Q12-Q13.1
Patrick Concannon, Virginia Mason Research Center	2001	R01 DK046635	Susceptibility Genes in Type 1 Diabetes
Stephen Rich, Wake Forest University Health Sciences	2002	U01 DK062418	Type 1 Diabetes Genetics Consortium
Johns Hopkins University	2002	N01 HG065403	Center for Inherited Disease Research
Repository Services for T1DGC			
Rutgers University	2005	N01 DK032610	Repository Services for T1DGC
Fine Mapping and Function of Genes for Type 1 Diabetes (DP3) (RFA DK08-006)			
Zhibin Chen, University of Miami School of Medicine	2009	DP3 DK085696	The Quantitative Biology of CTLA4 Splice Variants in T1D
Patrick Concannon, University of Virginia, Charlottesville	2009	DP3 DK085678	Expression and Proteomic Characterization of Risk Loci in Type 1 Diabetes
Hakon Hakonarson, Children's Hospital (Philadelphia)	2009	DP3 DK085708	Fine Mapping and Functional Evaluation of Selected Type 1 Diabetes Loci
Art Petronis, Centre for Addiction and Mental Health	2009	DP3 DK085698	DNA Methylome Study in Type 1 Diabetes
Stephen Rich, University of Virginia, Charlottesville	2009	DP3 DK085695	The Role of Copy Number Variants (CNV) in Type 1 Diabetes
13th International Histocompatibility Working Group			
John Hansen, Fred Hutchinson Cancer Research Center	2001	U24 AI049213	13th International Histocompatibility Working Group
The Environmental Determinants of Diabetes in the Young (TEDDY) (RFA DK02-029)			
William Hagopian, Pacific Northwest Research Institute	2003	U01 DK063829	Diabetes Evaluation in Washington (DEW-IT) Clinical Center
Jeffrey Krischer, Moffitt Cancer Center and Research Institute	2002	U01 DK063790	Data Coordinating Center
Ake Lernmark, University of Washington	2003	U01 DK063861	Diabetes Prediction in Skane (DiPiS)
Marian Rewers, University of Colorado Health Sciences Center	2003	U01 DK063821	Environmental Causes of Type 1 Diabetes
Jin-Xiong She, Medical College of Georgia	2003	U01 DK063865	Consortium for Identification of Environmental Triggers
Olli Simell, Turku University Central Hospital	2003	U01 DK063863	Environmental Triggers of Type 1 Diabetes
Anette Ziegler, Diabetes Research Institute	2003	U01 DK063836	Type 1 Diabetes Triggers: Diet Modification in Neonates

Footnotes for Table A2:

* In most cases, the year represents the first year that the project received support from the *Special Diabetes Program*. In some cases, grants are listed more than once because the grantee successfully recompeted for continued funding. For example, if a grant was initially funded in 2001, it will be listed under the relevant funding opportunity as starting in that year. If it successfully recompeted for continued funding under a new funding opportunity (*e.g.*, RFA) in 2006, the same grant number will again be listed under that funding opportunity, with 2006 listed as the start date of the new funding period.

‡ Institutional affiliations at the time of the grant award are listed. Some Principal Investigators (PIs) have moved to new institutions.

	Year	Project No.	Project Title
Limited Competition: The Environmental Determinants of Diabetes in the Young (TEDDY) Study (U01) (RFA DK07-500)			
William Hagopian, Pacific Northwest Research Institute	2008	U01 DK063829	The Environmental Determinants of Diabetes in Youth: Washington Clinical Center
Ake Lernmark, University of Washington	2008	U01 DK063861	The Environmental Triggers of Diabetes (TEDDY) in Sweden
Marian Rewers, University of Colorado Health Sciences Center	2008	U01 DK063821	The TEDDY Study - Colorado Clinical Center
Jin-Xiong She, Medical College of Georgia	2008	U01 DK063865	The TEDDY study: Georgia/Florida clinical center
Olli Simell, Turku University Central Hospital	2008	U01 DK063863	The Environmental Determinants of Diabetes in Young (TEDDY)
Anette Ziegler, Diabetes Research Institute	2008	U01 DK063836	The Environmental Determinants of Diabetes in the Young (TEDDY) Consortium
The Environmental Determinants of Diabetes in the Young (RFP NIH-NIDDK-07-01)			
University of South Florida	2007	HHSN267200700014C	The Environmental Determinants of Diabetes in the Young
Repository Services for TEDDY			
Fisher Scientific	2008	HHSN267200800015C	Repository Services for TEDDY
Uniform Population-based Approach to Case Ascertainment, Typology, Surveillance and Research on Childhood Diabetes: SEARCH for Diabetes in Youth Study (PA 00097)			
Lawrence Dolan, Children's Hospital Medical Center, Cincinnati	2001	U48 CCU919219	Search for Diabetes in Youth
Richard Hamman, University of Colorado Health Sciences Center	2001	U48 CCU81924	Search for Diabetes in Youth
Elizabeth Mayer-Davis, University of South Carolina	2001	U48 CCU419249	Search for Diabetes in Youth
Diana Pettiti, Kaiser Permanente Southern California	2001	U48 CCU919219	Search for Diabetes in Youth
Catherine Pihoker, Children's Hospital and Regional Medical Center, Seattle	2001	U58 CCU019235	Search for Diabetes in Youth
Beatriz Rodriguez, Pacific Health Research Institute	2001	U58 CCU019235	Search for Diabetes in Youth
Incidence, Natural History, and Quality of Life of Diabetes in Youth (SEARCH for Diabetes in Youth Study) (RFA DP05-069)			
Ronny Bell, Wake Forest University Health Sciences	2005	U01 DP000250	SEARCH for Diabetes in Youth Coordinating Center
Dana Dabelea, University of Colorado at Denver Health Sciences Center	2005	U01 DP000247	SEARCH for Diabetes in Youth 2: Colorado Center
Lawrence Dolan, Children's Hospital Medical Center, Cincinnati	2005	U01 DP000248	SEARCH for Diabetes in Youth 2: Ohio Center
Jean Lawrence, Kaiser Permanente Southern California	2005	U01 DP000246	SEARCH for Diabetes in Youth 2: California Center
Elizabeth Mayer-Davis, University of South Carolina	2005	U01 DP000254	SEARCH for Diabetes in Youth 2: South Carolina Center
Catherine Pihoker, Children's Hospital and Regional Medical Center, Seattle	2005	U01 DP000244	SEARCH for Diabetes in Youth 2: Washington Site
Beatriz Rodriguez, Pacific Health Research Institute	2005	U01 DP000245	Search for Diabetes in Youth 2: Hawaii Center
Type 1 Diabetes Mouse Resource			
Muriel Davisson, The Jackson Laboratory	2001	P40 RR009781	Transgenic and Targeted Mutant Preservation
Cadaveric Pancreas of Autoantibody Positive Individuals—Supplement to Diabetes Center			
John Hutton, Barbara Davis Center for Childhood Diabetes	2004	P30 DK057516	UCHSC Diabetes and Endocrinology Research Center
Bioinformatics Integration Support Contract (RFP NIAID-DAIT-02-016)			
Northrop Grumman	2002	N01 AI025487	Bioinformatics Integration Support Contract
Research Triangle Institute	2002	N01 AI025486	Bioinformatics Integration Support Contract

	Year	Project No.	Project Title
Mammalian Gene Collection			
Science Applications International Corporation	2001	N01 CO012400	Mammalian Gene Collection
Sequence the NOD Mouse for Immune System Genes for Type 1 Diabetes			
University of California, San Francisco	2001	N01 AI015416	Collaborative Network for Clinical Research on Immune Tolerance
Biotechnology Resource Centers (RFA DK00-002)			
Jin-Xiong She, University of Florida	2000	U24 DK058778	NIDDK Biotechnology Center at the University of Florida
Functional Genomics of the Developing Endocrine Pancreas (RFA DK99-007)			
Klaus Kaestner, University of Pennsylvania	1999	R24 DK056947	Functional Genomics of the Developing Endocrine Pancreas
Marshall Permutt, Washington University	1999	R24 DK056954	Functional Genomics of the Developing Endocrine Pancreas

GOAL II: PREVENT OR REVERSE TYPE 1 DIABETES

	Year	Project No.	Project Title
Type 1 Diabetes TrialNet (RFA DK01-004)			
John Lachin, George Washington University	2001	U01 DK061055	Type 1 Diabetes TrialNet: Operations Coordinating Center
Jay Skyler, University of Miami	2002	U01 DK061041	Type 1 Diabetes TrialNet
Type 1 Diabetes TrialNet: Clinical Centers (RFA DK01-003)			
Dorothy Becker, Children's Hospital of Pittsburgh	2005	U01 DK061058	Prediction and Prevention of Type 1 Diabetes
Jennifer Marks, University of Miami	2005	U01 DK061037	Diabetes TrialNet
Antoinette Moran, University of Minnesota	2005	U01 DK061036	Type 1 Diabetes--A Proposal for Prevention & Intervention
Tihamer Orban, Joslin Diabetes Center	2005	U01 DK061040	Type 1 Diabetes TrialNet: Clinical Centers
Henry Rodriguez, Indiana University School of Medicine	2005	U01 DK061038	Type 1 Diabetes TrialNet Indiana University Clinical Center
Darrell Wilson, Stanford University	2005	U01 DK061042	Type 1 Diabetes TrialNet at Stanford
Type 1 Diabetes TrialNet (RFP NIH-NIDDK-07-03)			
University of South Florida	2008	HHSN267200800019C	The Type 1 Diabetes TrialNet Data Coordinating Center
Type 1 Diabetes TrialNet: Clinical Centers (U01) (RFA DK08-011)			
Dorothy Becker, Children's Hospital of Pittsburgh	2009	U01 DK061058	Prediction and Prevention of Type 1 Diabetes
Stephen Gitelman, University of California, San Francisco	2009	U01 DK061010	UCSF Trialnet: A Phase II Trial of Imatimib in New Onset Type I Diabetes
Robin Goland, Columbia University	2009	U01 DK085504	Type 1 Diabetes TrialNet: Clinical Center at Berrie Center, Columbia University
Peter Gottlieb, University of Colorado, Denver	2009	U01 DK085509	Trainet: Diabetes Type 1 Prevention
Carla Greenbaum, Benaroya Research Institute at Virginia Mason	2009	U01 DK061034	Northwest Clinical Center for Type 1 Diabetes - TrialNet
Kevan Herold, Yale University	2009	U01 DK085466	Type 1 Diabetes TrialNet: Clinical Center at Yale University (U01)
Jennifer Marks, University of Miami	2009	U01 DK085499	Type 1 Diabetes TrialNet Clinical Center: Effects of Alefacept in New Onset T1D
Antoinette Moran, University of Minnesota, Twin Cities	2009	U01 DK085476	Type 1 Diabetes-A Proposal for Prevention & Intervention
Philip Raskin, University of Texas Southwestern Medical Center	2009	U01 DK085453	Pioglitazone preserves insulin secretion in type 1 diabetes
Henry Rodriguez, Indiana University	2009	U01 DK085505	Type 1 Diabetes TrialNet at Indiana University Clinical Center
William Russell, Vanderbilt University	2009	U01 DK085465	Vanderbilt University: Clinical Center Application, Type 1 Diabetes TrialNet
Desmond Schatz, University of Florida	2009	U01 DK085461	TrialNet: University of Florida Clinical Center and Network
Diane Wherrett, Hospital for Sick Children (Toronto)	2009	U01 DK085463	Type 1 Diabetes TrialNet: Toronto Clinical Centre
Darrell Wilson, Stanford University	2009	U01 DK061042	Type 1 Diabetes TrialNet at Stanford
Immune Tolerance Network - Immunomodulation (RFP NIAID-99-30)			
University of California, San Francisco	2001	N01 AI015416	Collaborative Network for Clinical Research on Immune Tolerance

	Year	Project No.	Project Title
Social & Scientific Systems	2007	N01 AI040089	Immune Tolerance Network support
Eminent Services Corporation	2007	N01 AI040090	Immune Tolerance Network support
PPD Development	2007	N01 AI040070	Immune Tolerance Network support
Rho Federal Systems	2008	N01 AI080029	Immune Tolerance Network support

Recruitment for Clinical Research Studies

	Year	Project No.	Project Title
Matthews Media	2004	N02 DK032625	Media Support Services for Type 1 Diabetes Mellitus Consortia
Matthews Media	2004	N02 DK042680	Media Support Services for Type 1 Diabetes Mellitus Consortia

Type 1 Diabetes-Rapid Access to Intervention Development (Projects Relevant to Prevention)

	Year	Project No.	Project Title
Jeffrey Bluestone, Tolerance Therapeutics, Inc.	2005	N01 CO12400	GMP Manufacturing of hOKT3gamma1 (Ala-Ala) Monoclonal
Jerry Nadler, DiaKine Therapeutics, LLC	2005	N02 CM37005/ N02 CM27005	Purification of Lisofylline Drug Substance and Manufacture of Lisofylline Drug Product
Terry Strom, Beth Israel Deaconess Medical Center	2005	N01 CO12400	IL-2/Fc-IL15/Fc Fusion Proteins Components of the "Power Mix" Immune Modulator

Repository Services for Type 1 Diabetes-Rapid Access to Intervention Development (Projects Relevant to Prevention)

	Year	Project No.	Project Title
Fisher Scientific	2007	N02 CM62200	Repository Services for T1D-RAID

Type 1 Diabetes-Preclinical Testing Program: Preclinical Efficacy in Prevention or Reversal of Type 1 Diabetes in Rodent Models (RFP DK05-005)

	Year	Project No.	Project Title
Biomedical Research Models	2006	N01 DK062909	Preclinical Study of Efficacy in Animal Models

Cooperative Study Group for Autoimmune Disease Prevention (RFA AI00-016)

	Year	Project No.	Project Title
Teodor-Doru Brumeanu, Mount Sinai School of Medicine	2001	R01 DK061927	Prevention of Type 1 Diabetes by Soluble, MHC-II Peptide
George Eisenbarth, University of Colorado Health Sciences Center	2001	U19 AI050864	Virginia Mason/UCHSC Autoimmune Prevention Center
C.Garrison Fathman, Stanford University	2001	U01 DK061934	Strategies for Prevention of Autoimmunity
C.Garrison Fathman, Stanford University	2001	U19 DK061925	CD25+ Regulator CD4+ T Cells
David Hafler, Brigham and Women's Hospital	2001	U01 DK061926	Role of Regulatory CD4+/CD25+ T Cells in Diabetes
Matthias Von Herrath, La Jolla Institute for Allergy & Immunology	2001	U19 AI051973	How Does Blockade of CD40/CD40L Prevent Autoimmunity?

Cooperative Study Group for Autoimmune Disease Prevention (RFA AI05-026)

	Year	Project No.	Project Title
George Eisenbarth, University of Colorado Health Sciences Center	2006	U19 AI050864	Benaroya Research Institute/UCDHSC Autoimmune Cooperative Study Group
C. Garrison Fathman, Stanford University	2006	U01 DK078123	Immunoregulation of Autoimmunity
Aldo Rossini, University of Massachusetts Medical School	2006	U01 AI073871	Adaptive Immunity in Virus-induced Diabetes in BBDR Rats
Linda Sherman, Scripps Research Institute	2006	U01 AI070351	Effects of Insulin-dependent Diabetes Resistance Alleles on CD8 Tolerance in NOD
Matthias Von Herrath, La Jolla Institute for Allergy & Immunology	2006	U01 DK078013	Achieving Therapeutic Antigent-Specific Tolerance in Type 1 Diabetes

Trial to Reduce the Incidence of Type 1 Diabetes in the Genetically-At-Risk (TRIGR)

	Year	Project No.	Project Title
Hans Akerblom, University of Helsinki	2001	U01 HD040364	Trial to Reduce IDDM in the Genetically At-Risk Study
Dorothy Becker, Children's Hospital (Pittsburgh)	2001	U01 HD042444	Nutritional Primary Prevention of Type 1 Diabetes
Jeff Krischer, University of South Florida	2006	U01 HD051997	Trial to Reduce IDDM in the Genetically at Risk (TRIGR) Data Management Unit

Gene Therapy Approaches for Diabetes and Its Complications (RFA DK01-006)

	Year	Project No.	Project Title
George Christ, Yeshiva University	2001	R21 DK060204	Gene Therapy for Bladder Hyperactivity in Diabetic Rats
Chih-Pin Liu, Beckman Research Institute	2001	R21 DK060190	Regulation of Type 1 Diabetes Using Ribozymes

	Year	Project No.	Project Title
William Osborne, University of Washington	2001	R21 AI051637	Autoantigen Delivery to Induce Tolerance in Diabetes
Manikkam Suthanthiran, Weill Medical College	2001	R21 DK060186	Gene Therapy for Islet Transplantation
Jide Tian, University of California, Los Angeles	2001	R21 DK060209	Genetic Modification of DCs as Immunotherapy for IDDM
Roland Tisch, University of North Carolina Chapel Hill	2001	R21 AI051638	The Use of VEE Replicons Encoding GAD65 to Treat IDDM
Keith Webster, University of Miami	2001	R21 HL069812	Therapeutic Angiogenesis to Treat Ischemic Disorders

Innovative Grants in Immune Tolerance (RFA AI00-006)

	Year	Project No.	Project Title
Adam Adler, University of Connecticut School of Med/Dnt	2001	R21 AI049813	Comparing Toleragenic Versus Immunogenic APC Function
Lin Chen, University of Colorado	2001	R21 AI049905	Develop Peptide Inhibitors of the NFAT/AP-1 Complex
Mark Crew, University of Arkansas	2001	R21 AI049885	Tolerated Xenografts Using Virus Stealth Technology
Joanna Davies, Scripps Research Institute	2001	R21 DK061334	Transplantation Tolerance Induced by Linked Suppression
Nicholas Gascoigne, Scripps Research Institute	2001	R21 DK061329	Real-Time Molecular Interactions in Tolerance Induction
Irving Goldschneider, University of Connecticut School of Med/Dnt	2001	R21 AI049882	Induction Acquired Thymic Tolerance by Regulatory APCs
Hidehiro Kishimoto, Scripps Research Institute	2001	R21 DK061332	Tolerance in NOD Mice
Mark Poznansky, Massachusetts General Hospital	2001	R21 AI049858	Movement of Recipient T-Cells Away from an Allograft
Haval Shirwan, University of Louisville	2001	R21 DK061333	Apoptosis: A Means of Immune Regulation to Treat Diabetes
Dario Vignali, St. Jude's Children's Research Hospital	2001	R21 DK061330	Tolerance Induction by Targeted Expression of GAD

Innovative Grants in Immune Tolerance (RFA AI03-010)

	Year	Project No.	Project Title
Andrea Sant, University of Rochester	2004	R21 AI059898	Selective Presentation of Autoantigens by B Cells
Matthias Von Herrath/Douglas Green, La Jolla Institute for Allergy & Immunology	2004	R21 AI059850	Immune Tolerance Induction By Apoptotic Bodies
Chen Dong, University of Texas, MD Anderson Cancer Center	2004	R21 DK069278	Costimulatory Regulation of CD8 T Cell Tolerance

Pilot Studies for New Therapies for Type 1 Diabetes and Its Complications (RFA DK99-013)

	Year	Project No.	Project Title
Steinunn Baekkeskov, University of California, San Francisco	1999	R21 DK055977	Generation of a Non-Human Primate Model of Type 1 Diabetes
Kevin Breuel, East Tennessee State University	1999	R21 DK057115	NF-Kappa B as a Therapeutic Target for IDDM
Alan Escher, Loma Linda University	1999	R21 DK057113	APC-Targeting Vaccine for Prevention of Type 1 Diabetes
Daniel Kaufman, University of California, Los Angeles	1999	R21 AI047773	Rational Design of Antigen-Based Immunotherapeutics
William Langridge, Loma Linda University	1999	R21 DK057206	A Targeted Plant-Based Vaccine for Type 1 Diabetes
Jon Mabley, Inotek Corporation	1999	R21 DK057239	Poly(ADP) Ribose Synthetase and Autoimmune Diabetes
Noel MacLaren, Louisiana State University Medical Center	1999	R21 DK057122	A Vaccine for Immune Mediated Diabetes
James Thomas, Vanderbilt University	1999	R21 AI047763	Selection and Regulation of B Lymphocytes in IDDM

Immunopathogenesis of Type 1 Diabetes Mellitus (RFA DK98-010)

	Year	Project No.	Project Title
Cheong-Hee Chang, University of Michigan Ann Arbor	1998	R21 AI044454	Tolerance and Autoreactivity by Self Antigen
Patrick Concannon, Virginia Mason Research Center	1998	R01 DK055970	Immunological Candidate Genes for IDDM Susceptibility
John Corbett, St. Louis University	1998	R01 AI044458	Mechanisms of Viral-Induced Beta Cell Damage
George Eisenbarth, University of Colorado Health Sciences Center	1998	R01 DK055969	In Vivo NOD Evaluation of a Pathogenic Insulin Peptide
Christopher Goodnow, Australian National University	1998	R01 AI044392	Mechanisms Regulating Islet Destruction by CD4 T cells
David Hafler, Brigham and Women's Hospital	1998	R01 AI044447	The Role of Invariant T Cells and IL-4 in Type 1 Diabetes
Kathryn Haskins, University of Colorado Health Sciences Center	1998	R01 AI044482	Immunoregulation in the NOD Mouse
Jonathan Katz, Washington University	1998	R01 AI044416	Role of I-AG7 on Selecting Autoreactive T Cells
William Kwok, Virginia Mason Research Center	1998	R01 AI044443	Structure and Immunobiology of an IDDM-Protective Molecule
Paul Lehmann, Case Western Reserve University	1998	R21 AI044484	Human/Humanized T Cell Response to Islet Cell Antigens
Chih-Pin Liu, Beckman Research Institute	1998	R21 AI044429	Regulatory Mechanisms in Type 1 Diabetes
Ali Naji, University of Pennsylvania	1998	R01 HD037754	Autoimmune Diabetes-Maternal Immunoglobulin
Alberto Pugliese, University of Miami	1998	R01 AI044456	Proinsulin Expression in the Immune System
Eric Simone, University of Colorado Health Sciences Center	1998	R01 AI044466	NOD T Cell Receptors for Specific Islet Autoantigens
Grete Sonderstrup, Stanford University	1999	P01 DK055364	Autoimmune T and B Cell Responses in Type 1 Diabetes
Matthias Von Herrath, Scripps Research Institute	1998	R01 AI044451	Regulation and Immunotherapy of IDDM
Li Wen, Yale University	1998	R01 AI044427	Development of a Novel Humanized Animal Model of IDDM

	Year	Project No.	Project Title

Biomarkers of Autoimmunity in Type 1 Diabetes (RFA DK06-002)

	Year	Project No.	Project Title
Steven Cahndy, University of California, Irvine	2006	R21 DK077553	Kv1.3 Channels: Functional Biomarker and Therapeutic Target for Type-1 Diabetes
Sofia Casares, Henry M. Jackson Foundation for the Advancement of Military Medicine	2006	R21 DK077521	Immunokinetics of Autoreactive CD4 T Cells in Blood as Biomarker for T1D
George Chessler, University of California, San Diego	2006	R21 DK077466	Serum GAD65 as a Biomarker of Islet Injury, Insulitis, and Transplant Rejection
Debra Counts, University of Maryland, Baltimore	2006	R21 DK077529	Zonulin and Cytokines as Markers of Autoimmunity in Type 1 Diabetes
Teresa Dilorenzo, Albert Einstein College of Medicine	2006	R21 DK077500	CD8 T Cell Reactivity to IGRP as an Autoimmunity Marker in Type 1 Diabetes
Daniel Geraghty, Fred Hutchinson Cancer Research Center	2006	R21 DK077531	Diabetes and Recombination in the 8.1 MHC Haplotype
William Kwok, Benaroya Research Institute at Virginia Mason	2006	R21 DK077525	Functional HLA-A*201-peptide and DR0401-peptide Microarrays for Type 1 Diabetes
Mikael Knip, University of Helsinki	2006	R21DK077506	Identification of Biomarkers of Autoimmunity in T1D by Novel Tools
Jerry Palmer, University of Washington	2006	R21 DK077545	Identification of Islet Proteins Stimulatory to T Cells from Autoimmune Diabetic
Alberto Pugliese, University of Miami	2006	R21 DK077491	Evaluation of MicroRNA Expression in CD4 T cells in Type 1 Diabetes

Diabetes Prevention Trial-Type 1 Diabetes (DPT-1) - Supplements

	Year	Project No.	Project Title
Nathaniel Clark, University of Vermont	1998	M01 RR000109	General Clinical Research Center: Diabetes Prevention Trial
George Eisenbarth, University of Colorado Health Sciences Center	1998	R01 AI039213	Antibodies to Recombinant Autoantigens- Prediction/Immunogenetics
Richard Jackson, Joslin Diabetes Center	1998	U01 DK046601	Diabetes Prevention Trial -Type 1
Noel MacLaren, University of Florida	1998	U01 DK046636	Diabetes Prevention Trial -Type 1
Alvin Powers, Vanderbilt University	1998	M01 RR000095	General Clinical Research Center: Diabetes Prevention Trial
Susan Ratzan, University of Connecticut Health Center	1998	M01 RR006192	General Clinical Research Center: Diabetes Prevention Trial
David Schade, University of New Mexico	1998	M01 RR000997	General Clinical Research Center: Diabetes Prevention Trial
Desmond Schatz, University of Florida	1998	M01 RR000082	General Clinical Research Center: Diabetes Prevention Trial
Stuart Weinzimer, Children's Hospital (Philadelphia)	1998	M01 RR000240	General Clinical Research Center: Diabetes Prevention Trial

Repository Services for DPT-1

	Year	Project No.	Project Title
Fisher Scientific	2009	HHSN267200800015C	Repository Services for DPT-1

One Year Supplements to Ongoing Projects

	Year	Project No.	Project Title
Mark Atkinson, University of Florida	1998	P01 AI042288	Immune Function and Low Risk Genotypes in IDD
Mark Atkinson, University of Florida	1998	R01 AI039250	Mechanisms of Immunotherapy in IDD Prevention Trials
William Hagopian, Pacific Northwest Research Institute	1998	P51 RR000166	Controlled Transfer Model for Autoimmune Diabetes
Laurence Turka, University of Pennsylvania	1998	P01 AI041521	Costimulation and Cytokines in Tolerance
Don Wiley, Children's Hospital (Boston)	1998	P01 AI039619	MHC Linked Susceptibility to Autoimmunity - Structure and Biology

GOAL III: DEVELOP CELL REPLACEMENT THERAPY

Beta Cell Biology Consortium (RFA DK01-014)

	Year	Project No.	Project Title
Michael German, University of California, San Francisco	2001	U19 DK061245	Molecular Control of Pancreatic Islet Development
Joel Habener, Massachusetts General Hospital	2001	U19 DK061251	Restoration of Endocrine Pancreas Function
John Hutton, University of Colorado Health Sciences Center	2001	U19 DK061248	Development and Regeneration of the Endocrine Pancreas
Mark Magnuson, Vanderbilt University	2001	U19 DK042502	Genes of Pancreas Function and Development
Catherine Verfaillie, University of Minnesota	2001	U19 DK061244	Characterization of Beta Cell Stem Cells

Beta Cell Biology Consortium (U19) (RFA DK04-017)

	Year	Project No.	Project Title
Mark Magnuson, Vanderbilt University	2005	U19 DK042502	Mechanisms of Pancreas Development
Palle Serup, Hagedorn Research Institute	2005	U19 DK072495	Pancreatic Endocrine Development and Regeneration

Beta Cell Biology Consortium (U01) (RFA DK04-018)

	Year	Project No.	Project Title
Markus Grompe, Oregon Health Sciences University	2005	U01 DK072477	Novel Reagents for Beta Cell Biology
Pedro Herrera, University of Geneva	2005	U01 DK072522	Transgenic Model of Inducible Diabetes
Gordon Keller, Mount Sinai School of Medicine	2005	U01 DK072513	Endoderm Induction and Pancreatic Specification from ES Cells

	Year	Project No.	Project Title
Douglas Melton, Harvard University	2005	U01 DK072505	Mechanisms of Pancreatic Beta Cell Regeneration
Lori Sussel, University of Colorado Health Science Center	2005	U01 DK072504	Defining the Roles of Nkx2.2 and NeuroD in Regulating Islet Cell Fate
Kenneth Zaret, Institute for Cancer Research, Fox Chase Cancer Center	2005	U01 DK072503	Gene Regulatory Signals for Beta Cell Development

Beta Cell Biology Consortium (Coordinating Center) (RFA DK04-500)

	Year	Project No.	Project Title
Mark Magnuson, Vanderbilt University	2005	U01 DK072473	Coordinating Center for Beta Cell Biology Consortium

Clinical Islet Transplantation Consortium (Data Coordinating Center) (RFA DK04-004)

	Year	Project No.	Project Title
William Clarke, University of Iowa	2004	U01 DK070431	Clinical Islet Transplantation: Data Coordinating Center

Clinical Islet Transplantation Consortium (Clinical Centers) (RFA DK04-005)

	Year	Project No.	Project Title
Bernhard Hering, University of Minnesota	2004	U01 AI065193	Advancing Islet Transplants for Type 1 Diabetes Care
Olle Korsgren, Uppsala University	2004	U01 AI065192	Innate Immunity in Clinical Islet Transplantation
Ali Naji, University of Pennsylvania	2004	U01 DK070430	B-Lymphocyte Immunotherapy in Islet Transplantation
Camillo Ricordi, University of Miami	2004	U01 DK070460	Strategies to Improve Long Term Islet Graft Survival
Andrew Shapiro, University of Alberta	2004	U01 AI065191	Islet Transplant - Costimulatory Blockade with LEA29Y

Limited Competition: Continuation of the Clinical Islet Transplantation (CIT) Consortium (U01) (RFA DK09-501)

	Year	Project No.	Project Title
William Clarke, University of Iowa	2009	U01 DK070431	Clinical Islet Transplantation: Data Coordinating Center
Dixon Kaufman, Northwestern University	2009	U01 AI089316	Clinical Islet Transplantation at Northwestern
Christian Larsen, Emory University	2009	U01 AI089317	Clinical Refinement of Islet Transplantation
Ali Naji, University of Pennsylvania	2009	U01 DK070430	B-Lymphocyte Immunotherapy in Islet Transplantation
Andrew Posselt, University of California, San Francisco	2009	U01 DK085531	Advancing Islet Transplant for Type 1 Diabetes Care
Camillo Ricordi, University of Miami	2009	U01 DK070460	Strategies to Improve Long Term Islet Graft Survival

Pilot and Feasibility Program in Human Islet Biology (RFA DK03-021)

	Year	Project No.	Project Title
John Corbett, St. Louis University	2004	R21 DK068839	Unfolded Protein Response as a Regulator of Human Beta-Cell Viability
Peter Drain, University of Pittsburgh	2004	R21 DK068833	Human Beta Cell Parameters for Islet Engraftment Success
Adolfo Garcia-Ocana, University of Pittsburgh	2004	R21 DK068836	Protein Kinase B/Akt in the Human Islet
Regina Kuliawat, Albert Einstein College of Medicine	2004	R21 DK068843	Beta-Cell Granule Protein Profile by Split Reporter Assay
Alvin Powers, Vanderbilt University	2004	R21 DK068854	Pdx-1 and Maf Proteins in Human Islets
Michael Roe, University of Chicago	2004	R21 DK068822	Real-Time Analyses of Apoptosis in Human Beta Cells
Rupangi Vasavada, University of Pittsburgh	2004	R21 DK068831	Parathyroid Hormone Related Protein in the Human Islet
Luis Fernandez, University of Wisconsin	2005	R21 DK071218	Donation After Cardiac Death for Isolated Pancreatic Islet Transplantation: Biology and Predicting Factors for Success
Klaus Kaestner, University of Pennsylvania	2005	R21 DK071216	Expression Profiling of Human Islets
Charles King, University of California, San Diego	2005	R21 DK071228	Proteomic Analysis of PI 3-Kinase Signaling in Islet
Brad Marsh, University of Queensland	2005	R21 DK071236	3D Structural Biology of the Human Islet
Anna Moore, Massachusetts General Hospital	2005	R21 DK071225	Labeling Human Pancreatic Islets for Multi-Modal Imaging
John Thompson, University of Alabama-Birmingham	2005	R21 DK071300	Effects of Brain-death on Islet Recovery and Function

Comprehensive Programs in Beta Cell Biology (RFA DK02-014)

	Year	Project No.	Project Title
Vincenzino Cirulli, University of California, San Diego	2002	R01 DK063443	Role of Connexins in Beta Cell Development and Function
Roger Davis, University of Massachusetts Medical School	2002	R01 DK063368	Functional Analysis of the Beta Cell
Peter Dempsey, Pacific Northwest Research Institute	2002	R01 DK063363	Endogenous Betacellulin Signaling in Beta Cell Biology
Kathleen Dunlap, New England Medical Center Hospitals	2002	R01 DK063344	GABA-B Receptors as Regulators of Islet Biology
Claudia Kappen, University of Nebraska Medical Center	2002	R01 DK063336	Genome-Wide Discovery of Beta Cell Gene Control Elements
Jeffrey Pessin, University of Iowa	2002	R01 DK063332	Beta Cell Insulin Granule Docking, Priming, and Fusion
Fredric Wondisford, University of Chicago	2002	R01 DK063349	Control of Beta Cell Function by Co-Activators

	Year	Project No.	Project Title
Beta Cell Regeneration for Diabetes Therapy (RFA DK05-007)			
Susan Bonner-Weir, Joslin Diabetes Center	2006	R01 DK074879	Strategies to Identify *In Vitro* Islet Progenitors
Lawrence Chan, Baylor College of Medicine	2006	R21 DK075002	Induced Islet Neogenesis Therapy *In Vivo*
Non-Human Primate Transplantation Tolerance Cooperative Study Group (RFA AI01-006)			
Hugh Auchincloss, Massachusetts General Hospital	2002	U01 AI051706	Tolerance Induction for Primate Islet Transplantation
Bernhard Hering, University of Minnesota	2002	U01 DK062932	Mixed Chimerism in Haploidentical Non-Human Primates
Christian Larsen, Emory University	2002	U19 AI051731	Transplant Tolerance
Greg Westergaard, Alpha Genesis	2000	U01 AI049916	Specific Pathogen Free Rhesus Macaque Breeding Program
Greg Westergaard, Alpha Genesis	2005	N01 AI050048	
Non-Human Primate Islet/Kidney Transplantation Tolerance (U01, U19) (RFA AI06-018)			
David Rothstein, Yale University	2007	U01 AI074676	Induction of Renal Allograft Tolerance in Monkeys with Anti-CD45RB Based Therapy
David Sachs, Massachusetts General Hospital	2007	U01 DK080653	Tolerance to Composite Islet-Kidney Transplants in Baboons
Terry Strom, Beth Israel Deaconess Medical Center	2007	U19 DK080652	Inflammation and T Cell Memory: Inter-related Barriers to Allograft Tolerance
Immune Tolerance Network - Islet Transplantation (RFP-NIAID-99-30)			
University of California, San Francisco	2001	N01 AI015416	Collaborative Network for Clinical Research on Immune Tolerance
Islet Cell Resource Centers (RFA RR01-002)			
A. Osama Gaber, University of Tennessee Health Sciences Center	2001	U42 RR016602	Standardization and Procedure on Islet Isolation
Ronald Gill, University of Colorado Health Sciences Center	2001	U42 RR016599	Islet Cell Resources Facility at the University of Colorado
Mark Hardy, Columbia University of Health Sciences	2001	U42 RR016629	New York Regional Islet Isolation Facility
Bernhard Hering, University of Minnesota	2001	U42 RR016598	Human Pancreatic Islet Cell Resources (ICRs)
Thalachallour Mohanakumar, Washington University	2001	U42 RR016597	Human Islet Isolation Program at Washington University
Ali Naji, University of Pennsylvania	2001	U42 RR016600	Isolation/Distribution of Human Pancreatic Islets
Jo Reems, Puget Sound Blood Center	2001	U42 RR016604	Human Islet Isolations in Seattle
Camillo Ricordi, University of Miami	2001	U42 RR016603	Islet Cell Resources for Diabetes Research and Treatment
Arthur Riggs, Beckman Research Institute	2001	U42 RR016607	Islet Cell Resources of Southern California
Gordon Weir, Joslin Diabetes Center	2001	U42 RR016606	Human Pancreatic Islet Cell Resources
Islet Cell Resource Centers: Administrative and Bioinformatics Coordinating Center (RFA RR02-002)			
Joyce Niland, City of Hope National Medical Center	2002	U42 RR017673	National Islet Cell Consortium Coordinating Center
Human Pancreatic Islet Cell Resources (ICRs) (RFA RR05-003)			
Luis Fernandez, University of Wisconsin, Madison	2006	U42 RR023240	Multi-Parametric Characterization of Human Islets: Predictor of Islet Quality
Bernhard Hering, University of Minnesota, Twin Cities	2006	U42 RR016598	Human Pancreatic Islet Cell Resources
Ali Naji, University of Pennsylvania	2006	U42 RR016600	Isolation and Distribution of high quality human pancreatic islets
Jose Oberholzer, University of Illinois, Chicago	2006	U42 RR023245	Chicago Islet Consortium ICR at UIC
Camillo Ricordi, University of Miami	2006	U42 RR016603	Human Pancreatic Islet Cell Resource to Catalyze Collaborative Diabetes Research
Arthur Riggs, City of Hope/Beckman Research Center	2006	U42 RR016607	Southern California Islet Cell Resources (SCI-ICR) Center
Islets for Basic Research - NIDDK Islet Cell Distribution Coordinating Center (RFP DK 08-99SB)			
Beckman Research Institute of City of Hope	2009	PUR276200900006C1	NIDDK Islet Cell Distribution Coordinating Center

	Year	Project No.	Project Title

Collaborative Islet Transplant Registry (RFP NIDDK-00-002)

	Year	Project No.	Project Title
EMMES Corporation	2001	N01DK012472	Islet/Beta Cell Transplant Registry

Immunobiology of Xenotransplantation Cooperative Research Program (RFA AI04-042)

Simon Robson, Beth Israel Deconess Medical Center	2005	U01 AI066331	Thromboregulatory Strategies to Prolong Xenografts

Islet Encapsulation Research - Pilot and Feasibility Supplements to Existing Centers

John Hutton, University of Colorado Health Sciences Center	2002	P30 DK057516	Diabetes Endocrinology Research Center
Jerry Palmer, University of Washington	2002	P30 DK017047	Diabetes Endocrinology Research Center
Robert Sherwin, Yale University	2002	P30 DK045735	Diabetes Endocrinology Research Center
Donald Steiner, University of Chicago	2002	P60 DK020595	Diabetes Research and Training Center

Gene Transfer Approaches To Enhance Islet Transplantation (RFA DK02-020)

Mark Cattral, Toronto General Hospital	2002	R21 AI055024	Immunomodulation of Pancreatic Islets by Adenoviral Genes
Lieping Chen, Mayo Clinic Rochester	2002	R21 AI055028	Novel Strategies to Prevent Islet Transplantation Rejection
Christiane Ferran, Beth Israel Deaconess Medical Center	2002	R21 DK062601	Gene Transfer with A20 to Improve Islet Transplantation
Donald Kohn, Children's Hospital (Los Angeles)	2002	R21 DK062649	Gene Expression in Beta Cells by Lentiviral Vectors
Joseph LeDoux, Georgia Institute of Technology	2002	R21 DK062616	Induction of Stem Cells to Adopt an Endocrine Fate
Adrian Morelli, University of Pittsburgh	2002	R21 AI055027	Dendritic Cells with Galectin-1 to Enhance Islet Grafts
Alvin Powers, Vanderbilt University	2002	R21 DK062641	Gene Transfer and Revascularization of Transplanted Islets
Paul Robbins, University of Pittsburgh	2002	R21 AI055026	Inhibition of NF-KB to Facilitate Islet Transplantation
Daniel Salomon, Scripps Research Institute	2002	R21 DK062598	Lentiviral-Transduced Endothelium for Islet Transplants
Sihong Song, University of Florida	2002	R21 DK062652	Anti-Inflammatory Serpin (AAT and Elafin) Gene Transfers
Jide Tian, University of California, Los Angeles	2002	R21 AI055025	Genetic Modification of Mouse Islets for Transplantation
Zandong Yang, University of Virginia, Charlottesville	2002	R21 DK062610	Induction of Suppression for Islet Transplantation

Imaging Pancreatic Beta Cell Mass, Function, Engraftment, or Inflammation (RFA DK02-002)

Paul Harris, Columbia University Health Sciences	2002	R01 DK063567	Human Islet Antigen Discovery and Imaging
Dixon Kaufman, Northwestern University	2002	R01 DK063565	Bioluminescent Imaging of Pancreatic Islet Transplants
Wen-Hong Li, University of Texas Southwestern Medical Center	2002	R01 DK063525	Image Beta Cell Mass and Function in Implants and Pancreas
Anna Moore, Massachusetts General Hospital	2002	R01 DK063572	In Vivo Imaging of Autoimmune Attack in Type 1 Diabetes
Louis Philipson, University of Chicago	2002	R01 DK063493	Imaging Beta Cell Function with Biosensors
Massimo Trucco, Children's Hospital (Pittsburgh)	2002	R01 DK063335	Optical Imaging of Beta Cell Function and Engraftment

Toward Imaging the Pancreatic Beta Cell in People (RFA DK06-003)

Thierry Berney, University of Geneva	2006	R01 AI074225	Islets of Langerhans Graft Monitoring by Magnetic Resonance Imaging
Jeff Bulte, Johns Hopkins University	2006	R01 DK077537	MR-Guided Delivery and Monitoring of Magnetocapsules Immunoprotecting Islet Cells
Barjor Gimi, University of Texas Southwestern Medical Center	2006	R01 EB07456	Imaging Islets in Implantable Microcapsules
Martin Gotthardt, Radboud University Nijmegen	2006	R01 AG030328	Non-invasive Beta-cell Imaging using a Ga-68-labeled Glucagone-like Peptide-1
Paul Harris, Columbia University Health Sciences	2006	R01 DK077493	PET Imaging of Human Beta Cell Mass
Eba Hathout, Loma Linda University	2006	R01 DK077541	In vivo Dynamic Imaging of Angiogenesis in Transplanted Islets

New Strategies for Treatment of Type 1 Diabetes Mellitus (RFA DK00-001)

Paul Gores, Carolinas Medical Center	2000	R01 DK059070	Islet Transplantation in Non-Uremic Diabetic Patients
Peter Gottlieb, University of Colorado Health Sciences Center	2000	R01 DK059097	Immunotherapy Trial in New-onset Type 1 Diabetes
A. Shapiro, University of Alberta	2000	R01 DK059101	Trial of Anti-TNFalpha in Islet Transplantation

	Year	Project No.	Project Title

Pilot Studies for New Therapies for Type 1 Diabetes and its Complications (RFA DK99-013)

	Year	Project No.	Project Title
Geoffrey Block, University of Pittsburgh	1999	R21 DK057143	Bioengineered Primary Islets for Transplantation
George Gittes, New York University School of Medicine	1999	R21 DK057224	Mesenchymal Inducers of Beta Cell Differentiation
Lawrence Olson, Michigan State University	1999	R21 DK057173	Pluripotent Human Pancreatic Ductal Cells
Vijayakumar Ramiya, Ixion Biotechnology, Inc.	1999	R21 DK057121	Islets from Islet Progenitor/Stem Cells for Implantation
Raymond Steptoe, Walter and Eliza Hall Institute	1999	R21 DK057228	Proinsulin Gene Transfer Via Bone Marrow to Prevent IDDM
Hei Sul, University of California, Berkeley	1999	R21 DK057217	Pref-1 Function in Islet Growth and Differentiation

Cellular and Molecular Approaches for Achieving Euglycemia (RFA DK98-007)

	Year	Project No.	Project Title
Kenneth Brayman, University of Pennsylvania	1998	R21 DK055353	Adenoviral Mediated Islet Gene Transfer
Michael Brownlee, Albert Einstein College of Medicine	1998	R01 DK055299	Genetic Engineering of Beta Cells for Transplantation
Sylvia Christakos, University of Med/Dnt of New Jersey	1998	R21 DK055050	Preservation of Beta Cell Function by Calbindin-D28K
Joanna Davies, Scripps Research Institute	1998	R01 AI045488	Allograft Induced IL-4 in Pancreas Graft Protection
Herbert Gaisano, University of Toronto	1998	R21 DK055160	SNARE Regulation of B-Cell KCA and SUR Potentiates Secretion
Lakshmi Gaur, Puget Sound Blood Center and Program	1998	R01 AI045487	Induction of Tolerance to Islet Allografts in Primates
Ivan Gerling, University of Tennessee	1998	R21 DK055263	Human Leukocyte Response to Human Islets in SCID mice
Marvin Gershengorn, Cornell University of Medical College	1998	R21 DK055087	Dynorphin and Beta Cell Sensitization
Ronald Gill, University of Colorado Health Sciences Center	1998	R01 DK055333	T Cell Mediated Injury to Islet Allografts
Suzanne Ildstad, Allegheny University of Health Sciences	1998	R01 AI045486	Hematopoetic Stem Cell Chimerism to Treat Diabetes
Karen Kover, University of Kansas Medical Center	1998	R21 AI045490	The Effects of Anti-Rat CD40L on Islet Allograft Survival
Fred Levine, University of California, San Diego	1998	R01 DK055065	Inhibition of Apoptosis in Pancreatic Beta Cells
Andreas Martin, Mount Sinai School of Medicine	1998	R21 DK055277	An In Vivo Model of Pancreatic Islet Organoids
Albee Messing, University of Wisconsin Madison	1998	R21 DK055309	New Method for Purifying Islets from Transgenic Pancreas
Jerry Nadler, City of Hope Medical Center	1998	R01 DK055240	Lipid Mediators in Induced Pancreatic Islet Dysfunction
Christopher Newgard, University of Texas Southwestern Medical Center	1998	R01 DK055188	Engineering of Immunoprotection in Beta Cell Lines
Colin Nichols, Washington University	1998	R01 DK055282	Genetic Engineering of Glucose Regulation
Camillo Ricordi, University of Miami	1998	R01 DK055347	Immunomodulation for Islet Transplantation in Diabetes
David Rothstein, Yale University	1998	R01 AI045485	Role of CD45 in Generation of Islet Allograft Tolerance
Thomas Steinberg, Washington University	1998	R01 HD037799	P2 Receptors, Extracellular ATP, and Islet Function

Beta Cell Proteomics (PAR-00-101)

	Year	Project No.	Project Title
Joshua LaBaer, Harvard University Medical School	2001	R01 DK061906	Manipulating the Proteome

One Year Supplements to Ongoing Projects

	Year	Project No.	Project Title
Hugh Auchincloss, Massachusetts General Hospital	1998	R01 AI038397	Pathways of Alloreactivity
Jeffrey Bluestone, University of Chicago	1998	P01 AI029531	Immunomodulation of Transplant Rejection
Kenneth Polonsky, University of Chicago	1998	P01 DK044840	Molecular Mechanisms/Beta Cell Dysfunction in Diabetes
Daniel Salomon, Scripps Research Institute	1998	R01 AI042384	Importance of Islet Structure in Islet Transplantation
Nora Sarvetnick, Scripps Research Institute	1998	R01 HD029764	Model of Islet Regeneration and Neogenesis
Ming-Jer Tsai, Baylor College of Medicine	1998	R37 HD017379	In Vitro Expression of Hormone-Regulated Genes

GOAL IV: PREVENT OR REDUCE HYPOGLYCEMIA IN TYPE 1 DIABETES

Diabetes Research in Children Network (DirecNet) (RFA HD01-009)

	Year	Project No.	Project Title
Roy Beck, Jaeb Center for Health Research, Inc.	2001	U01 HD041890	Coordinating Center - Glucose Sensors in Type 1 Diabetes
Peter Chase, University of Colorado Health Sciences Center	2001	U10 HD041919	Glucose Sensors in Children with Type 1 Diabetes
William Tamborlane/Stuart Weinzimer, Yale University	2001	U10 HD041906	Yale's Center in the Children's Glucose Sensor Network
Eva Tsalikian, University of Iowa	2001	U10 HD041915	Glucose Sensors and Hypoglycemia in Children with DM
Darrell Wilson/Bruce Buckingham, Stanford University	2001	U10 HD041908	Near-Continuous Glucose Monitoring in Pediatrics
Tim Wysocki, Nemours Children's Hospital	2001	U10 HD041918	Continuous Glucose Sensors in Youth: a Biobehavioural Study

	Year	Project No.	Project Title

Cooperative Multicenter Diabetes Research Network for Hypoglycemia Prevention (U10) (RFA HD06-020)

	Year	Project No.	Project Title
Roy Beck, Jaeb Center for Health Research, Inc.	2007	U01 HD041890	Cooperative Multicenter Diabetes Research Network for Hypoglycemia Prevention
Bruce Buckingham, Stanford University	2007	U10 HD041908	Prevention of Nocturnal Hypoglycemia: Effect on Neurologic Outcome in Toddlers
Stuart Weinzimer, Yale University	2007	U10 HD041906	Yale Study of Closed-Loop Automated Glucose Control for Hypoglycemia Prevention
Eva Tsalikian, University of Iowa	2007	U10 HD041915	Prevention of Hypoglycemia and Associated Complications in Type 1 Diabetes
Nelly Mauras, Nemours Children's Hospital	2007	U10 HD041918	Hypoglycemia in Children and Adolescents with T1DM: Mechanisms and Prevention
Neil White, Washington University in St. Louis	2007	U10 HD056526	Diabetes Research in Children Network (DirecNet)

Hypoglycemia in Patients with Type 1 Diabetes (RFA DK03-017)

	Year	Project No.	Project Title
Stephen Davis, Vanderbilt University	2004	R01 DK069803	Hypoglycemia Associated Autonomic Failure in Type 1 DM
Rory McCrimmon, Yale University	2004	R01 DK069831	Role of AMPK in Hypoglycemia-Sensing in the VMH
Charles Mobbs, Mount Sinai School of Medicine	2004	R01 DK070057	Adenosine Receptors and Hypoglycemic Responses
Douglas Rothman, Yale University	2004	R01 NS051854	MRS Studies of Brain Metabolic Adaptations in Diabetes
Raymond Swanson, University of California, San Francisco	2004	R01 NS051855	Hypoglycemic Neuronal Death
Cornelis Tack, University Medical Center St. Radboud	2004	R21 DK069881	Brain Glucose Metabolism and Hypoglycemia Unawareness
Dennis Turner, Duke University Medical Center	2004	R01 NS051856	Lifespan Metabolic Neuroprotection During Hypoglycemia

Effects of Hypoglycemia on Neuronal and Glial Cell Function (RFA NS02-008)

	Year	Project No.	Project Title
James Mandell, University of Virginia, Charlottesville	2002	R21 NS045300	Hypoglycemic Signaling Targets in Astrocytes
Jullie Pan, Yeshiva University	2002	R21 DK064565	Cerebral Activation in Hypoglycemia and Hyperketonemia
Scott Rivkees, Yale University	2002	R21 NS045310	The Role of Adenosine in Hypoglycemic Brain Injury
Vanessa Routh, University of Med/Dnt of New Jersey	2002	R01 DK064566	Glucosensing Neurons in Euglycemia, Hypoglycemia, and HAAF
Stephen Salton, Mount Sinai School of Medicine	2002	R01 NS045305	Mechanisms of Neuronal Hypoglycemic Injury
Dennis Turner, Duke University	2002	R21 NS045304	Lifespan Neuronal/Glial Metabolism During Hypoglycemia

Sensor Development and Validation (RFA EB02-002)

	Year	Project No.	Project Title
Mark Arnold, University of Iowa	2002	R01 DK064569	Continuous Near Infrared Glucose Sensor
David Gough, University of California, San Diego	2002	R01 DK064570	Validation of Long-Term Glucose Sensor in Tissues
Myra Lipes, Joslin Diabetes Center	2002	R01 DK064568	A Cell-Based Glucose Sensing and Insulin Delivery System
Garry Steil, Medtronic Minimed	2002	R01 DK064567	Long Term Glucose Sensing and Physiologic Insulin Delivery

Understanding Hypoglycemia Unawareness in Patients with Type 1 Diabetes (RFA DK01-031)

	Year	Project No.	Project Title
Casey Donovan, University of Southern California	2002	R01 DK062471	Portal Vein Glucose Sensors in Hypoglycemia
Rolf Gruetter, University of Minnesota Twin Cities	2002	R21 NS045519	NMR Measurements of Human Brain Glycogen Metabolism
Lauren Jacobson, Albany Medical College	2002	R21 DK062442	Role of Glucocorticoids in Hypoglycemia Unawareness
Dianne Lattemann, University of Washington	2002	R21 DK062446	CNS Stress Pathways and the Development of Acute HAAF
Yijun Liu, University of Florida	2002	R21 NS045518	Dynamic FMRI Analyses of Hypoglycemia Unawareness
S. Ritter, Washington State University	2002	R01 NS045520	Hindbrain Mechanisms of Hypoglycemia Unawareness
Elizabeth Seaquist, University of Minnesota	2002	R01 DK062440	Cerebral Responses to Insulin-Induced Hypoglycemia
Harry Shamoon, Yeshiva University	2002	R01 DK062463	Modulation of Hypoglycemic Counterregulatory Responses

	Year	Project No.	Project Title
Pilot Studies for New Therapies for Type 1 Diabetes and its Complications (RFA DK99-013)			
David Gough, University of California San Diego	1999	R21 DK057109	Key Parameters for Artificial Pancreas Controller
Glucose Sensors in the Treatment of Diabetes (RFA DK98-008)			
Mark Arnold, University of Iowa	1998	R21 DK055255	Solid-State Optics for Non-Invasive Glucose Monitors
Sanford Asher, University of Pittsburgh	1998	R01 DK055348	Development of (Non) Invasive Real-Time Glucose Sensors
Katherine Crothall, Animas Corporation	1998	R01 DK055246	An Implantable Near IR Glucose Sensor
Casey Donovan, University of Southern California	1998	R01 DK055257	Portal Glucosensors in Hypoglycemic Detection
Dale Drueckhammer, State University of New York Stony Brook	1998	R21 DK055234	New Approaches to Fluorescence-Based Glucose Sensors
Johannes Everse, Texas Tech University	1998	R21 RR014174	Enzyme-Thermistors as Glucose Sensors
David Gough, University of California San Diego	1998	R01 DK055064	Tissue Response to Implanted Glucose Sensor
Joseph Izatt, Case Western Reserve University	1998	R21 RR014172	Pathlength-Resolved Non-Invasive Optical Glucose Sensors
John Mastrototaro, Minimed, Inc.	1998	R01 DK055242	Transdermal Glucose Sensing with Optical Amplification
Francis Moussy, University of Connecticut	1998	R01 RR014171	Control of Sensor/Tissue Interact for Extended Lifetime
Govind Rao, University of Maryland	1998	R01 RR014170	Protein Engineered Glucose Sensor
Kerstin Rebrin, Minimed, Inc.	1998	R01 DK055337	Interstitial Glucose Dynamics Using a Glucose Sensor
Christopher Saudek, Johns Hopkins University	1998	R01 DK055132	Clinical Research Toward Closed-Loop Insulin Delivery
Gary Sayler, University of Tennessee	1998	R21 RR014169	Eukaryotic Bioluminescent Integrated Circuit Sensors
Binghe Wang, North Carolina State University	1998	R21 DK055062	Glucose-Sensitive Artificial Receptors for Insulin
Joseph Wang, New Mexico State University Las Cruces	1998	R01 RR014173	Oxygen-Independent Interference-Free Glucose Sensors
George Wilson, University of Kansas Lawrence	1998	R01 DK055297	Evaluation of a Continuous Glucose Monitoring System
Developing New Tools for Detecting and Monitoring Low Blood Glucose for People with Diabetes (CDC PA #99151)			
Robert Langer, Massachusetts Institute of Technology	1999	R08/CCR117792	Ultrasound Mediated Transdermal Glucose Monitoring
Kenneth Ward, National Applied Science	1999	R08/CCR017796	Development of a Continuous Hypoglycemia Monitor
Suzanne Gebhart, SpectRx, Inc.	1999	R08/CCR417812	Continuous Interstitial Fluid Glucose Monitoring
Closed Loop Technologies: Clinical and Behavioral Approaches to Improve Type 1 Diabetes Outcomes (RFA DK08-012)			
Boris Kovatchev, University of Virginia, Charlottesville	2009	R01 DK085623	Modular Bio-behavioral closed-loop control of type 1 diabetes
Edward Damiano, Boston University	2009	R01 DK085633	Clinical Trials of a Closed-loop Control System for Type 1 Diabetes Management
Yogish Kudva, Mayo Clinic College of Medicine, Rochester	2009	R01 DK085516	Integrated Approaches To Close the Loop in Type 1 Diabetes
Roman Hovorka, University of Cambridge	2009	R01 DK085621	Home Testing of 24/7 Closed-loop Control in Children and Adolescents with Type 1 Diabetes
Roy Beck, Jaeb Center for Health Research	2009	R01 DK085591	In Home Closed Loop Reduction of Nocturnal Hypoglycemia and Daytime Hyperglycemia
Francis Doyle, University of California, Santa Barbara	2009	R01 DK085628	Closed-loop Artificial Pancreas: Algorithm Engineering and Clinical Evaluation
Ali Cinar, Illinois Institute of Technology	2009	R01 DK085611	Multivariable Closed Loop Technologies for Physically Active Young Adults
Stuart Weinzimer, Yale University	2009	R01 DK085618	Closed-Loop Effectiveness and Ambulatory Regimens (CLEAR)
Rubina Heptulla, Baylor College of Medicine	2009	R01 DK085597	Novel Glucagon Modulators and the Closed Loop System
Closed Loop Technologies: Pilot and Exploratory Clinical and Behavioral Approaches to Improve Type 1 Diabetes Outcomes (RFA DK08-013)			
Marc Breton, University of Virginia, Charlottesville	2009	R21 DK085641	Introduction of Heart Rate Monitoring to the Closed-loop Control of T1DM
Development of Surrogate Markers for Clinical Trials: Supplements			
University of Iowa	2001	N01 MH120006	Brain Molecular Anatomy Project (BMAP)

	Year	Project No.	Project Title
One Year Supplements to Ongoing Projects			
Peter Havel, University of California Davis	1998	R01 DK050129	ANS Hypoglycemia Induced Glucagon Secretion in Diabetes
Govind Rao, University of Maryland	1998	R01 RR010955	Minimally Invasive Glucose Monitoring

GOAL V: PREVENT OR REDUCE THE COMPLICATIONS OF TYPE 1 DIABETES

Epidemiology of Diabetes Interventions and Complications: Measurement of Cardiovascular Disease

	Year	Project No.	Project Title
William Dahms, Case Western Reserve University	1998	N01 DK062203	Coordinating Center - Diabetes Interventions/Complications
John Lachin, George Washington University	1998	N01 DK062204	Epidemiology of Diabetes Interventions and Complications

Epidemiology of Diabetes Interventions and Complications: Uropathy and Autonomic Neuropathy

	Year	Project No.	Project Title
William Dahms, Case Western Reserve University	1998	N01 DK062203	Coordinating Center - Diabetes Interventions/Complications

Epidemiology of Diabetes Interventions and Complications: Genetics Study

	Year	Project No.	Project Title
William Dahms, Case Western Reserve University	2001	N01 DK062203	Coordinating Center - Diabetes Interventions/Complications
John Lachin, George Washington University	2001	N01 DK062204	Epidemiology of Diabetes Interventions and Complications

Epidemiology of Diabetes Interventions and Complications: Genetics Repository

	Year	Project No.	Project Title
Rutgers University	2006	N01 DK032610	Repository Services for EDIC Genetics

Family Investigation of Nephropathy and Diabetes Study (FIND) (RFA DK99-005)

	Year	Project No.	Project Title
EMMES Corporation	2001	N01 EY062112	Clinical Trials and Statistical Study Monitoring and Coordination
Hanna Abboud, University of Texas Health Sciences Center	2001	U01 DK057295	Genetics of Diabetic Nephropathy in Mexican Americans
Sharon Adler, Harbor-UCLA Research and Education Institute	2001	U01 DK057249	Identification of Diabetic Nephropathy Risk Genes
Robert Elston/Sudha Iyengar, Case Western Reserve University	2004	U01 DK057292	Linkage Consortium for End-Stage Renal Disease
Barry Freedman, Wake Forest University	2001	U01 DK057298	Renal Failure Genes in the Southeastern U.S.
Susanne Nicholas/Mohammed Saad, University of California, Los Angeles	2001	U01 DK057303	Genetics of Diabetic Nephropathy in Hispanics
John Sedor, Case Western Reserve University	2001	U01 DK057329	Genetic Regulation of Renal Disease Progression
Philip Zager, University of New Mexico Albuquerque	2001	U01 DK057300	Zuni Kidney Project- Family Studies

Diabetic Retinopathy Clinical Research Network (RFA EY01-001)

	Year	Project No.	Project Title
Roy Beck, Jaeb Center for Health Research, Inc.	2002	U10 EY014231	Diabetic Macular Edema Clinical Research Network

Animal Models of Diabetic Complications Consortium (RFA DK01-009, HL01-010)

	Year	Project No.	Project Title
Erwin Bottinger, Yeshiva University	2001	U01 DK060995	Mouse Models for Human Diabetic Nephropathy
Matthew Breyer, Vanderbilt University	2004	U01 DK061018	Generating Mouse Mutants with Diabetic Nephropathy
Jan Breslow, Rockefeller University	2001	U01 HL070524	Animal Models of Diabetic Vascular Disease
David Clemmons, University of North Carolina, Chapel Hill	2001	R01 HL069364	Atherosclerosis in Insulin-Resistant, Hyperlipidemic PTS
Thomas Coffman, Duke University	2001	U01 HL070523	Duke-UNC-Stanford AMDC Unit
Willa Hsueh, University of California, Los Angeles	2001	U01 HL070526	Novel Models of Cardiovascular Complications of Diabetes
Donald McClain, University of Utah	2001	U01 HL070525	Animal Models of Diabetic Cardiovascular Complications

Animal Models of Diabetic Complications Consortium (RFA DK05-011)

	Year	Project No.	Project Title
Erwin Bottinger, Yeshiva University	2006	U01 DK060995	Mouse Models for Human Diabetic Nephropathy
Matthew Breyer/Raymond Harris, Vanderbilt University	2006	U01 DK061018	Generating Mouse Mutants with Diabetic Nephropathy
Evan Dale Abel, University of Utah	2006	U01 HL087947	Modeling Diabetic Cardiomyopathy and Microangiopathy
Richard Davis, University of California, Los Angeles	2006	U01 HL087944	Atherosclerosis and other complications in the hyperlipidemic BKS diabetic mouse

	Year	Project No.	Project Title
Kumar Sharma, University of California, San Diego	2006	U01 DK076133	Adiponectin and Nox 4 in Diabetic Kidney Disease
Firouz Daneshagri, Case Western Reserve University	2006	U01 DK076162	Diabetic Uropathy Pathobiology Site
Thomas Coffman, Duke University	2006	U01 DK076136	Angiogenic Signals in Diabetic Complications
Oliver Smithies, University of North Carolina, Chapel Hill	2006	U01 DK076131	Bradykinin, Nitric Oxide and Mitochondrial DNA Damage in Diabetic Complications
Frank Brosius, University of Michigan	2006	U01 DK076139	Recapitulating transcriptional pathways of human diabetic nephropathy in mice
Eva Feldman, University of Michigan	2006	U01 DK076160	Mitochondrial SOD as a Target for Diabetic Neuropathy
Moshe Levi, University of Colorado, Denver	2006	U01 DK076134	Novel Models of Diabetic Nephropathy

Animal Models of Diabetic Complications Consortium: Mouse Metabolic Phenotyping Centers (RFA DK05-008)

	Year	Project No.	Project Title
David Wasserman, Vanderbilt University	2006	U24 DK059637	Vanderbilt Mouse Metabolic Physiology Center
Patrick Tso, University of Cincinnati	2006	U24 DK059630	Cincinnati Mouse Metabolic Phenotyping Center
Renee LeBouef, University of Washington	2006	U24 DK076126	MMPC: Diabetes and Diabetic Complications

Coordinating and Bioinformatics Unit for the Mouse Metabolic Phenotyping Centers and Animal Models of Diabetic Complications Consortium (RFA DK05-012)

	Year	Project No.	Project Title
Richard McIndoe, Medical College of Georgia	2006	U24 DK076169	Coordinating and Bioinformatics Unit for the AMDCC/MMPC

Animal Models of Diabetic Complications Consortium Mouse Generation and Husbandry Core

	Year	Project No.	Project Title
Jackson Laboratories	2007	N01 DK075000	AMDCC Mouse Generation and Husbandry Core

Genetics of Kidneys in Diabetes Study

	Year	Project No.	Project Title
Stacey Gabriel, Massachusetts Institute of Technology	2007	U54 RR020278	An NCRR Center for High Throughput SNP Genotyping and Analysis

Repository Services for Genetics of Kidneys in Diabetes Study

	Year	Project No.	Project Title
Rutgers University	2006	N01 DK032610	Repository Services for GoKinD

Biomarkers for Diabetic Complications (RFA DK06-004)

	Year	Project No.	Project Title
Fred Prior, Washington University	2007	R21 DK079457	Biomarkers for Charcot Arthropathy in Diabetic Patients
Kelvin Davies, Yeshiva University	2007	R21 DK079594	Vcsa1 (hSMR3A) as a Marker for Diabetes
Solomon Tesfaye, Sheffield Teaching Hospital NHS Trust	2007	R21 DK079657	Can dynamic pupillography and/or spectral analysis of heart rate variability prov
Matthias Kretzler, University of Michigan	2007	R21 DK079441	Identification of Biomarkers for Progressive Diabetic Nephropathy
David Sell, Case Western Reserve University	2007	R21 DK079432	Biochemical Nature and Significance of Skin Autofluorescence in Diabetes
Subramaniam Pennathur, University of Michigan	2007	R21 HL092237	Mass Spectrometry platform for Oxidative Biomarker Discovery in Type 1 Diabetes
Ho-Jin Park, Tufts University	2007	R21 DK079622	A Molecular Marker for Cardiac Autonomic Dysfunction

Collaborative Studies on Angiogenesis and Diabetic Complications (RFA DK04-022)

	Year	Project No.	Project Title
Matthew Breyer/Chuan-Ming Hao, Vanderbilt University Medical Center	2005	R01 DK074116	Role of Cyclooxygenase Stimulated Neovascularization in Diabetic Nephropathy
Ambra Pozzi, Vanderbilt University School of Medicine	2005	R01 DK074359	Role of Cyclooxygenase Stimulated Neovascularization in Diabetic Nephropathy
Robert Cohen, University of Cincinnati	2005	R01 DK074361	Endothelial Progenitor Cell Biology in Type 1 Diabetes
Timothy Crombleholme, Cincinnati Children's Hospital	2005	R01 DK074055	Endothelial Progenitor Cell Biology in Type 1 Diabetes
Patricia Parson-Wingerter, NASA Glenn Research Center	2005	R01 EY017529	Vascular Remodeling and Effects of Angiogenic Inhibition in Diabetic Retinopathy
Peter Kaiser, Cleveland Clinic Foundation	2005	R01 EY017528	Vascular Remodeling and Effects of Angiogenic Inhibition in Diabetic Retinopathy
Geoffrey Gurtner, New York University School of Medicine	2005	R01 DK074095	Progenitor Cell Dysfunction and Impaired Vasculogenesis
Michael Brownlee, Albert Einstein College of Medicine	2005	R01 DK074153	Progenitor Cell Dysfunction and Impaired Vasculogenesis

	Year	Project No.	Project Title
Progression of Cardiovascular Disease in Type 1 Diabetes (RFA HL04-013)			
Zixi Cheng, University of Louisville	2004	R01 HL079636	Cardiac Neuropathy in Type 1 Diabetic and Aging Mice
Barry Goldstein, Thomas Jefferson University	2004	R01 DK071360	Adiponectin Improves Vascular Function In High Glucose
Catherine Hedrick, University of Virginia	2004	R01 HL079621	Sphingolipids and Cardiovascular Disease Type I Diabetes
George King, Joslin Diabetes Center	2004	R01 DK071359	PKC Activation and Cardiovascular Disease in Diabetes
William Mayhan, University of Nebraska Medical Center	2004	R01 HL079587	Cerebrovascular Disease in Type 1 Diabetes
Trevor Orchard, University of Pittsburgh	2004	R01 DK071487	Progression of Cardiovascular Disease in TID: CADRE/EDC
Marian Rewers, University of Colorado Health Sciences Center	2004	R01 HL079611	Determinants of Accelerated CVD in Type 1 Diabetes
Ming-Hui Zou, University of Oklahoma	2004	R01 HL079584	Reactive Nitrogen Species and Accelerated Atherosclerosis
Type 1 Diabetes-Rapid Access to Intervention Development (Projects Relevant to Complications)			
Bo Hedlund, Biomedical Frontiers, Inc.	2005	N01 CO12400/ N02 CM27010	Starch-Deferoxamine (S-DFO) for Diabetic Neuropathy
Type 1 Diabetes-Preclinical Testing Program: Preclinical Efficacy in Prevention or Reversal of Diabetic Complications in Rodent Models (RFP DK05-004)			
Nigel Calcutt, University of California, San Diego	2006	N01 DK062889	Preclinical Study of Efficacy in Animal Models of Diabetic Complications
Administrative Supplements for a Drug Screening Program for Diabetic Complications (NOT-DK-05-017)			
Yuqing Chen, University of Michigan	2006	R01 HL068878	PPARgamma and Vascular Lesion Formation
David Clemmons, University of North Carolina, Chapel Hill	2006	R01 HL056850	Mechanisms by which IGF-I Stimulates Smooth Muscle Cells
Michael Brownlee, Yeshiva University	2006	R01 DK033861	Intracellular Glycation and Diabetic Complications
Ross Cagan, Washington University	2006	R21 DK069940	Drosophila Screens for Diabetes and Glucose Toxicity
Royce Mohan, University of Kentucky	2006	R21 NS053593	Novel High Content Vascular Patterning Assay(RMI)
George King, Harvard University	2006	R01 DK071359	PKC Activation and Cardiovascular Disease in Diabetes
Rosario Scalia, Thomas Jefferson University	2006	R01 DK064344	Role of Calpain in Diabetic Endothelial Dysfunction
Fred Levine, University of California, San Diego	2006	R01 DK055283	Growth Versus Differentiation in Human Beta Cells
Friedhelm Schroeder, Texas A&M University	2006	R01 DK041402	Fatty Acid Binding Proteins-Ligand Specificity
Genetics of Diabetic Complications			
Fisher BioServices Inc.	2007	N01 DK032608	
High-Density Genotyping of Diabetes and Diabetic Complications Sample Collections (RFA DK06-005)			
Nancy Cox, University of Chicago	2006	R01 DK077489	Genetic Studies of Diabetic Complications
Andrew Paterson, Hospital for Sick Children	2006	R01 DK077510	Genome-wide association of common alleles with long-term diabetic complications
Andrzej Krolewski, Harvard University	2006	R01 DK077532	Mapping Genes for End-Stage Renal Disease in Type 1 Diabetes
Feasibility Projects To Test Strategies for Preventing or Slowing the Progression of Diabetic Nephropathy (RFA DK02-025)			
Timothy Meyer, Stanford University	2002	R01 DK063011	Maximizing the Benefit of Ras Blockade in Diabetic Nephropathy
Kumar Sharma, Thomas Jefferson University	2002	R01 DK063017	Pirfenidone: Novel Anti-Scarring Therapy for Diabetic Nephropathy
Robert Toto, University of Texas SW Medical Center	2002	R01 DK063010	Improving Outcomes in Diabetic Nephropathy
Surrogate Endpoints for Diabetic Microvascular Complications (RFA DK02-016)			
Paul Beisswenger, Dartmouth College	2002	R01 DK062995	Enzymatic Controls of Nonenzymatic Glycation
Andrew Boulton, Victoria University of Manchester	2002	R01 NS046259	Non-Invasive Surrogate Markers for Diabetic Neuropathy
Robert Cohen, University of Cincinnati	2002	R01 DK063088	The Glycosylation Gap and Diabetic Complications
Jose Halperin, Harvard University Medical School	2002	R01 DK062994	Complement in the Vascular Complications of Diabetes
George King, Joslin Eye Institute	2002	R21 DK063000	Monocyte VEGF and PKC, Markers for Diabetic Complications

	Year	Project No.	Project Title
Oliver Lenz, University of Miami	2002	R21 DK063083	Clonal Selection in Diabetic Nephropathy
Mara Lorenzi, Schepens Eye Research Institute	2002	R01 EY014812	Retinal Blood Flow and Microthrombi in Type 1 Diabetes
Lois Smith, Children's Hospital (Boston)	2002	R21 EY014811	Surrogate Markers for Early Stage Diabetic Retinopathy
Kathryn Thrailkill, Arkansas Children's Hospital	2002	R01 DK062999	Matrix Metalloproteinases and Diabetic Nephropathy
Lance Waller, Emory University	2002	R21 NS046258	Assessing Spatial Patterns of Epidermal Nerve Fibers

Imaging Early Markers of Diabetic Microvascular Complications in Peripheral Tissues (RFA DK02-001)

	Year	Project No.	Project Title
Abass Alavi, University of Pennsylvania	2002	R01 DK063579	FDG-PET Imaging in Complicated Diabetic Foot
Randall Barbour, SUNY Downstate Medical Center	2002	R21 DK063692	Functional Imaging of the Vascular Bed
Pierre Carlier, Laboratoire RMN-CEA-AFM	2002	R21 DK063496	NMR of Muscle Perfusion and Oxygenation in Diabetes
George King, Joslin Diabetes Center	2002	R21 DK063511	Retinal Imaging Tests for Microvascular Functions
Jonathan Lindner, University of Virginia, Charlottesville	2002	R01 DK063508	Contrast Ultrasound and Diabetic Microvascular Disease
Ronald Meyer, Michigan State University	2002	R21 DK063497	Functional MRI of Diabetic Peripheral Vascular Disease

Oral Microbiology/Immunology of Type 1 Diabetes (RFA DE01-001)

	Year	Project No.	Project Title
Ashraf Fouad, University of Connecticut School of Med/Dnt	2001	R21 DE014476	Endodontic Infections in Type 1 Diabetic Hosts
Evanthia Lalla, Columbia University	2001	R21 DE014490	Periodontal Microbiota, Serum Antibody Response, and IDDM
Paul Moore, University of Pittsburgh	2001	R21 DE014472	Microbiology/Immunology of Periodontal Disease in Type 1 Diabetes
Maria Ryan, State University of New York Stony Brook	2001	R21 DE014491	Host Modulation/Periodontal Therapy Effects on Diabetes
Thomas Van Dyke, Boston University	2001	R21 DE014478	Periodontal Inflammation in Type 1 Diabetes

Functional Genomics Approaches to Diabetic Complications - IHWG SNPs: Supplements

	Year	Project No.	Project Title
Maynard Olson, University of Washington	2001	P50 HG002351	Center for the Study of Natural Genetic Variation
Richard Spielman, University of Pennsylvania	2001	R01 HG002386	Genome-Wide Analysis of Genetic Variation and Expression

Neurobiology of Diabetic Complications (RFA NS00-002)

	Year	Project No.	Project Title
Joseph C. Arezzo, Yeshiva University	2000	R01 NS041194	Electrophysiologic Measures in Diabetic Neuropathy
Thomas K. Baumann, Oregon Health Sciences University	2000	R21 NS041157	Dorsal Root Ganglion as Source of Neuropathic Pain
Joseph Beverly, University of Illinois	2000	R01 DK059755	Glucose Mediation of Noradrenergic Activity in VMH
Scott T. Brady, University of Texas SW Medical Center	2000	R01 NS041170	Regulation of Fast Axonal Transport Diabetic Neuropathy
Rick Dobrowsky, University of Kansas Lawrence	2000	R21 DK059749	Role of Caveolin in Schwann Cell Signal Transduction
Charlene Hafer-Macko, University of Maryland Baltimore	2000	R01 DK059758	Endothelial Dysfunction in Human Diabetic Neuropathy
Lynn Heasley, University of Colorado Health Sciences Center	2000	R01 DK059756	MAP Kinases as Mediators of Diabetic Neuropathy
William R. Kennedy, University of Minnesota Twin Cities	2000	R01 NS041163	A Thermal Probe Method for Staging Diabetic Neuropathy
Kathy J. LePard, Midwestern University	2000	R21 NS039768	Synaptic Transmission in Diabetic Enteric Nervous System
Jill Lincoln, University of London	2000	R01 DK058010	Oxidative Stress: Roles in Diabetic Autonomic Neuropathy
Charles V. Mobbs, Mount Sinai School of Medicine	2000	R01 NS041183	Autonomic Diabetic Neuropathy in Mice
Hui-Lin Pan, Pennsylvania State University	2000	R21 NS041178	Spinal Plasticity in Diabetic Neuropathic Pain
Marise B. Parent, Georgia State University Research Foundation	2000	R01 NS041173	Neurochemical and Behavioral Effects of Hyperglycemia
David C. Randall, University of Kentucky Research Foundation	2000	R01 NS039774	Sympathetic Function in Diabetes
Judith A. Richter, Indiana University	2000	R21 NS041162	Hyperglycemia-Induced Neuronal Sensitization
Nancy Tkacs, University of Pennsylvania	2000	R21 DK059754	Counterregulatory Failure and the Arcuate Nucleus
Vickery Trinkaus-Randall, Boston University	2000	R21 DK059753	Role of Growth Factors on Epidermal and Neuronal Injury
Jeffrey Twiss, University of California, Los Angeles	2000	R21 DK059752	Neurotrophic Factor Responsiveness in Diabetic Neuropathy

Pilot Studies for New Therapies for Type 1 Diabetes and Its Complications (RFA DK99-013)

	Year	Project No.	Project Title
Maria Alexander-Bridges, Massachusetts General Hospital	1999	R21 DK057200	DAF16 Homologues and Mediating Complications of Diabetes
Deborah Ellis, Wayne State University	1999	R21 DK057212	Therapy in IDDM Adolescents in Poor Metabolic Control
Patrizia Marchese, Scripps Research Institute	1999	R21 HL065146	Mechanisms of Thrombus Formation in Type 1 Diabetes
N. Nahman, Ohio State University	1999	R21 DK057223	Alpha-Sense of Therapy of Diabetic Glomerulosclerosis
Csaba Szabo, Inotek Corporation	1999	R21 HL065145	Poly Ribose Synthetase and Endothelial Dysfunction
Benjamin Szwergold, Dartmouth College	1999	R21 DK057146	Nonenzymatic Glycation: Enzymatic Mechanism for Control
Helen Vlassara, Mount Sinai School of Medicine	1999	R21 DK057126	Gene Transfer and Diabetic Complications
Ian Zagon, Pennsylvania State University Hershey Medical Center	1999	R21 EY013086	Regulation of Corneal Wound Healing in Type 1 Diabetes

	Year	Project No.	Project Title
Neurological Complications of Diabetes (RFA NS99-005)			
Nigel Calcutt, University of California, San Diego	1999	R01 NS038855	Prosaposin and Prosaptides in Diabetic Neuropathy
Nicole Gibran, University of Washington	1999	R01 DK058007	Diabetic Neuropathy: Implications for Wound Repair
Rolf Gruetter, University of Minnesota	1999	R21 DK058004	In Vivo Studies of Brain Glycogen in Hypoglycemia
Jean Jew, University of Iowa	1999	R01 NS039771	Diabetic Autonomic Neuropathy and Mitral Valve Dysfunction
Phillip Low, Mayo Clinic Rochester	1999	R01 NS039722	Diabetic Autonomic Neuropathy
Anthony McCall, Oregon Health Sciences University	1999	R01 DK058006	Glucocorticoids, Hypoglycemia, and Brain Glucose Transport
Jose Ochoa, Emanual Hospital and Health Center	1999	R01 NS039761	New Approaches to C Nociceptors in Diabetic Neuropathy
Kaushik Patel, University of Nebraska Medical Center	1999	R01 NS039751	Altered Nitric Oxide Mechanisms in PVN During Diabetes
Timothy Raabe, St. Mary's University	1999	R21 NS039748	Role of Neuregulin on Axon/Glia Interactions in Diabetes
Mark Yorek, University of Iowa	1999	R01 DK058005	Vascular Disease in Diabetic Neuropathy
Pathogenesis and Therapy of Complications of Diabetes (RFA DK98-009)			
Evan Abel, Beth Israel Deaconess Medical Center	1998	R21 HL062886	The Role of GLUT4 in the Pathogenesis of Diabetic Cardiomyopathy
Lloyd Aiello, Joslin Diabetes Center	1998	R01 EY012603	Systemic VEGF and Diabetic Retinopathy: Clinical Trials
Mark Alliegro, Louisiana State University	1998	R01 EY012602	Control of VEGF-Stimulated Endothelial Proliferation
Karin Bornfeldt, University of Washington	1998	R01 HL062887	Hyperglycemia, Protein Kinases, and Smooth Muscle Growth
Marshall Corson, University of Washington	1998	R21 HL062885	Endothelial-Fibronectin Interactions in Diabetes
Arup Das, University of New Mexico Albuquerque	1998	R01 EY012604	Extracellular Proteinases in Retinal Neovascularization
Eva Feldman, University of Michigan, Ann Arbor	1998	R01 NS038849	Glucotoxicity Mediates Apoptosis in Diabetic Neuropathy
Martin Friedlander, Scripps Research Institute	1998	R01 EY012599	Cell-Based Ocular Delivery of Anti-Angiogenics for PDR
Kenneth Gabbay, Baylor College of Medicine	1998	R01 DK055137	Species Susceptibility to Diabetic Complications
Gary Gibbons, Brigham and Women's Hospital	1998	R01 HL062884	Diabetic Macrovascular Disease: Role of Apoptosis
Jonathan Glass, Emory University	1998	R01 NS038848	Calpains in the Pathogenesis of Diabetic Neuropathy
Maria Grant, University of Florida	1998	R01 EY012601	Nitric Oxide in the Pathogenesis of Diabetic Retinopathy
Jose Halperin, Harvard University	1998	R01 DK052855	The Role of Complement in the Complications of Diabetes
William Haynes, University of Iowa	1998	R21 NS038846	Sympathetic Neurovascular Function in Diabetes Mellitus
Cinda Helke, Henry M. Jackson Foundation	1998	R01 NS038845	Neurotrophins and Visceral Afferent Neurons in Diabetes
Michael Humphreys-Beher, University of Florida	1998	R01 DE013290	Factor Effects on Oral Complications of Diabetes
Claudia Kappen, Mayo Foundation	1998	R01 HD037804	Molecular Mechanisms in Diabetic Embryopathy
Francis Kappler, Fox Chase Cancer Center	1998	R21 DK055079	Isolation of a Novel Enzymatic Activity
Alexander Ljubimov, Cedars-Sinai Medical Center	1998	R01 EY012605	Growth-Factor Induced Tenascin-C in Diabetic Retinopathy
Jian-Xing Ma, Medical University of South Carolina	1998	R01 EY012600	Retinal Capillaries in Diabetic Retinopathy
Ramesh Nayak, Tufts University	1998	R21 EY012607	Immunogenetic Mechanisms in Diabetic Retinopathy
Ted Reid, Texas Tech University	1998	R21 NS038847	Role of Substance P in Diabetes-Impaired Wound Healing
David Sane, Wake Forest University	1998	R21 HL062891	Role of Vitronectin in the Vascular Complications of Diabetes
Richard Schaeffer, University of Arizona	1998	R01 DK055151	VEGF-Induced Modulation of Endothelial Structure and Function
Gina Schatteman, University of Iowa	1998	R01 DK055965	Adult Angioblasts in Vascular Maintenance and Repair
Richard Spielman, University of Pennsylvania	1998	R01 DK055227	Genetic Studies of Diabetic Nephropathy
James Beach/James Tiedeman, University of Virginia	1998	R01 EY012606	Role of Vascular Autoregulation in Diabetic Retinopathy
Philip Tsao, Stanford University	1998	R01 HL062889	Signaling Mechanisms in Glucose-Induced MCP-1 Expression
Gordon Williams, Brigham and Women's Hospital	1998	R01 HL062888	Mechanisms Underlying Cardiovascular Risks in Diabetes
Douglas Wright, University of Kansas Medical Center	1998	R21 NS038844	GDNF and Nociceptive Primary Sensory Neurons in Diabetes
Development of Clinical Markers for Kidney Disease: Supplements			
Erwin Bottinger, Yeshiva University	2001	U24 DK058768	Albert Einstein Biotechnology Center
Alfred George, Vanderbilt University	2001	U24 DK058749	Vanderbilt NIDDK Biotechnology Center
Steven Gullans, Brigham and Women's Hospital	2001	U24 DK058849	DNA Microarray Biotechnology Center
Raymond Harris, Vanderbilt University	2001	P50 DK039261	Biology of Progressive Destruction
Arthur Matas, University of Minnesota	2001	P01 DK013083	Organ Transplantation in Animals and Man
Richard Quigg, University of Chicago	2001	U24 DK058820	Massively Parallel Gene Expression Analysis
John Sedor, Case Western Reserve University	2001	P50 DK054178	CWRU O'Brien Renal Research Center
Development of Surrogate Markers for Clinical Trials: Supplement			
Christopher Bradfield, University of Wisconsin	2001	R01 ES005703	Characterization of the AH Receptor Signaling Pathway

	Year	Project No.	Project Title

One Year Supplements for Ongoing Projects

	Year	Project No.	Project Title
Robert Eckel, University of Colorado Health Sciences Center	1998	R01 DK042266	Nutrition, Lipoprotein Lipase, and Body Weight Regulation
Martin Friedlander, Scripps Research Institute	1998	R01 EY011254	Integrins and Ocular Angiogenesis
Anthony Iacopino, Texas A & M Baylor College of Dentistry	1998	R29 DE011553	Impaired Wound Signaling in Diabetic Periodontitis
Timothy Kern, Case Western Reserve University	1998	R01 EY000300	Diabetic Retinopathy
George King, Joslin Diabetes Center	1998	R01 EY005110	Cell Biology Approach to Diabetic Retinopathy
Trevor Orchard, University of Pittsburgh	1998	R01 DK034818	Epidemiology of Diabetic Complications
Ann Schmidt, Columbia University	1998	R01 DE011561	Glycation, Receptors, Cytokines in Periodontal Disease
William Tamborlane, Yale University	1998	R01 HD030671	Effects of Puberty on Metabolism and Body Composition
Russell Tracy, University of Vermont and St. Agric College	1998	R01 HL058329	Epidemiology of Impaired Coagulant Balance in Diabetes

GOAL VI: ATTRACT NEW TALENT AND APPLY NEW TECHNOLOGIES TO RESEARCH ON TYPE 1 DIABETES

Training Programs in Diabetes Research for Pediatric Endocrinologists (RFA DK02-024)

	Year	Project No.	Project Title
Silva Arslanian, Children's Hospital of Pittsburgh	2003	T32 DK063686	Research and Academic Training in Pediatric Diabetes
		K12 DK063704	Academic Career Development in Pediatric Diabetes (K12)
Morey Haymond, Baylor College of Medicine	2002	T32 DK063873	Baylor Pediatric Diabetes Research Training Program
		K12 DK063691	Baylor Mentored Diabetes Investigator Award
Georgeanna Klingensmith, University of Colorado Health Sciences Center	2002	T32 DK063687	Training Program in Diabetes Research
		K12 DK063722	Diabetes Research for Pediatric Endocrinologists
Lori Laffel/Joseph Majzoub, Joslin Diabetes Center	2002	T32 DK063702	Training Grant in Diabetes for Pediatric Endocrinologists
		K12 DK063696	Career Development in Diabetes for Pediatric Endocrinologists
Charles Stanley, Children's Hospital (Philadelphia)	2002	T32 DK063688	Ped Endocrine Fellowship Training in Diabetes Research
		K12 DK063682	Ped Endocrine Career Development in Diabetes Research
William Tamborlane, Yale University	2002	T32 DK063703	Training in Pediatric Endocrinology/Diabetes Research
		K12 DK063709	Pediatric Endocrine/Diabetes Physician Scientists
Neil White, Washington University, St. Louis	2003	T32 DK063706	Fellowship Training in Pediatric Diabetes at WUMS
		K12 DK063683	Career Development in Pediatric Diabetes at WUMS

Innovative Partnerships in Type 1 Diabetes (RFA DK02-023)

	Year	Project No.	Project Title
Pamela Carmines, University of Nebraska Medical Center	2002	R21 DK063416	Renal Cortical Oxidative and Nitrosative Stress in IDDM
Alexander Chervonsky, The Jackson Laboratory	2002	R21 DK063452	Role of Innate Immunity in Type 1 Diabetes
Craig Crews, Yale University	2002	R21 DK063404	Pancreatic Stem Cell Induction by Small Molecules
Maria Grant, University of Florida	2002	R21 EY014818	CXCR4/SDF-1 Axis in Proliferation of Diabetic Retinopathy
Wayne Hancock, Children's Hospital (Philadelphia)	2002	R21 DK063591	Modulation of Chemokine-Dependent Islet Injury
William Langridge, Loma Linda University	2002	R21 DK063576	Vaccinia Virus Vaccine for Type 1 Diabetes
Sigurd Lenzen, Hannover Medical School	2002	R21 AI055464	Pathophysiological and Genetic Characterization of IDDM Rats
Diane Mathis, Joslin Diabetes Center	2002	R21 DK063660	Diabetes Susceptibility Genes through Zebrafish Genetics
Jaime Modiano, AMC Cancer Research Center	2002	R21 DK063410	Role of Negative Regulation in Development of Diabetes
Marcus Peter, University of Chicago	2002	R21 AI055465	Fas Internalization and Beta Cells
Alvin Powers, Vanderbilt University	2002	R21 DK063439	Molecular Determinants of Vascularization in Islets
Marian Rewers, University of Colorado Health Sciences Center	2002	R21 AI055466	Viral Triggers of Type 1 Diabetes
Alexander Rudensky, University of Washington	2002	R21 AI055463	Role of Cathepsins S, L, and B in Type 1 Diabetes
Doris Stoffers, University of Pennsylvania	2002	R21 DK063467	cAMP Signaling in the Pancreatic Beta Cell
Michael Uhler, University of Michigan, Ann Arbor	2002	R21 DK063340	Postgenomic Approaches to Diabetic Complications
Elena Zhukova, University of California, Los Angeles	2002	R21 DK063607	Models of Insulin Production in Enteroendocrine Cells

Innovative Partnerships in Type 1 Diabetes (RFA DK03-015)

	Year	Project No.	Project Title
Stelios Andreadis, State University of New York at Buffalo	2004	R01 DK068699	Regulated Insulin Delivery From Tissue Engineered Skin for Treatment of Type 1 Diabetes
David Antonetti, Pennsylvania State University	2004	R01 EY016413	Drug Discovery for Diabetic Retinopathy
Anil Bhushan, University of Southern California	2004	R01 DK068763	Cell Cycle Control of Beta-Cell Mass
Jeffery Chalmers, Ohio State University	2004	R01 DK068757	Magnetic Separation of Liberated Islets During Isolation
Gay Crooks, Children's Hospital, Los Angeles	2004	R01 DK068719	Cell Cycle Control of B-Cell Mass
Nika Danial/Stanley Korsmeyer, Dana Farber Cancer Institute	2004	R01 DK068781	Dissecting the Death Pathway in the Islet beta cell
Teresa Dilorenzo, Albert Einstein College of Medicine	2004	R01 AI064422	Prevention of Diabetes with Lipid Immunomodulators
Francis Doyle, University of California, Santa Barbara	2004	R01 DK068706	A Run-to-Run Algorithm for Glucose Regulation

	Year	Project No.	Project Title
John Gore, Vanderbilt Universtiy	2004	R01 DK068751	Pancreatic Islet Imaging and Blood Flow
Kevan Herold, Columbia University	2004	R01 DK068678	Islet Growth in NOD Mice Tolerant to Autoimmune Diabetes
Lois Jovanovic, Sansum Medical Research Institute	2004	R01 DK068663	A Run-to-Run Algorithm for Glucose Regulation
Keith Kirkwood, University of Michigan	2004	R01 DK068673	Regulated Insulin Delivery From Tissue Engineered Skin for Treatment of Type 1 Diabetes
Rohit Kulkarni, Joslin Diabetes Center	2004	R01 DK068721	Dissecting the Death Pathway in Islet Beta Cells
Suzanne Laychock, State University of New York at Buffalo	2004	R01 DK068700	Regulated Insulin Delivery From Tissue Engineered Skin for Type 1 Diabetes
Fred Levine, University of California, San Diego	2004	R01 DK068754	Small Molecular Regulation of Beta-Cell Differentiation
Mark Mercola, Burnham Institute	2004	R01 DK068715	Small Molecule Regulators of Beta-Cell Differentiation
Virginia Papaioannou, Columbia University	2004	R01 DK068661	Islet Growth in NOD Mice Tolerant to Autoimmune Diabetes
Klearchos Papas, University of Minnesota	2004	R01 DK068717	Magnetic Separation of Liberated Islets During Isolation
Steven Porcelli, Albert Einstein College of Medicine	2004	R01 AI064424	Prevention of Diabetes with Lipid Immunomodulators
Alvin Powers, Vanderbilt University	2004	R01 DK068764	Pancreatic Islet Imaging and Blood Flow
Charles Smith, Pennsylvania State University	2004	R01 EY016448	Drug Discovery for Diabetic Retinopathy
Richard Young, Whitehead Institute for Biomedical Research	2004	R01 DK068655	Transcriptional Regulatory Networks in Pancreatic Islets

Bench to Bedside Research on Type 1 Diabetes (RFA DK02-022)

	Year	Project No.	Project Title
Christophe Benoist, Joslin Diabetes Center	2002	R21 AI055467	High Sensitivity Detection of Autoimmune T Cells in Type 1 DM
David Bleich, Beckman Research Institute	2002	R21 DK063351	Prevention of Type 1 Diabetes with MMP Inhibitors
Michael Clare-Salzler, University of Florida	2002	R21 DK063422/ R33 DK063422	Dendritic Cells and the Prevention of Type 1 Diabetes
C. Fathman, Stanford University	2002	R21 AI055468/ R33 AI055468	Adoptive Cellular Gene Therapy in Type 1 Diabetes
Peter Gottlieb, University of Colorado Health Sciences Center	2002	R21 DK063518	Human TCR/HLA Transgenic Mice to Prevent Type 1 Diabetes
Zhiguang Guo, University of Minnesota	2002	R21 AI055469	A Strategy to Cure Type 1 Diabetes
Kevin Lemley, Stanford University	2002	R21 DK063456	Urinary Podocyte Excretion Using FACS Methodology
Jerry Nadler, University of Virginia, Charlottesville	2002	R21 DK063521	New Anti-Inflammatory Agents to Prevent Damage to Islets
Gerald Nepom, Virginia Mason Research Center	2002	R21 DK063423	Treatment of Type 1 Diabetes with hGAD65 Altered Peptide Ligand
David Sachs, Massachusetts General Hospital	2002	R21 DK063503	Islet-Kidney Transplants for Treatment of Diabetic ESRD
Massimo Trucco, Children's Hospital (Pittsburgh)	2002	R21 DK063499/ R33 DK063499	Gene-Engineered Dendritic Cell Therapy for Diabetics

Bench to Bedside Research on Type 1 Diabetes (RFA DK03-001)

	Year	Project No.	Project Title
Sofia Casares, Mount Sinai School of Medicine	2003	R21 DK066421	HLA Chimeric-Based Interventions in Type 1 Diabetes
Alessio Fasano, University of Maryland	2003	R21 DK066630	Gut Permeability in the Pathogenesis of Type 1 Diabetes
Ronald Gill, University of Colorado Health Sciences Center	2003	R21 AI060349	Correcting Dysregulated Peripheral Tolerance in NOD Mice
Raimund Hirschberg, University of California, Los Angeles	2003	R21 DK063360	Prevention of Diabetic Nephropathy by BMP7
Jian-Xing Ma, University of Oklahoma Health Sciences Center	2003	R21 EY015650/ R33 EY015650	A New Therapy for Diabetic Macular Edema
Alvin Powers, Vanderbilt University	2003	R21 DK066636/ R33 DK066636	GLP-1 to Enhance Islet Transplantation
Bellur Prabhakar, University of Illinois at Chicago	2003	R21 AI060386	Induction of Tolerance to Islet Cell Transplants
Nora Sarvetnik, Scripps Research Institute	2003	R21 DK066511	Engraftment of Pancreatic Progenitors
Andrew Shapiro, University of Alberta	2003	R21 DK066512	ICOS-B7h in Islet Transplant Rejection and Autoimmunity
Andrew Stewart, University of Pittsburgh	2003	R33 DK066127	Islet Allograft Gene Therapy for Primate Diabetes

Bench to Bedside Research on Type 1 Diabetes (RFA DK03-019)

	Year	Project No.	Project Title
Sridevi Devaraj, University of California, Davis	2004	R21 DK069801	Cellular Pathways of Inflammation in Type 1 Diabetes
Francis Doyle, University of California, Santa Barbara	2004	R21 DK069833	Model-Based Advanced Control of Insulin in T1DM
Kevan Herold, Columbia University	2004	R21 DK069872	Combination of Anti-CD3 and Ag-Specific Immunotherapy
Daniel Kaufman, University of California, Los Angeles	2004	R21 DK069839	Noninvasive PET Imaging of Islet Grafts
David Kurnit, University of Michigan	2004	R21 DK069877	Detection and Treatment of Nephropathy in DM Type 1
Timothy Lyons, University of Oklahoma Health Sciences Center	2004	R21 HL080921	Apolipoproteins and the Complications of Type 1 Diabetes
Ali Naji, University of Pennsylvia	2004	R33 AI065356	B Cell Immunomodulation in Islet Transplantation
David Sachs, Massachusetts General Hospital	2004	R33 DK069827	Islet-Kidney Transplants for Treatment of Diabetic ESRD
Jin-Xiong She, Medical College of Georgia	2004	R21 DK069878	Development of Microarray-Based Biomarkers for Type 1 Diabetes
Rusung Tan, BC's Children's Hospital	2004	R21 AI065179	Detecting Beta Cell Specific T Cells in Type 1 Diabetes
Ian Zagon, Pennsylvania State University	2004	R21 EY016666	Naltrexone as a Novel Treatment for Diabetic Keratopathy

	Year	Project No.	Project Title
Type 1 Diabetes Pathfinder Award (RFA DK08-001)			
Brian Brown, Mount Sinai School of Medicine of NYU	2008	DP2 DK083052	Novel Strategy to Induce Islet Protective Regulatory T Cells and Prevent Diabetes
Deyu Fang, Northwestern University	2008	DP2 DK083050	A Novel Target for Type 1 Diabetes
John Hollander, West Virginia University	2008	DP2 DK083095	Mechanisms of Diabetic Cardiomyopathy: Mitochondria Subpopulations Brought to Foc
Kenneth Liechty, University of Mississippi	2008	DP2 DK083085	Extracellular matrix structure and function in diabetic wound healing
Xunrong Luo, Northwestern University	2008	DP2 DK083099	ECDI Coupled Cells for Tolerance in Allogeniec Islet Cell Transplantation for T1D
Edward Mitre, Uniformed Services University of Health Sciences	2008	DP2 DK083131	Protection against Type I diabetes by parasitic helminths
Cherie Stabler, University of Miami	2008	DP2 DK083096	Functionalized, Nanoscale Coatings for Islet Encapsulation
Ben Stanger, University of Pennsylvania	2008	DP2 DK083111	An *In Vivo* Approach to Cell-Based Therapy for Type 1 Diabetes
Bridget Wagner, Massachusetts Institute of Technology	2008	DP2 DK083048	Small-molecule approaches to restore glycemic control in type 1 diabetes
Xingxing Zang, Yeshiva University	2008	DP2 DK083076	New T Cell Coinhibitory Pathway and Type 1 Diabetes
SBIR and STTR RFA in Type 1 Diabetes and Its Complications (RFA DK03-020)			
William Beschorner, Ximerex, Inc.	2004	R44 DK057986	Islet Transplantation with Chimeric Donor Pigs
John Centanni, Stratatech Corporation	2004	R44 DK069924	Antimicrobial, Angiogenic Skin Substitutes for Diabetic Ulcers
Jenny Freeman, HyperMed, Inc.	2004	R41 DK069871	Hyperspectral Imaging to Predict and Assess Foot Ulcers
Joseph Lucisano, Glysens, Inc.	2004	R44 EB005174	Robust Signal Processing for Tissue Glucose Sensor
Uwe Staerz, Isogenis, Inc.	2004	R43 DK069618	Protecting Pancreatic Islet Grafts from Rejection
Rebecca Tirabassi, Biomedical Research Models, Inc.	2004	R43 DK069733	Neurogenic Compounds for Treating Diabetic Complications
John Wilson, Wilson Wolf Manufacturing Corp.	2004	R43 DK069865	Islet Culture, Shipping, and Infusion Device
Todd Zion, Smartcells, Inc.	2004	R43 DK069870	Glucose-Responsive Self-Regulated Insulin Delivery
SBIR: Measurement Tools For Altered Autonomic Function In Spinal Cord Injury And Diabetes (RFA HD04-018)			
Firouz Daneshgari, Neurotron, Inc.	2005	R41 DK074987	Assessment of Altered Function in Diabetic Bladder
SBIR and STTR: New Therapeutics and Monitoring Technologies for Type 1 Diabetes and its Complications (RFA DK05-015, DK05-016)			
Robert Van Buskirk, Cell Preservation Services Inc.	2006	R43 DK077240	Improving Pancreas/Islets Preservation HTS/CryoStor
Shay Soker, Plureon Corporation	2006	R41 DK077256	Cell therapy of diabetes using broad spectrum multipotent stem cells
Mark Arnold, ASL Analytical	2007	R41 DK077252	Noninvasive Nocturnal Hypoglycemic Alarm
Joseph Lucisano, GlySens, Inc.	2007	R43 DK077254	Pre-Clinical Validation & Ultimate Lifetime of Long Term Implanted Glucose Sensor
Ernest Guignon, Ciencia, Inc.	2007	R43 DK077291	MHC Array T Cell Assay System for Monitoring Immune Status in Type 1 Diabetes
Cathy Swindlehurst, NovoMedix	2007	R43 DK077285	Discovery and Development of Compounds to Enhance b-cell Number and Function
Todd Zion, SmartCells, Inc.	2007	R43 DK077292	Multimeric RNA Aptamers for Glucose-Responsive Insulin Formulations
Uwe Staerz, Isogenis, Inc.	2006	R44 DK069618	Protecting Pancreatic Islet Grafts from Rejection
Omnibus Solicitation of the NIH, CDC, and FDA for Small Business Innovation Research Grant Applications (Parent SBIR [R43/R44]) (PA07-280, PA07-281)			
William Beschorner, Ximerex, Inc.	2008	R43 DK082122	Ex Vivo Induction of Tolerance for Autoimmune Diabetes
Meera Saxena, Luminomics Inc.	2009	R41 DK082060	Type I Diabetes Model in Zebrafish
Omnibus Solicitation of the NIH for Small Business Technology Transfer Grant Applications (Parent STTR [R41/R42]) (PA08-051)			
Michael Weiss, Thermalin Diabetes Incorporated	2009	R41 DK081292	Clinical Testing of an Insulin Analog

	Year	Project No.	Project Title

SBIR and STTR: New Therapeutics and Monitoring Technologies for Type 1 Diabetes and its Complications (RFA DK09-001)

	Year	Project No.	Project Title
Joseph Lucisano, GlySens, Inc.	2009	R43 DK077254	Pre-Clinical Validation & Ultimate Lifetime of Long Term Implanted Glucose Sensor
Ioannis Tomazos, Biorasis, Inc.	2009	R43 EB011886	Needle-Implantable, Wireless Multi-Sensor for Continuous Glucose Monitoring
Ralph Ballerstadt, Biotex, Inc.	2009	R43 DK085892	Assay for Monitoring Glycemic Control in Diabetics
David Vachon, Aegis Biosciences LLC	2009	R43 DK085957	Novel Approaches to Extending Glucose Sensor Lifespan

SBIR: Innovative Patient Outreach Programs and Ocular Screening Technologies to Improve Detection of Diabetic Retinopathy (RFA EY09-001)

	Year	Project No.	Project Title
Peter Soliz, Visionquest Biomedical LLC	2009	R43 EY020015	Automated Diabetic Retinopathy Screening System
Matthew Muller, Aeon Imaging, LLC	2009	R44 EY020017	System for Increasing Patient Access to Eye Exams for Diabetic Retinopathy
Kevin Hsu, Micron Optics, Inc.	2009	R44 EY017212	OCT Imaging of Diabetic Retinopathy in 1060nm Spectral Range
Gary Gregory, Advanced Diagnostics, LLC	2009	R43 EY020028	Innovative Systems & Educational Tools to Advance an Established Diabetic Retinopathy
Randal Chinnock, Optimum Technologies, Inc.	2009	R43 EY020034	Easy-to-Use, Low-Cost, Handheld Retinal Camera for Screening for Diabetic Retinopathy

Proteomics and Metabolomics in Type 1 Diabetes and Its Complications (RFA DK03-024)

	Year	Project No.	Project Title
M. Amin Arnaout/Darryl Palmer-Toy, Massachusetts General Hospital	2004	R21 DK070212	Metabolomic Analysis of Type 1 Diabetic Nephropathy
Helene Bour-Jordan, University of California, San Francisco	2004	R21 NS052132	Autoimmune Basis of Diabetic Neuropathy
Mark Chance, Albert Einstein College of Medicine	2004	R21 DK070229	Proteomic Approaches to Type I Diabetes Progression
Paul Harris, Columbia University	2004	R21 DK070192	Soluble Protein Markers of T1D Progression
Kathryn Haskins, University of Colorado Health Sciences Center	2004	R21 AI065355	Proteomics Analysis of T Cell Autoantigens in TID2
Michael Mauer, University of Minnesota	2004	R21 DK070210	Proteomics in Type 1 Diabetes and its Complications
Sreekumaran Nair, Mayo Clinic	2004	R21 DK070179	Plasma Protein Synthesis and Abundance in T1 Diabetes
Mark Nicolls, University of Colorado	2004	R21 DK070203	Viability Assay for Human Islet Transplantation
Jin-Xiong She, Medical College of Georgia	2004	R21 HD050196	Proteomic Changes/Progression of Human Type 1 Diabetes
Richard Smith, Battelle Pacific Northwest National Laboratory	2004	R21 DK070146	Proteomics and Metabolomics Studies of Type 1 Diabetes
Forest White, Massachusetts Institute of Technology	2004	R21 AI065354	Proteomics of Central Tolerance in NOD vs B6 Mice

Phased Innovation Partnerships - Supplements to Centers

	Year	Project No.	Project Title
Yaakov Barak, University of Massachusetts Medical School	2001	P30 DK032520	PPAR Gamma KO and Insulin Resistance
Giacomo Basadonna, Yale University	2001	P30 DK045735	Glucose Responsive Transgene
James Callis, University of Washington	2001	P30 DK017047	Islet Purification
Shaoping Deng, University of Pennsylvania	2001	P30 DK019525	Gene Therapy with PDX
Denise Faustman, Massachusetts General Hospital	2001	P30 DK057521	TNF Apoptosis
Eva Feldman, University of Michigan, Ann Arbor	2001	P60 DK020572	Postgenomic Approaches to Complications
Yang-Xin Fu, University of Chicago	2001	P60 DK020595	Lymphotoxin
Mark Geraci, University of Colorado Health Sciences Center	2001	P30 DK057516	RNA Profile of Islet Development
Wouter Hoff, University of Chicago	2001	P60 DK020595	Glucose Sensing Fusion Proteins
Shin-Ichiro Imai, University of Washington	2001	P30 DK017047	Sir2a in Beta Cell Differentiation
Klaus Kaestner, University of Pennsylvania	2001	P30 DK019525	Islet Stem Cells
Myra Lipes, Joslin Diabetes Center	2001	P30 DK036836	Optimize Gene Expression in Surrogate Beta Cells
Diane Mathis, Joslin Diabetes Center	2001	P30 DK036836	Imaging Inflammation
Ruslan Medzhitov, Yale University	2001	P30 DK045735	Innate Immunity in Type 1 Diabetes
Mark Nicolls, University of Colorado Health Sciences Center	2001	P30 DK057516	Proteomics and Transplantation

	Year	Project No.	Project Title
William Osborne, University of Washington	2001	P30 DK017047	Glucose Regulated Insulin Delivery
Sunhee Park, University of Massachusetts Medical School	2001	P30 DK032530	ART2 Ligands
Alvin Powers, Vanderbilt University	2001	P60 DK020593	*In Vivo* Assessment of Transplanted Islets
Alexander Rudensky, University of Washington	2001	P30 DK017047	Cathespins
Jaromir Ruzicka, University of Washington	2001	P30 DK017047	GAD Assay
Harry Shamoon, Yeshiva University	2001	P60 DK020541	Liver Glycogen Metabolism/Hypoglycemia
Li Wen, Yale University	2001	P30 DK045735	Dendritic Cell Therapy
Burton Wice, University of Washington	2001	P30 DK017047	Gut Stem Cells
John Wiley, University of Michigan, Ann Arbor	2001	P60 DK020572	Neuropathy
Kelvin Yamada, University of Washington	2001	P30 DK017047	Hypoglycemia

Type 1 Diabetes Pilot & Feasibility Studies Through Diabetes Centers

	Year	Project No.	Project Title
Aldo Rossini, University of Massachusetts Medical School	2006	P30 DK032520	Diabetes Endocrinology Research Center
Willa Hsueh, University of California, Los Angeles	2006	P30 DK063491	Diabetes Endocrinology Research Center
Robert Sherwin, Yale University	2006	P30 DK045735	Diabetes Endocrinology Research Center
William Herman, University of Michigan	2006	P60 DK020572	Michigan Diabetes Research and Training Center

Description of Non-consortia Research Efforts Supported by the Special Diabetes Program (FY 2006-2009)

In addition to supporting numerous consortia focused on type 1 diabetes and its complications, which are discussed in the main section of this document and in Appendix C, funds for the *Special Diabetes Program* were deployed to support numerous other initiatives. These initiatives have promoted a broad spectrum of research projects in areas identified as of particular opportunity or challenge to complement the efforts of the research consortia. This Appendix includes descriptions of non-consortia initiatives from March 1, 2006 through September 30, 2009. Initiatives released prior to March 1, 2006 can be found in the 2007 *"Evaluation Report"* on the *Special Diabetes Program* (http://www.T1Diabetes.nih.gov/evaluation).

Goal I: Identify the Genetic and Environmental Causes of Type 1 Diabetes

Fine Mapping and Function of Genes for Type 1 Diabetes (DP3) RFA DK-08-006

This program brings together investigators with experience in genetics, immunology, and biochemistry to pinpoint the exact genes in regions of DNA that are known to influence type 1 diabetes and to study their biological role in health and disease. This research may allow future health care to be more personalized, based on a patient's genetic profile. Grants were awarded in 2009.

Goal II: Prevent or Reverse Type 1 Diabetes

Agents To Be Tested for Pre-clinical Efficacy in Prevention or Reversal of Type 1 Diabetes in Rodent Models. Type 1 Diabetes Pre-clinical Testing Program (T1D-PTP) RFP DK-05-05

This Pre-clinical Testing Program was established to provide the means to perform pre-clinical efficacy testing of promising agents for type 1 diabetes prevention or reversal. The program is supporting the Type 1 Diabetes-Rapid Access to Intervention Development (T1D-RAID) program, which independently provides more advanced pre-clinical studies and drug manufacturing services, and for which a need to test compounds after manufacturing was predicted. In addition, the contract is supporting NIH clinical trials networks considering drug therapies deemed promising for clinical development, but which require additional pre-clinical testing in animals. Finally, the scientific community has been invited to propose promising drug candidates that require additional animal testing (http://grants.nih.gov/grants/guide/notice-files/NOT-DK-09-006.html).

Testing for Pre-clinical Efficacy in Prevention or Reversal of Diabetic Complications in Rodent Models RFP DK-05-04

The objective of this contract is to support NIDDK in its mission to develop safe and effective drugs for the prevention and treatment of the complications of diabetes. The contractor performs pre-clinical studies of potential new therapeutics for the prevention or treatment of diabetic complications. The contract assesses the efficacy of new drugs that are under consideration for further development by the T1D-RAID program, and new drugs being developed by the diabetes complications research community at-large (http://grants.nih.gov/grants/guide/notice-files/NOT-DK-09-009.html).

Biomarkers of Autoimmunity in Type 1 Diabetes (R21) RFA DK-06-002

This initiative was developed to promote progress in the development of biomarkers of autoimmunity in type 1 diabetes, which are critically needed in three areas: to predict disease risk; to monitor disease initiation or progression in people at high risk for developing the disease; and to monitor autoimmune responses during therapeutic intervention. Grants were awarded in 2006.

Goal III: Develop Cell Replacement Therapy

Toward Imaging the Pancreatic Beta Cell in People (R01) RFA DK-06-003

The ability to image or otherwise directly monitor beta cells in people would greatly enhance understanding of the causes and progression of diabetes and the life cycle of the islet. Furthermore, it would also improve the ability of clinicians to study the beta cell in human health and disease, as well as to monitor therapy, particularly islet transplantation. This initiative was designed to provide resources to propel research progress on imaging the pancreatic beta cell, beta cell function, or inflammation *in vivo*, using approaches that would be clinically applicable. Grants were awarded in 2006.

Goal IV: Prevent or Reduce Hypoglycemia in Type 1 Diabetes

Small Business Innovation Research To Develop New Therapeutics and Monitoring Technologies for Type 1 Diabetes Towards an Artificial Pancreas (SBIR [R43/R44]) RFA DK-09-001

Clinical trials have demonstrated significant reductions in rates of complications of type 1 diabetes through intensive control of blood glucose levels. However, despite the availability of increasingly effective treatments, a substantial proportion of people with type 1 diabetes cannot achieve optimal blood glucose control despite enormous efforts. A promising therapeutic option for the treatment of diabetes is a system (termed an artificial pancreas or closed-loop) that can mimic normal pancreatic beta cell function. However, important technological obstacles exist, such as glucose-sensing inaccuracies, imperfect algorithms for calculating the appropriate dose of insulin taking into consideration diet and physical activity, insulin pump mechanical problems, time delay from subcutaneous insulin infusion to pharmacologic effect, and biocompatibility issues that impede a long-term use of invasive or minimally invasive devices. The broad scope of this solicitation encompassed research to further address these obstacles. Grants were awarded in 2009.

Closed-Loop Technologies: Clinical and Behavioral Approaches To Improve Type 1 Diabetes Outcomes (R01) RFA DK-08-012

Closed-Loop Technologies: Pilot and Exploratory Clinical and Behavioral Approaches To Improve Type 1 Diabetes Outcomes (R21) RFA DK-08-013

These programs support development of tools for glucose sensing and insulin delivery in order to provide automated glucose control. These studies are focused on enhancing the application of new technology to improve glucose control and reduce hypoglycemia in people with type 1 diabetes by considering clinical and behavioral factors that may enhance or constrain their sustained use. Grants were awarded in 2009.

Goal V: Prevent or Reduce the Complications of Type 1 Diabetes

Innovative Patient Outreach Programs and Ocular Screening Technologies To Improve Detection of Diabetic Retinopathy (SBIR [R43/R44]) RFA EY-09-001

Diabetes is the leading cause of blindness in working age adults in the United States.[29] This program supports the development of: (1) educational outreach programs to create a greater awareness of the risk of diabetic retinopathy in people with type 1 and type 2 diabetes; and (2) tools and systems to be used for increasing patient access to eye exams for detecting diabetic retinopathy. Grants were awarded in 2009.

High-density Genotyping of Diabetes and Diabetic Complications Sample Collections (R01) RFA DK-06-005

This initiative supports large-scale studies using samples from the Diabetes Control and Complications Trial (DCCT)/Epidemiology of Diabetes Interventions and Complications (EDIC) study or the Genetics of Kidneys in Diabetes (GoKinD) study to identify genes and specific genetic variants that confer susceptibility or resistance to diabetic complications. Grants were awarded in 2006.

Biomarker Development for Diabetic Complications (R21) RFA DK-06-004

Recent advances in understanding the mechanisms of diabetic complications have led to the potential development of new therapeutics that delay or reverse the complications. A significant obstacle in developing drugs that modulate these targets is the paucity of biomarkers for diabetic complications. Biomarkers are needed as surrogate end-points for pilot studies on new therapeutics. Biomarkers could also be used in patient care to determine an individual's risk of developing certain complications and response to interventions. This initiative supports studies to develop and validate biomarkers and surrogate endpoints for the complications of diabetes. Grants were awarded in 2007.

---

[29] Centers for Disease Control and Prevention. National diabetes fact sheet: national estimates and general information on diabetes and prediabetes in the United States 2011. Atlanta, GA: U.S. Department of Health and Human Services, Centers for Disease Control and Prevention, 2011.

Goal VI: Attract New Talent and Apply New Technologies to Research on Type 1 Diabetes

Type 1 Diabetes Pathfinder Award (DP2)
RFA DK-08-001

The Type 1 Diabetes Pathfinder Award supports exceptional new investigators who proposed highly innovative new research approaches that have the potential to produce a major impact on important problems in biomedical and behavioral research related to type 1 diabetes and its complications. Grants were awarded in 2008.

Small Business Innovation Research To Develop New Therapeutics and Monitoring Technologies for Type 1 Diabetes and its Complications (SBIR [R43/R44])
RFA DK-05-016

Small Business Technology Transfer To Develop New Therapeutics and Monitoring Technologies for Type 1 Diabetes and its Complications (STTR [R41/R42])
RFA DK-05-015

These parallel initiatives support innovative research on type 1 diabetes and its complications in the biotechnology industry. Grants were awarded in 2006.

APPENDIX B

ASSESSMENT OF THE *SPECIAL STATUTORY FUNDING PROGRAM FOR TYPE 1 DIABETES RESEARCH*

EVALUATION OBJECTIVES

In designating special set-aside funds to "provide for research into the prevention and cure of type 1 diabetes," the Congress recognized the opportunity to finally overcome this devastating, long-standing disease and its complications. The intent of this congressionally mandated evaluation report is not only to highlight and assess the significant progress made by the *Special Statutory Funding Program for Type 1 Diabetes Research* (*Special Diabetes Program* or *Program*) toward this goal, but also to describe and analyze the innovative process by which the U.S. Department of Health and Human Services (HHS) approached this challenge. The multipronged scientific structure of the *Program*; the establishment of large collaborative research consortia and clinical trials networks; the incentives to promote high-risk, pioneering research; and the major investments in translational research, clinical investigator training, scientific infrastructure, and technology and resource development represent a significant departure from traditional mechanisms of funding smaller-scale research in type 1 diabetes. This appendix describes the multiple evaluation approaches used to assess the scientific and clinical outcomes of the research; it also explains the decision process used in developing the scientific emphases and allocating the resources of the *Special Diabetes Program*.

This evaluation has been guided by the following questions:

- What impact has the *Special Diabetes Program* made on the field of type 1 diabetes? How has the field progressed since the *Program's* inception?

- What objective measures can be used to benchmark the progress of the *Special Diabetes Program*, both scientifically and programmatically?

- To what extent has the scientific progress already benefited patients, and what additional anticipated outcomes could affect the lives of patients living with the disease or at risk of developing it?

- How appropriate is the scientific focus of the *Special Diabetes Program* and to what extent has the program been able to adapt to emerging research opportunities and input from external experts?

- To what extent has the planning process for the *Special Diabetes Program* relied on perspectives of various scientific and lay stakeholders?

- How effectively has the *Special Diabetes Program* been administered by NIDDK, which was delegated this responsibility by the Secretary, HHS? To what extent do the scientific initiatives and distribution of resources reflect a coordinated strategic plan?

- In which ways could the research supported by the *Special Diabetes Program* be enhanced?

- How are the collaborative research consortia and clinical trial networks perceived by scientists not affiliated with these projects?

- Has the creation of large, collaborative consortia enabled unique research opportunities and enhanced research in type 1 diabetes?

- Has there been added value in supporting collaborative consortia tackling specific major barriers to progress in type 1 diabetes research, rather than supporting individual researchers tackling those particular areas?

- To what extent has the *Special Diabetes Program* stimulated high-risk, high-impact research, or diabetes research in new fields that have not previously addressed diabetes?

- How successful has the *Special Diabetes Program* been in cultivating cross-disciplinary interactions and coordination?

- How successful has the *Special Diabetes Program* been in recruiting new investigators to apply their talents to type 1 diabetes research? What impact has it had on their careers?

- How effectively have strategies promoted clinical and translational research?

Evaluation Approaches

Multiple approaches were taken to evaluate the planning and implementation processes involved in administration of the *Special Diabetes Program*, and the scientific accomplishments of initiatives supported by this *Program*. It must be emphasized that achievement in biomedical research is a process that reflects the progressive accumulation of knowledge; the incremental building of scientific knowledge can therefore be a long-term process. Although many promising scientific findings have begun to emerge from research initiated by the *Special Diabetes Program*, the public health impact of this program is not yet fully manifest and thus cannot yet be fully assessed.

Type 1 diabetes is a chronic disease often diagnosed in childhood, adolescence, or young adulthood, with complications sometimes appearing decades later. From the *Special Diabetes Program*, new insights into the biology of this disease and its therapy are continuing to develop. For example, the *Special Diabetes Program* has initiated long-term prospective clinical studies, including one that has enrolled newborns who will be followed until they reach age 15; it has also supported infrastructure development to facilitate future research, such as the creation of animal models and the invaluable collections of genetic and tissue samples that are being stored in a repository for later analysis. Thus, many results from the evaluation approaches described in this report represent only a preliminary assessment of the advances that can be expected to flow from the *Special Diabetes Program*.

The major parameters that guided the evaluation process include:

- *Research Accomplishments:* Review of scientific advances and technological developments that have had positive impacts on patients or enabled future basic and clinical research. These data are primarily obtained from research publications, as well as from research advances included in *"Advances and Emerging Opportunities in Diabetes Research: A Strategic Planning Report of the DMICC."*

- *Professional Assessment:* Scientific judgment of external experts in the type 1 diabetes field garnered from specific assessments of clinical and pre-clinical consortia supported by the *Program* at meetings convened in April 2008 and June 2009 respectively. Additionally, each individual consortium or project has ongoing assessment.

- *Bibliometric Analysis:* Compendium of *Program*-associated publications in peer-reviewed scientific journals and the impact of these publications as determined by a citation analysis.

- *Grant Portfolio Analysis:* Use of NIH archival databases to determine program effectiveness in terms of dimensions such as recruitment of new investigators and stimulation of clinical research.

- *Interviews with Consortia Investigators:* Sample consortia investigators provided input on the importance and value of consortia supported by the *Special Diabetes Program.*

- *Other Metrics of Progress:* Outcome measures including patents, research resources (*e.g.*, microarray chips, antibodies, genetic and tissue samples, Internet-accessible data sets, animal models), and progress toward patient recruitment goals. These data are primarily obtained from annual progress reports or meetings of external review committees.

Cut-off Dates

In order to prepare this evaluation to meet the statutory deadline, data collection on research progress was terminated in spring 2010. Although there have been notable scientific advances between the cut-off date and the publication of this report, the cut-off date has been maintained, and these examples have not been included to ensure that data reporting is consistent from project to project. Budget data in Appendix A are reported

through the end of Fiscal Year (FY) 2009. However, the collection of references for scientific journal publications was limited to articles published prior to January 1, 2010.

Data Sources

Several sources were used to collect data needed to evaluate the *Special Diabetes Program*:

➤ **electronic Scientific Portfolio Assistant (e-SPA):** The NIDDK utilized NIAID's electronic Scientific Portfolio Assistant (e-SPA) to collect data on a portfolio of grants (see below) supported by the *Special Diabetes Program.* The data collected through e-SPA included: *Program*-associated publications in peer-review journals and the number of times those publications were cited in other papers; patent activity resulting from the *Special Diabetes Program*; the number of new investigators recruited to research; and the number of grants coded as clinical research supported by the *Program.* e-SPA was also utilized to capture NIH-wide comparison data. e-SPA is an application that combines modern search and business intelligence reporting tools to provide indicators on quality, relevance, and impact using data from IMPAC II (Information for Management, Planning, Analysis, and Coordination), iEdison, NIH Intramural Database, NLM MEDLINE, Thomson Reuters Web of Science and Journal Citation Reports, and U.S. Patent and Trademark Office (USPTO) Patent Applications and Grants. The initial production system was launched in 2008.

➤ ***Special Diabetes Program* Grant Portfolio:** The total portfolio of grants and contracts supported by the *Special Diabetes Program* for FY 1998-2009 is found in Appendix A. A subset of these projects was included in the e-SPA analyses. The following award types were excluded: (1) contracts, because the e-SPA tool does not capture complete data on contracts; (2) supplements to existing grants or centers, because it would not be possible to determine if the data collected related to the supplement portion of the grant or only to the primary grant.

➢ **Other NIH Archival Databases**: In addition to e-SPA, NIDDK used other NIH archival databases to collect data for this evaluation, including IMPAC II, Research Portfolio Online Reporting Tools Expenditures and Results (NIH RePORTER), and PubMed.

➢ **Reports on Progress**: The NIDDK used progress reports prepared for planning and evaluation meetings on the *Special Diabetes Program* and Web sites of the research consortia to obtain data on outcome measures such as development of research resources, progress toward patient recruitment goals, and scientific accomplishments.

➢ **2007 *"Evaluation Report"* on the *Special Statutory Funding Program for Type 1 Diabetes Research*:** A previous evaluation was published in 2007 to meet a congressional reporting requirement (www.T1Diabetes.nih.gov/evaluation). The NIDDK used data collected for the 2007 evaluation to supplement or verify data collected for this Report.

Changes in Data Sources Since the 2007 Evaluation of the *Special Diabetes Program*: For the 2007 Report, the data collection was performed manually, with database searches to obtain data on metrics such as publications resulting from the *Special Diabetes Program*. Data to supplement the manual searches, such as information on patent activity, was obtained through a survey of grantees supported by the *Program*.

Since that time, NIAID developed e-SPA, which automates data collection on a variety of metrics, as described above. The new availability of e-SPA enabled NIDDK to collect data that was only available via grantee survey for the 2007 evaluation. Because of the availability of e-SPA, NIDDK did not administer another grantee survey.

EMPLOYMENT OF AN INNOVATIVE PARADIGM FOR TRANS-HHS, CROSS-DISCIPLINARY, AND TRANSPARENT RESEARCH PLANNING AND MANAGEMENT

As designated by the Secretary of HHS, NIDDK has coordinated the development of a sound planning, implementation, and evaluation process for the *Special Diabetes Program*. The allocation of funds has been performed in a scientifically competitive manner in cooperation with multiple Institutes and Centers of NIH, CDC, and other components of HHS with expertise in type 1 diabetes. A series of planning meetings—involving these agencies, Institutes and Centers, and members of the diabetes patient-advocacy community—resulted in administrative plans for allocation of funds of the *Special Diabetes Program*. These plans, released in 1998 and 2001, established the framework for initiatives and research priorities to be pursued.

Since that time, critical sources of input that have informed program planning have included a variety of scientific workshops and conferences; meetings of the statutory Diabetes Mellitus Interagency Coordinating Committee (DMICC); a series of planning and evaluation meetings in which NIDDK convened panels of external scientific and lay experts to provide input on the *Special Diabetes Program* and future directions; and strategic planning processes, with broad external input, that have culminated in the publication of two reports: "*Advances and Emerging Opportunities in Type 1 Diabetes Research: A Strategic Plan*" and "*Advances and Emerging Opportunities in Diabetes Research: A Strategic Planning Report of the DMICC*." Notably, the *Special Diabetes Program* ties a set of HHS-wide research planning and evaluation efforts to the deployment of a specified amount of budgetary resources in a highly effective and efficient research management process.

Type 1 diabetes is a systemic disease that requires a multidisciplinary research approach and therefore is addressed by multiple components of NIH and HHS. The disease involves the body's endocrine and metabolic functions (NIDDK) and immune system (NIAID); complications affecting the heart and arteries (NHLBI), eyes (NEI), kidneys and digestive and urologic tracts (NIDDK), nervous system (NINDS, NIMH), and oral cavity (NIDCR); the special problems of a disease diagnosed primarily in children and adolescents (NICHD); complex genetic (NHGRI) and environmental (NIEHS) factors; the need for novel imaging technologies (NIBIB); data on disease incidence and prevalence in the United States (CDC); development of research resources (NCRR); and services for pre-clinical testing of therapeutics (NCI).

The *Special Diabetes Program* supports a spectrum of research within these NIH and HHS components, making it a model trans-NIH and trans-HHS program. In addition to the components listed above, the NIH Office of Research on Women's Health, NIH Office of Dietary Supplements, National Institute on Aging, National Center on Minority Health and Health Disparities, National Center for Complementary and Alternative Medicine, and National Institute of Nursing Research have also participated in the *Special Diabetes*

Program. Thus, the *Special Diabetes Program* has catalyzed and synergized the efforts of a wide range of HHS components to combat type 1 diabetes and its complications.

Pursuit of a Scientifically Focused, but Flexible, Budgeting Process

Six major, scientific research Goals that offer exceptional promise for the treatment and prevention of type 1 diabetes form the basis of the planning and allocation processes of the *Special Diabetes Program*:

- Goal I: Identify the Genetic and Environmental Causes of Type 1 Diabetes

- Goal II: Prevent or Reverse Type 1 Diabetes

- Goal III: Develop Cell Replacement Therapy

- Goal IV: Prevent or Reduce Hypoglycemia in Type 1 Diabetes

- Goal V: Prevent or Reduce the Complications of Type 1 Diabetes

- Goal VI: Attract New Talent and Apply New Technologies to Research on Type 1 Diabetes

More information on each Goal, and the research supported under those Goals, is found in the main body of the report. The annual funding levels by Goal for FY 1998-2009 are shown in Table B1. The total budget distribution of the *Program* by Goal from FY 1998-2009 is displayed in Figure B1. A detailed budget analysis is found in Appendix A.

The professional judgment of scientific and lay expert panels has repeatedly endorsed the structure of these Goals as an appropriate and effective framework to manage the *Special Diabetes Program* (see section later in this Appendix on the "Broadly Consultative Planning

Process for Priority Setting and Resource Distribution"). One challenge in managing large-scale science is the time required to accelerate or decelerate research programs in response to the availability of funds. The dynamic interdependence of the efforts of government program managers and the external scientific and diabetes voluntary communities has helped the scientific priorities develop to reflect the changing needs of research.

Table B1: Budget of the *Special Diabetes Program* by Goal (FY 1998-2009)[a]

	Goal I	Goal II	Goal III	Goal IV	Goal V	Goal VI	Administrative (e.g., personnel, conferences)	TOTAL
1998	493,436	9,247,235	6,379,977	3,470,740	10,339,294	0[b]	69,318	30,000,000
1999	2,070,192	6,211,806	6,293,237	3,672,012	11,725,416	0[b]	27,337	30,000,000
2000	4,463,743	5,615,924	5,881,222	2,579,693	11,344,751	0[b]	114,667	30,000,000
2001	22,535,131	25,888,609	25,204,681	2,674,074	19,435,977	4,049,000	212,528	100,000,000
2002	16,378,537	21,934,292	19,346,899	8,993,845	21,402,845	11,793,551	150,031	100,000,000
2003	19,717,454	21,631,424	19,701,970	7,643,699	15,017,921	16,130,672	156,860	100,000,000
2004	34,808,000	19,367,709	47,148,270	8,389,536	16,359,078	23,789,681	137,726	150,000,000
2005	45,084,403	15,176,867	41,716,120	7,680,901	17,748,844	22,056,018	536,847	150,000,000
2006	37,706,975	15,090,798	53,200,058	4,425,237	26,948,806	11,825,222	802,904	150,000,000
2007	63,186,097	26,064,134	29,809,919	4,301,484	15,322,431	10,611,551	704,384	150,000,000
2008	21,179,111	60,227,685	21,567,125	3,845,729	11,514,911	31,077,754	587,685	150,000,000
2009	59,761,987	37,755,958	33,859,097	7,461,138	6,130,362	4,167,000	864,458	150,000,000
Total	327,385,066	264,212,441	310,108,575	65,138,088	183,290,636	135,500,449	4,364,745	1,290,000,000

[a] Please see Appendix A for detailed budget analysis.
[b] In addition to solicitations focused exclusively on attracting new talent to type 1 diabetes research, Goal VI was addressed by solicitations for research projects that encouraged the participation of new investigators and the submission of applications for pilot and feasibility awards, as well as the development of new technology in the context of Goals I-V. These early efforts relative to Goal VI are thus embedded in other Goals during the FY 1998-2000 period of the *Program*. Starting in FY 2001, specific initiatives were also launched relative to Goal VI.

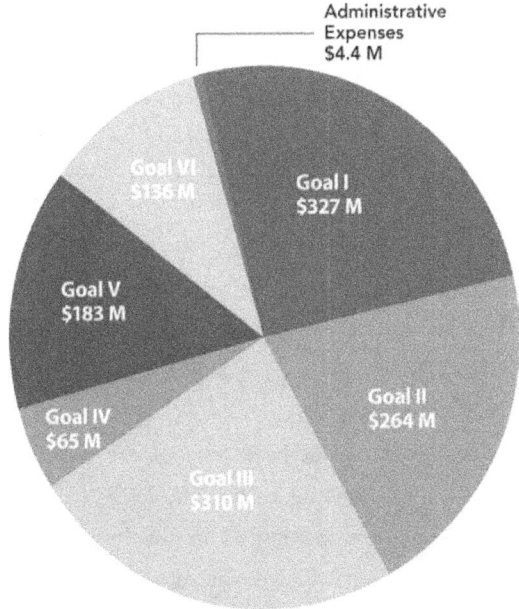

Figure B1: Total budget distribution by Goal, FY 1998-2009

Based on this scientific framework, a comprehensive management strategy has been used to: promote maximum flexibility; respond to new scientific opportunities; and plan and initiate broad, multidisciplinary projects that would not have been undertaken without the *Special Diabetes Program*. The *Special Diabetes Program* has included both short-term and long-term initiatives. Short-term grant supplements and pilot and feasibility grants have enabled the *Program* to capitalize quickly on emerging research opportunities of high priority. Longer-term research grants and consortia and research infrastructure initiatives have been pursued to initiate unique, ambitious, large-scale research projects of critical importance. Because of the uncertainty of future funding of a time-limited *Program*, the NIH has employed novel funding mechanisms to support new research projects in later years of the *Program* in order to capitalize on new and emerging research opportunities.

The *Special Diabetes Program* has also established targeted type 1 diabetes-relevant components within initiatives that are supported in part by regularly appropriated funds. This strategy has maximized NIH and CDC's investment in type 1 diabetes research by building upon and realizing the greatest potential benefits from existing research infrastructure and ongoing clinical trials. Conversely, now that numerous clinical research studies and clinical trials networks have been established through support from the *Special Diabetes Program*, scientists are taking advantage of the existing infrastructure to conduct ancillary studies to maximize the research investment. Ancillary studies have been supported by the *Special Diabetes Program* or other sources (*e.g.*, regular NIH appropriations, the American Recovery and Reinvestment Act, diabetes voluntary organizations), which saves resources by building upon established studies and using data that have already been collected. Samples from ongoing studies are also being stored in the NIDDK Central Repositories, so that they can serve as a resource to the scientific community for additional research on type 1 diabetes and its complications, which maximizes the investment into these unique research studies. Moreover, several initiatives launched by the *Special Diabetes Program* have attracted investment from private foundations, industry, or other non-federal government sources with an interest in type 1 diabetes research.

Establishment of Large-Scale, Collaborative, and Infrastructural Initiatives

In the first years (FY 1998-2000), the *Special Diabetes Program* primarily supported initiatives soliciting research from independent investigators on topics of urgent and unmet need. When the *Program* was augmented in FY 2001, the additional funds enabled the creation of unique, innovative, and collaborative research consortia and clinical trials networks. The *Special Diabetes Program* enabled the initiation of these high-impact research efforts at a scientifically optimal scale. The majority of the funds since 2001 have supported these collaborative research efforts, with a goal of promoting progress in type 1 diabetes research that could not be achieved by a single laboratory. The collaborative initiatives, which have become a hallmark of the *Special Diabetes Program*, include genetics consortia, long-term epidemiological efforts, a beta cell biology consortium, animal models consortia, a clinical islet transplantation consortium, and clinical trials networks. Such projects are significantly different in size, scope, duration, and nature from investigator-initiated type 1 diabetes research efforts supported through the *Special Diabetes Program* or regular NIH appropriations. Most NIH research takes the form of 3- to 5-year hypothesis-driven research grants, either initiated by investigators in the field or submitted in response to NIH research solicitations. Such grants and funding initiatives often involve only a single NIH funding component and are carried out in a single, academic research laboratory. In contrast, the infrastructural and other large-scale research initiatives of the *Special Diabetes Program* represent a new paradigm in that overt trans-NIH and NIH-CDC collaborations are integral and essential to their successful operation, and the involvement of multiple research groups is

required. For examples of the infrastructure that has been established to support research consortia, please see the main body of the report: "Critical Investment in Infrastructure for Type 1 Diabetes Research" feature (Goal I) and "The Beta Cell Biology Consortium: An Experiment in Team Science" feature (Goal III).

This approach has yielded remarkable progress. For example, collecting DNA from thousands of volunteers through the Type 1 Diabetes Genetics Consortium has resulted in the identification of over 40 new genes and gene regions associated with type 1 diabetes. Researchers working together in the Beta Cell Biology Consortium have made tremendous progress that can inform the development of cell replacement therapy for type 1 diabetes. Researchers collaborating in Type 1 Diabetes TrialNet have identified a new cellular target for possibly preventing or treating type 1 diabetes. Even more progress is expected in the future as research continues to build on this progress.

This Report describes several metrics for evaluating the scientific progress of the collaborative research consortia. One key metric was the evaluation of consortia by ad hoc groups of external scientific and lay experts in April 2008 and June 2009 (see descriptions of meetings later in this Appendix). These meetings provided critical sources of input for enhancing research being conducted by the consortia and future research directions. A second evaluation metric was obtaining input from scientists participating in research consortia to determine if there has been benefit in conducting the research as a collaborative endeavor. That input is found in "Investigator Profiles" in the main body of the report. Third, evaluation of major research consortia, networks, and resources is found in Appendix C. Finally, scientific output from the consortia is included in the bibliometric analysis found later in this Appendix.

IMPROVING PATIENTS' HEALTH

In the 89 years since the discovery of insulin, diabetes research and the medical treatment of people with diabetes have witnessed many "modern miracles." Yet, scientific research is both serendipitous and incremental, a process in which advances typically accrue and build upon each other over a relatively extensive time period. In the 12 years since its inception, the *Special Diabetes Program* has accelerated this process, uniting government and privately funded medical research with medical providers and biotechnology and pharmaceutical companies to bring about many improvements in the health and quality of life of people with type 1 diabetes. Examples of scientific advances follow.

Greatly Improved Prognosis for Americans with Type 1 Diabetes: Because of research progress over the last 2 decades, including research supported by the *Special Diabetes Program*, people with the disease are living longer and healthier lives than ever before and experiencing lower rates of disease complications. A recent study of the clinical course of type 1 diabetes concluded that starting intensive control of blood glucose as soon as possible after diagnosis greatly improves the long-term prognosis for patients. The study also found that the outlook for people with longstanding type 1 diabetes has greatly improved over the past 20 years due to a better understanding of the importance of intensive glucose control, as well as advances in insulin formulations and delivery, glucose monitoring, and the treatment of cardiovascular disease risk factors. These findings come from analyses of the long-term health outcomes for people who participated in NIDDK's

landmark Diabetes Control and Complications Trial (DCCT) and its ongoing, *Special Diabetes Program*-supported, follow-up study, the Epidemiology of Diabetes Interventions and Complications, which began in 1993. This study reinforced and extended the DCCT's initial findings that intensive blood glucose control dramatically reduces the risk of eye, kidney, and nerve damage due to diabetes. In particular, researchers found that, among DCCT participants who had received intensive glucose control during the trial, rates of vision loss and kidney failure had fallen to much lower levels than seen historically. Achieving and maintaining intensive glucose control is not easy for people with type 1 diabetes; the 21st century picture of clinical outcomes provided by this study can aid health care providers in discussing the tremendous health benefits of intensive control with their patients and reinforces the need for research to develop less burdensome approaches to help patients achieve these goals.

Newly Discovered Type 1 Diabetes Genes: Using new and emerging genetics technologies, scientists in the NIDDK-led and *Special Diabetes Program*-supported Type 1 Diabetes Genetics Consortium and their collaborators identified over 40 different genes or genetic regions that influence a person's risk of developing type 1 diabetes, bringing the total number of known regions to near 50—up from only three known genes a few years ago. Now, the challenge is to understand how those genes may influence disease development. Further research is ongoing to pinpoint the exact genes and understand their function in type 1 diabetes. Understanding the genetic underpinnings of type 1 diabetes can aid the ability to predict risk, as well as inform the development of new prevention and treatment strategies.

Adult Pancreas Cells Reprogrammed to Insulin-producing Beta Cells: Scientists in the NIDDK-led and *Special Diabetes Program*-supported Beta Cell Biology Consortium (BCBC) have made tremendous progress in understanding beta cell biology toward the goal of developing cell-based therapies for diabetes. For example, in order to promote the formation of new beta cells, BCBC scientists are determining when and how certain pancreatic progenitor cells become "committed" to developing into specific pancreatic cell types and discovering flexibility in these cells. In one study, scientists made an exciting discovery that a type of adult cell in the mouse pancreas, called exocrine cells, can be reprogrammed to become insulin-producing beta cells. Using a genetically engineered virus and a combination of just three transcription factors, the researchers were able to reprogram some of the exocrine cells into beta cells. The newly formed beta cells produced enough insulin to decrease high blood glucose levels in diabetic mice. If the same type of approach can be developed to work safely and effectively in humans, this discovery could have a dramatic impact on the ability to increase beta cell mass in people with diabetes.

In another study, scientists uncovered plasticity in another pancreatic cell type—the alpha cell. Using genetic techniques in mice, the researchers increased the levels of a protein called Pax4, which is known to be involved in promoting cells to develop into the pancreatic beta cell type. They found that mice with high levels of Pax4 had oversized clusters of beta cells, which resulted from alpha-beta precursor cells and established alpha cells being induced to form beta cells. In addition, in a mouse model of diabetes, high levels of Pax4 promoted

generation of new beta cells and overcame the diabetic state. In another study, BCBC scientists observed spontaneous conversion in beta cell-depleted mice of alpha cells to insulin-producing cells. These discoveries--that adult pancreatic cells have the potential to convert to beta cells--generate a fuller picture of pancreatic development and may pave the way toward new cell-based therapies for diabetes.

Hemoglobin A1c (HbA1c) Standardization Improves Care for People with Diabetes: HbA1c is a component of blood that is a good surrogate measure of long-term blood glucose control and, as such, reflects risk of diabetic complications. Clinical guidelines for controlling blood glucose to reduce diabetes complications set targets for control of blood glucose as assessed by this key test based on results from two landmark clinical trials: the DCCT for type 1 diabetes and the United Kingdom Prospective Diabetes Study for type 2 diabetes. To enable translation of these targets for control of blood glucose into common medical practice, the CDC and NIDDK, with support from the *Special Diabetes Program*, launched the HbA1c Standardization Program in 1998. This program improved the standardization and reliability in measures of HbA1c so that clinical laboratory results can be used by health care providers and patients to accurately and meaningfully assess blood glucose control and risks for complications. The standardization effort has been a great success and has facilitated national campaigns to improve control of blood glucose. As a result, the percentage of Americans with diabetes who had excellent glucose control increased from 37 percent in 1999-2000 to 56 percent in 2003-2004.[30] The American Diabetes Association (ADA) built on

---

[30]   Hoerger TJ, Segel JE, Gregg EW, et al: Is glycemic control improving in U.S. adults? Diabetes Care 31: 81-86, 2008.

the tremendous success of the HbA1c Standardization Program to set treatment goals for glucose control in all forms of diabetes based on the test and has recommended HbA1c as a more convenient approach to diagnose type 2 diabetes.

New Glucose Monitoring Tools for Controlling Blood Glucose Levels: Research supported by the *Special Diabetes Program* contributed to the development of U.S. Food and Drug Administration (FDA)-approved continuous glucose monitors, which reveal the dynamic changes in blood glucose levels. Alarms warn the patient if blood glucose becomes too high or too low, thereby reducing the need for invasive finger sticks to monitor blood glucose levels. This revolutionary technology can make it easier for patients to keep blood glucose at healthy levels and can enhance their ability to achieve the intensive control necessary to prevent or delay disease complications. In addition, this technology, when linked to insulin delivery (known as an "artificial pancreas"), has the potential to have a further positive impact on patients' health and quality of life, and alleviate an enormous amount of patient burden.

Novel Drugs for Treating Complications: The *Special Diabetes Program* has supported the development and clinical testing of new therapeutic agents for diabetic eye disease. For example, a recent comparative effectiveness research study, conducted by the National Eye Institute (NEI)-led Diabetic Retinopathy Clinical Research Network, found that a therapeutic called ranibizumab, in combination with laser therapy, was substantially better than laser therapy alone or laser therapy with a different drug, at treating diabetic macular edema, a swelling in the eye that often accompanies and aggravates diabetic retinopathy. Ranibizumab with laser therapy substantially improved vision among study patients, and could

become the new standard of care for diabetic macular edema.

Advances in Islet Transplantation as a Therapeutic Approach for People with Type 1 Diabetes: The *Special Diabetes Program* supported the first islet transplantation trial in the United States using a procedure referred to as the "Edmonton protocol" that dramatically improved islet survival and rendered many patients insulin-free. Through the Immune Tolerance Network (ITN), which is led by the National Institute of Allergy and Infectious Diseases (NIAID), the *Special Diabetes Program* also supported the first international, multicenter trial of islet transplantation using the protocol. Additionally, research supported by the *Program* laid the foundation for an unprecedented islet transplant to an American airman, sparing him from a life-long insulin requirement after pancreatic damage from wounds suffered while serving in Afghanistan. Improved approaches to islet transplantation are important not only as an alternative to whole pancreas transplantation for treatment of type 1 diabetes but also to avoid diabetes through auto-transplantation after removal of the pancreas due to pancreatitis or injury. The *Special Diabetes Program* is supporting multifaceted research efforts to overcome barriers to making islet transplantation a viable therapy, such as the shortage of available islets and the toxicity associated with the life-long immunosuppressive medication.

Promise of Therapies that Target Specific Lymphocytes in Preventing and Reversing Type 1 Diabetes: Previous clinical trials have suggested that preserving patients' remaining beta cell function can have dramatic, long-term health benefits. Researchers in NIDDK's Type 1 Diabetes TrialNet, which is supported by the *Special Diabetes Program*, reported that an immunosuppressive drug (rituximab), which destroys immune system cells called B lymphocytes, preserved the function of insulin-producing beta cells in people newly diagnosed with type 1 diabetes. Improved insulin production was maintained 1 year after the drug was administered, but the effect dissipated at 2 years. As drugs such as rituximab broadly deplete B lymphocytes, they can increase the risk of infection and therefore can have significant side effects. Nonetheless, the finding is very important because it will propel research to find drugs targeting the specific B lymphocytes involved in type 1 diabetes without the associated side effects of drugs like rituximab.

In another study, researchers in NIAID's ITN, also supported by the *Special Diabetes Program*, are building on an earlier study showing benefits of teplizumab, a humanized anti-CD3 monoclonal antibody that targets white blood cells known as "T cells" that are involved in the autoimmune attack on the beta cells. A pilot study of teplizumab showed that a single course of the antibody could delay progression of the disease over a 2-year period. The new trial is a larger follow-up study, in which two courses of the antibody are administered, one year apart, in an effort to extend its effects on beta cell preservation.

Testing Novel Type 1 Diabetes Prevention Strategies: Research supported by the *Special Diabetes Program* has enabled testing of new type 1 diabetes prevention strategies and demonstrated that it is possible to predict with great accuracy a person's risk of developing type 1 diabetes. Moreover, while an oral insulin type 1 diabetes prevention trial (now part of TrialNet) did not demonstrate protection in the entire study population, it suggested a possible effect in the subgroup with highest insulin antibody titers. This knowledge has set the stage for screening and enrolling patients into new type 1 diabetes prevention trials, including a new trial through TrialNet that is testing oral insulin in a subgroup of people with high levels of insulin autoantibodies.

Building on findings from successful trials in newly diagnosed patients, TrialNet has developed a new paradigm: therapeutics demonstrated to be effective in new-onset patients are then tested for their prevention potential. One such prevention trial was recently launched with teplizumab, a monoclonal antibody engineered to alter the balance between destructive and protective T cells. Based on promising results in preserving beta cell function in patients newly diagnosed with type 1 diabetes, teplizumab is now being studied in family members of type 1 diabetes who are at 80 percent risk of developing type 1 diabetes over the next 5 years. This effort builds not only on the earlier success with teplizumab but also on the proven accuracy of tests to predict type 1 diabetes risk.

SCIENTIFIC PRODUCTIVITY

Bibliometric Analysis

Compendium of *Special Diabetes Program*-supported Scientific Publications: Perhaps the most accepted metric for assessing scientific productivity is to look at peer-reviewed publications in scientific and medical journals. Peer-reviewed publication is the forum in which scientists report their discoveries and propound new ideas, and it is one means by which productivity is measured for NIH grant applications, faculty appointments, and tenure decisions. The NIDDK used e-SPA to search for scientific publications associated with grants funded through the *Special Diabetes Program*, and identified 2,793 unique articles published from January 1, 1998, and prior to January 1, 2010.

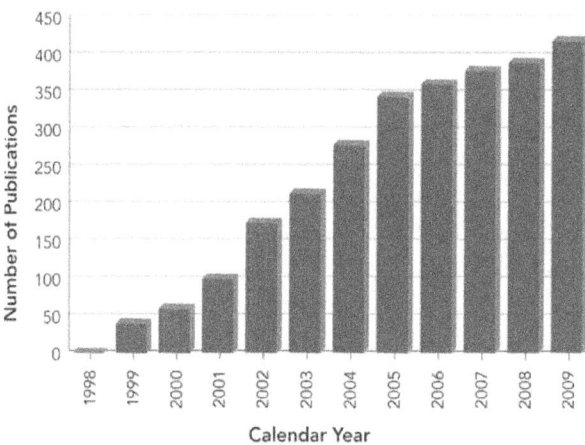

Figure B2: Number of Scientific Publications Supported by the Special Diabetes Program
The graph represents the number of papers published each calendar year. Data include the 2,793 papers published before January 1, 2010, produced from initiatives, clinical trials, or research consortia made possible by the *Special Diabetes Program*.

The identified set includes only publications from grants awarded through initiatives, clinical trials, or research consortia made possible through the *Special Diabetes Program*. Pre-existing grants that were augmented through the *Program* were not included in the bibliometric analysis. The final collection of papers analyzed in this evaluation report is almost certainly an underrepresentation of the actual publication output, because it is impossible to capture all published papers that do not give attribution to the grants that supported the research.

Figure B2 displays the number of articles published in each calendar year of the *Special Diabetes Program*. As would be expected, fewer articles were published in the early years of the *Program*; a scientific project can take many years from design of the project to publication of the results. The data show an increasing trend and in the

later years of the *Special Diabetes Program*, there is a robust output of scientific articles.

Citation Analysis for Scientific Papers: The 2,793 papers were analyzed to evaluate their impact on the scientific community (Table B2, Figure B2, Figure B3, and Figure B4). One of the most objective methods for assessing the scientific impact of a publication is to analyze how frequently the work has been cited in other scientific publications. A higher number of citations may indicate that the paper has had a particularly large influence on subsequent work in the field, introducing a new experimental technique, for example. However, it takes time to design and carry out new experiments, so there is typically a lag time of 3 to 5 years after a paper is published before most citations of it appear in the scientific literature. Therefore, papers published in more recent years will likely generate many more citations in the future than are reported here.

Citation data obtained from e-SPA was derived from the Thomson Web of Science database and includes citation activity that occurred through December 31, 2009. A few publications were not included in the Web of Science database and therefore citation data was not reported for a limited number of publications. These publications were not included in statistical analysis of citation data. Citation data are available for 2,574 publications and, therefore, missing for 219 papers. The citation data, therefore, are likely underreported and thus limit any conclusion of impact assessment from citation analysis.

Among the 2,574 papers for which citation data are available, there are 52,739 total citations prior to January 1, 2010 (Table B2). The number of citations ranged from

Table B2: Citation Analysis of Scientific Papers

Year	Total Papers	Papers with Available Citation Data	Maximum Citations	Mean Citations	Median Citations	Total Citations
1998	2	2	261	158	158	316
1999	38	38	111	43	38	1,638
2000	62	60	226	42	31	2,522
2001	102	93	222	39	26	3,610
2002	175	163	743	47	29	7,687
2003	216	196	489	39	23	7,576
2004	291	274	528	28	18	7,751
2005	346	318	166	23	15	7,409
2006	358	345	406	19	12	6,678
2007	390	370	248	14	8	5,089
2008	397	374	121	6	3	2,103
2009	416	341	27	1	0	360
1998-2009 Total	**2,793**	**2,574**	**743**	**38**	**21**	**52,739**

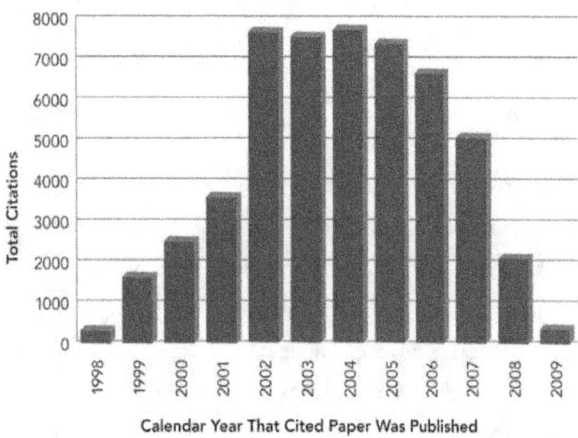

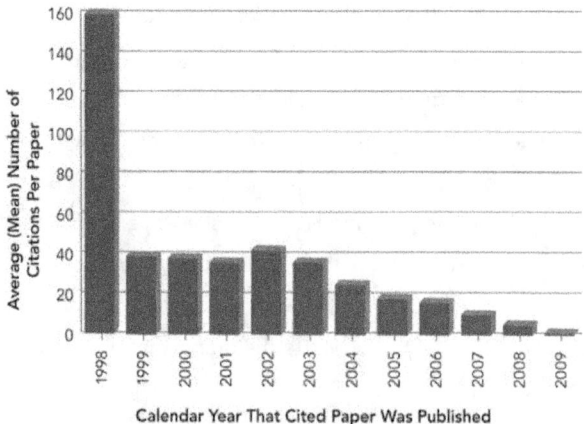

Figure B3: Total Citations of *Special Diabetes Program*-supported Research Publications

The cited papers are the subset of papers for which citation data are available. Citations appearing in papers published on January 1, 2010, or later were not included in this analysis.

Figure B4: Average Citations of *Special Diabetes Program*-supported Research Publications

Mean citations are grouped by the calendar year during which the cited papers were published. The cited papers are a subset of papers for which citation data are available. Citations appearing in papers published on January 1, 2010, or later were not included in this analysis. Because there is typically a lag time of 3-5 years after a paper is published before the majority of citations occur, the average number of citations is lower for more recently published papers.

0 to 743, with an average (mean) of 38 and a median of 21. The total number of citations per year is dramatically higher for the papers published a few years after the inception of the *Program* (Figure B3). This likely reflects the years necessary for the projects funded early in the *Program* to publish results, but also that a sufficient number of years have passed to achieve a high number of citations. As expected, the average number of citations per paper is higher for papers published early in the *Program* than for those published later (Figure B4).

Comparison to Data from 2007 Report: It is important to note that data reported here differ from the data previously reported in the 2007 *"Evaluation Report."* The bibliometric analysis previously conducted identified 4,755 articles published from January 1, 1998, and prior to January 1, 2006. This number included publications that cited pre-existing grants that were augmented through the *Special Diabetes Program*. Many of these grants supplemented existing research project grants or Diabetes Research Centers grants at academic institutions, allowing innovative pilot projects or development of resources relevant to type 1 diabetes. Because it was not possible to determine which of these publications were made possible by the additional funding, and which were more related to the prior award, they were eliminated from the bibliometric analysis for the 2007 report. Also for this reason, they were not included in the bibliometric analysis reported here. In 2007, a total of 1,552 publications from grants awarded through initiatives, clinical trials, or research consortia made possible through the *Special Diabetes Program* were collected and used for the citation analysis in the 2007 *"Evaluation Report."*

Two additional methods used to supplement the previous publications list were not used for the data collection in this report. This includes the investigator survey, which was used to collect additional publications. Additionally, for the 2007 report, the publications list was supplemented by scientific program directors at NIH responsible for management of *Special Diabetes Program* consortia and trial networks. In order to keep the eSPA the sole variable for data collection and to keep the data as consistent as possible, these methods were not employed for the bibliometric analysis reported here.

Patents

Patents represent an objective metric of productivity. The e-SPA tool was used to collect data on patent activity on the portfolio of research grants supported by the *Special Diabetes Program* from FY 1998-2009. e-SPA interfaced with the U.S. Patent and Trademark Office (USPTO) database to search issued patents for the inclusion of specified grant numbers. If the issued patent acknowledged support from a grant, it was identified by e-SPA as associated with that grant.

The e-SPA analysis yielded a total of 23 unique, issued patents that were tied to *Program* grants (see Table B3). A previous evaluation of the *Special Diabetes Program* published in 2007 identified 15 additional issued patents that were associated with the *Special Diabetes Program* but not identified by e-SPA. Those patents were captured through self-report data from a grantee survey. Further analysis revealed that the relevant grant numbers were not included in those 15 patents filed with the USPTO, which is why they were not identified by e-SPA. Combining datasets shows that there are at least 38 issued patents associated with the *Special Diabetes Program* (Table B3). Information on issued patents is shown in Table B4.

The estimate of 38 issued patents is likely an underestimation due to the limitations of using e-SPA. Because e-SPA is an automated system, if the patent did not cite a grant number, cited an incorrect grant number, or cited only the funding agency, it was not identified by e-SPA. However, because of the availability of the new automated e-SPA tool for identifying patent data, which was not available during the 2007 *Program* evaluation, NIDDK chose not to conduct a grantee survey. Thus, the two datasets were combined to obtain a conservative estimate of patent activity resulting from the *Special Diabetes Program*.

Research Resources

Research resources are research tools, technologies, biological samples, data, or other scientific materials that are produced or collected to enable scientific experimentation. A focus of the *Special Diabetes Program* has been to promote development of resources that can be used by the broad scientific community. Therefore, the resources are not only benefiting researchers funded by the *Program*, but the entire diabetes research enterprise. In addition, researchers outside of diabetes also use the resources. For example, scientists studying pancreatic cancer use resources developed by the Beta Cell Biology Consortium. Examples of available research resources are shown

Table B3: U.S. Patents

Patents Issued – e-SPA dataset	23
Patents Issued – identified in grantee survey from 2007 *"Evaluation Report"* (non-overlapping with e-SPA dataset)	15
TOTAL PATENTS ISSUED	38

in Table B5 (more information on resources generated by research consortia is found in Appendix C). Several consortia—such as SEARCH, TEDDY, and others—also make protocols, study forms, and publications available to the scientific community through a public Web site. Furthermore, some consortia were established specifically to serve as a resource to the scientific community, such as the T1D-RAID program that provides resources for pre-clinical drug development.

In addition to the numerous resources that have already been developed with support from the *Program*, other resources are expected to become available in the future. For example, several clinical consortia, such as TEDDY and TRIGR, are currently collecting biological samples that will be made available and serve as invaluable resources to scientists in their quest to understand the underlying mechanisms of type 1 diabetes and to identify environmental triggers of disease.

PROMOTION OF DIVERSE, INNOVATIVE, AND PATIENT-ORIENTED RESEARCH ON TYPE 1 DIABETES

Diverse Research Portfolio

Research proposals for support by the *Special Diabetes Program* are received through a variety of mechanisms, including Requests for Applications (RFAs) for grant and cooperative agreement awards, and requests for administrative supplements for pilot or ancillary studies related to ongoing projects. From FY 1998 through FY 2009, a total of 74 RFAs were issued for the support of focused research of critical importance to the prevention and cure of type 1 diabetes and its complications. RFAs solicit research on a specific scientific topic of high relevance to program goals; they are used to solicit individual research projects, or in some cases to

Table B4: Issued Patents*

U.S. Patent Number	Year Issued	Inventor(s)	Title
5,723,333	1998	Levine F, Wang S, Beattie G, Hayek A	Human Pancreatic Cell Lines: Developments and Uses
6,110,743	2000	Levine F, Wang S, Beattie G, Hayek A	Development and Use of Human Pancreatic Cell Lines
6,122,536	2000	Sun X, Joseph J, Crothall K	Implantable Sensor and System for Measurement and Control of Blood Constituent Levels
6,197,534	2001	Lakowicz J, Tolosa L, Eichhorn L, Rao G	Engineered Proteins for Analyte Sensing
6,348,429	2002	Lim D, Gough D, Rourke A	Polymers From Vinylic Monomers Peroxides and Amines
6,448,045	2002	Levine F, Dufayet D	Inducing Insulin Gene Expression in Pancreas Cells Expressing Recombinant PDX-1
6,497,729	2002	Moussy F, Kreutzer D, Burgess D, Koberstein J, Papadimitrakopoulos F, Huang S	Implant Coating for Control of Tissue/Implant Interactions
6,544,800	2003	Asher S	Polymerized Crystalline Colloidal Arrays
6,589,452	2003	Asher S, Kamenjicki M, Lednev I, Meier V	Photochemically Controlled Photonic Crystal Diffraction
6,592,746	2003	Schmid-Schoenbein G, Baker D, Gough D	Sensor Probe for Determining Hydrogen Peroxide Concentration and Method of Use Thereof
6,673,596	2004	Sayler GS, Simpson ML, Applegate BM, Ripp SA	In vivo Biosensor Apparatus and Method of Use
6,673,625	2004	Satcher, Jr. J, Lane S, Darrow C, Cary D, Tran J	Saccharide Sensing Molecules Having Enhanced Fluorescent Properties
6,682,938	2004	Satcher, Jr. J, Lane S, Darrow C, Cary D	Glucose Sensing Molecules Having Selected Fluorescent Properties
6,721,587	2004	Gough DA	Membrane and Electrode Structure for Implantable Sensor
6,753,191	2004	Asher SA, Reese CE	Polymerized Crystalline Colloidal Array Chemical Sensing Materials for Use in High Ionic Strength Solutions
6,766,183	2004	Walsh J, Heiss A, Noronha G, Vachon D, Lane S, Satcher, Jr. J, Peyser T, Van Antwerp W, Mastrototaro J	Long Wave Fluorophore Sensor Compounds and Other Fluorescent Sensor Compounds in Polymers
6,777,546	2004	Langridge W, Arakawa T	Methods and Substances for Preventing and Treating Autoimmune Disease
6,811,785	2004	Brumeanu T, Casares S, Bona C	Multivalent MHC Class II - Peptide Chimeras
6,835,545	2004	Halperin J	Methods, Products and Treatments for Diabetes
6,884,785	2005	von Herrath MG	Compositions and Methods for the Treatment or Prevention of Autoimmune Diabetes
6,884,585	2005	Levine F, Dufayet D	Induction of Beta Cell Differentiation in Human Cells by Stimulation of the GLP-1 Receptor
6,893,552	2005	Wang J, Zhang X, Lu F	Microsensors for Glucose and Insulin Monitoring
6,911,324	2005	Levine F, Gouty D, Itkin-Ansari P	Induction of Beta Cell Differentiation in Human Cells
6,916,660	2005	Wang B, Weston B, Yang W	Fluorescent Sensor Compounds for Detecting Saccharides
6,979,542	2005	Cheung VG, Spielman RS	Methods for Identifying Heterozygous Carriers of Autosomal Recessive Diseases
7,014,998	2006	Rothstein DM, Basadonna GP	Screening Immunomodulatory Agents by CTLA-4 Upregulation
7,026,294	2006	Fasano A, Watts T	Method of Use of Peptide Antagonists of Zonulin to Prevent or Delay the Onset of Diabetes
7,049,082	2006	Halperin J	Methods, Products and Treatments for Diabetes
7,059,719	2006	Asher S	Contact Lenses Colored With Crystalline Colloidal Array Technology
7,071,298	2006	Brown TR, Kappler F	Compounds and Methods for Treating Glycogen Storage Disease and other Pathological Conditions Resulting from Formation of Age-Proteins
7,094,555	2006	Kwok WW, Nepom G, Gebe J, Reijonen H, Liu A	Methods of MHC Class II Epitope Mapping, Detection of Autoimmune T Cells and Antigens, and Autoimmune Treatment
7,105,352	2006	Asher SA, Alexeev VL, Lednev IK, Sharma AC, Wilcox C	Intelligent Polymerized Crystalline Colloidal Array Carbohydrate Sensors
7,336,984	2008	Gough DA, Lucisano JY	Membrane and Electrode Structure for Implantable Sensor
7,402,153	2008	Steil GM, Rebrin K	Closed-loop Method for Controlling Insulin Infusion
7,439,330	2008	Halperin J	Anti-glycated CD59 Antibodies and Uses Thereof
7,491,389	2009	Scott EW, Grant M, May WS	Modulating Angiogenesis
7,615,528	2009	Brown TR, Keppler F	Methods for Alleviating Deleterious Effects of 3-Deoxyglucosone
7,622,117	2009	Tobia A, Kappler F	3-Deoxyglucosone and Skin

* Data obtained from the USPTO database (http://www.uspto.gov/patents/process/search/). Patents in light blue boxes were identified from 2007 self-reported survey data provided by grantees supported by the *Special Diabetes Program*; see Appendix 5 of the 2007 "*Evaluation Report*" (www.T1Diabetes.nih.gov/evaluation) for more information on the survey. Other patents were identified using e-SPA.

attract applications for participation in a consortium. Solicitations asked for creative approaches to solve particularly difficult problems. These solicitations encouraged high-risk, discovery research to overcome obstacles to research progress. Additionally, the *Special Diabetes Program* provided full or partial support for projects associated with Requests for Proposals (RFPs) and Program Announcements (PAs); notices were used to announce availability of funding or research resources (see Appendix A for a complete list of funding announcements and initiatives). A breakdown of activity in terms of the *Special Diabetes Program*'s funding mechanisms is provided in Table B6.

The *Special Diabetes Program* supported 648 grants and supplements and 29 contracts. Individual investigators predominantly received short-term or long-term research project grants. In some cases, the

Table B5: Examples of Available Research Resources*

CONSORTIUM	RESOURCE
Animal Models of Diabetic Complications Consortium	➢ Over 40 animal models of type 1 diabetes that closely mimic various aspects of the human complications of diabetes ➢ Standardized assays for phenotyping diabetic complications in animal models ➢ Validation criteria for animal models of diabetic complications ➢ Phenotype database ➢ Comprehensive Web site (www.amdcc.org) with public access to AMDCC resources and data
Type 1 Diabetes Mouse Resource	➢ Maintain over 199 stocks of mice important to diabetes research that are available to the scientific community ➢ Generated 19 new mouse strains that are sensitized to the development of diabetes complications for use by the research community.
Beta Cell Biology Consortium	➢ Public Web site (www.betacell.org) with over 300 unique and useful resources, of which 70 percent are publically available (those that are not remain in development and are released after validation and/or publication) ➢ 110 antibodies against markers expressed at different stages of stem cell to beta cell maturation ➢ Four PancChips (microarrays) for studying genes expressed in the pancreas/islets of both humans and mice, as well as over 36,000 gene promoter regions in mice ➢ 50 new lines of genetically engineered mice or mouse embryonic stem cells ➢ Genomics.betacell.org, which is a searchable database that provides search tools for genes, their transcripts, and their profiles in expression studies
Cooperative Study Group for Autoimmune Disease Prevention	➢ Class II human MHC tetramers ➢ NOD microarray database ➢ Antibody proteomic arrays
Type 1 Diabetes TrialNet	➢ DPT-1 dataset ➢ Biological samples
Collaborative Islet Transplant Registry	➢ Annual reports with international data on islet transplantation
Diabetic Retinopathy Clinical Research Network	➢ Study data
Diabetes Research in Children Network	➢ Study data
Type 1 Diabetes Genetics Consortium	➢ Study data ➢ Biological samples
Epidemiology of Diabetes Interventions and Complications	➢ Study data ➢ Biological samples
Genetics of Kidneys in Diabetes Study	➢ Study data ➢ Biological samples
Family Investigation of Nephropathy and Diabetes	➢ Study data ➢ Biological samples

* Data obtained from reports on progress of research consortia developed for planning and evaluation meetings, consortia Web sites, and/or NIDDK Central Repositories Web site.

Special Diabetes Program funded 1-year supplements to ongoing NIH grants for ancillary research. Research consortia and networks were funded either through cooperative agreement mechanisms, which allow NIH program officials to have significant involvement with the external scientists in the framing and achievement of a specified research goal, or with contracts or project grants (R01). The *Special Diabetes Program* established resource centers or provided supplements to established research centers to augment their type 1 diabetes research investments. These centers included animal model facilities, non-human primate centers, general clinical research centers, specialized centers, and centers that provided certain resources, such as islets for transplantation or basic research. The *Special Diabetes Program* also supported 28 grants to small businesses—Small Business Innovation Research grants (SBIR) and Small Business Technology Transfer Research grants (STTR)—to promote the development of innovative technologies such as sensors for continuous glucose monitors. Contracts were used for services such as coordinating trial networks, maintaining genetic and tissue sample repositories, supporting bioinformatics

integration, coordinating patient recruitment for clinical trials, and DNA sequencing.

NIH Involvement in Research Programs Supported by the *Special Diabetes Program*

Cooperative agreements (or U mechanism awards) are those in which NIH is significantly involved with the external scientists in the framing and achievements of the research program. As shown in Table B7, *Special Diabetes Program* support for cooperative agreements differs markedly from the NIH-wide pattern; the *Program* funded a significantly higher percentage of U awards in relationship to R awards than did NIH as a whole during the same time period. These data demonstrate that the funds of the *Special Diabetes Program* have been deployed so that NIH and the research community work in partnership to develop the research programs and ensure that progress is being made.

Clinical and Translational Research

The *Special Diabetes Program* has a clear focus on clinically relevant research that can improve the health and well-being of individuals with type 1 diabetes or at risk for developing the disease. This focus is consistent

Table B6: *Special Diabetes Program* Funding Mechanisms (FY 1998-2009)

Activity	New Awards	Supplements	Grants+Supplements
Research Project Grants (R01, R21, R24, R29, R33, R37)	379	28	407
Small Business Grants (STTR: R41; SBIR: R43, R44)	28	0	28
Research Programs and Centers (P01, P30, P40, P50, P51, P60, M01)	2	50	52
Cooperative Agreements (U01, U10, U19, U24, U42)	126	6	132
Training Awards (Career: K12; Institutional: T32)	14	0	14
Training Projects (DP2, DP3)	15	0	15
Contracts	28	1	29
TOTAL PROJECTS	592	85	677

Table B7: New Research Grants (FY 1998-2009)

* Data from e-SPA.

with the statutory language establishing the *Program*. An analysis was conducted (see methodology below) to determine the number of funded grants that were coded for human subject research (excluding research coded for human subject research, but that only involved human tissue samples). Of the 539 grants included in the analysis (R and U mechanisms), 225 (42 percent) were categorized as clinical research (see Table B8). By comparison, 40 percent of grants supported by NIH over the same time period matched the same definition of clinical research (42,554 of 105,000 grants using R or U mechanisms). A higher percentage of U grants supported by the *Special Diabetes Program* were categorized as clinical (63 percent, or 80 of 126 grants) compared to U grants supported by NIH during the same time period (56 percent, or 4,451 of 7,986). The *Special Diabetes Program* has had a particular focus on supporting clinical research through U mechanism grants. This focus is thus reflected in the high percentage of U mechanism grants supported by the *Program* that are clinically relevant. Furthermore, 23 of the grants supported by the *Special Diabetes Program* involved Phase III clinical trials, the final stage required before a therapy can be approved by FDA.

To complement the above grants analysis on the absolute number of grants supported by the *Program* that are categorized as clinical research, another analysis was performed to determine the percent of the overall budget that has supported clinical research projects. As shown in Figure B5, 63 percent of the budget of

the *Special Diabetes Program* from FY 1998-2009 was used to support clinical research. This budget analysis included not only R and U mechanism grants, but also contracts, training grants, and others (see methodology below). Using available data from NIH databases[31] showed that approximately one-third of the NIH budget in recent Fiscal Years (FY 2006-2009) has been categorized as clinical research. To be consistent with the statutory language establishing the *Program*, funds of the *Special Diabetes Program* have been deployed in a different way than regular NIH appropriations, which includes having a greater focus on clinical research and a correspondingly larger budget dedicated to it.

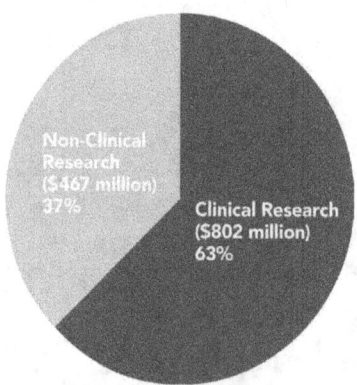

Figure B5: Budget of *Special Diabetes Program* Supporting Clinical Research, FY 1998-2009
Analysis includes R, U, T, K, DP2, and DP3 mechanism grants, as well as contracts; it excludes supplements to grants or centers because it would not be possible to determine if the categorization of the research as clinical related to the supplement portion of the grant or only to the primary grant. Thus, because the analysis excluded supplements, those budgets were also excluded from the denominator to calculate the percent clinical budget. The FY 1998-2009 budget used in the denominator of this calculation is $1.27 billion (rather than $1.29 billion, which is the total budget of the *Special Diabetes Program* over that time period).

---

[31] Analysis included data from: (1) NIH RePORTER (http://report.nih.gov/rcdc/categories/) for budget levels categorized as clinical research; and (2) the NIH almanac for historical total NIH budget figures (www.nih.gov/about/almanac/appropriations/index.htm).

In addition to clinical research, the *Special Diabetes Program* has also engendered significant research that translates basic research discoveries to the clinical setting. For example, animal models consortia—such as a consortium that evaluates the safety and efficacy of novel therapies to induce immune tolerance in non-human primate models of islet, kidney, heart, and lung transplantation—expedite the translation of promising therapies into clinical research. Indeed, one therapy that was tested by this consortium has been approved for testing in a human clinical trial. To further facilitate the pipeline of drug development, the Type 1 Diabetes—Rapid Access to Intervention Development (T1D–RAID) program was established to provide resources for the manufacture and pre-clinical development of drugs, natural products, and biologics that will be tested in type 1 diabetes clinical trials. Several agents have been manufactured through T1D-RAID and are being tested, or are planned for testing, in clinical trials. In addition, the Pre-clinical Testing Program associated with T1D-RAID has developed better methods for using rodent models for pre-clinical testing and has initiated testing of several new possible therapeutics. Overall, the *Special Diabetes Program* has supported a research continuum from basic to pre-clinical to clinical research, in which promising new therapeutic agents are being identified in the laboratory and subsequently tested in patients.

Methodology

- **Clinical Research Portfolio (analysis of R and U mechanism grants):** In this Report, clinical research was defined as all human subject research, excluding research labeled as human subject research but that only involved human tissue samples. To identify grants from FY 1998-2009 that fit this definition, the type 1 diabetes grant portfolio (as described under "Data Sources" earlier in this Appendix) was analyzed by e-SPA to obtain the IMPAC II human subject code for each grant application in order to classify projects as involving clinical research. Codes 10 and E4 were used to determine if a project was non-clinical; all other codes were considered clinical research. E4 projects were excluded because they involve the use of "human tissue samples," and this exclusion is consistent with the NIH decision to classify E4 projects as non-clinical research (described at http://grants.nih.gov/grants/policy/hs/faqs_specimens.htm; accessed May 19, 2010).

Table B8: Clinical Research Grants (FY 1998-2009)*

	Special Diabetes Program Grants		NIH-wide Grants	
	Fraction of Clinical Research Grants	Percent	Fraction of Clinical Research Grants	Percent
R Mechanism	145/413	35	38,089/97,307	39
U Mechanism	80/126	63	4,451/7,968	56
TOTAL (R+U)	225/539	42	42,554/105,400	40

* Data from e-SPA. This analysis included only R and U mechanism grants.

Sometimes, research grants in the NIH database were not flagged as clinical research in the first year or more of funding, but this flag was applied to the research in later years. Any research grant that was coded as clinical research at any point in its grant history was considered "clinical research" for the purpose of this analysis.

Data from the NIH comparison set was collected through e-SPA, using the same definitions for clinical research.

- **Phase III Clinical Trials:** *Special Diabetes Program* grants coded as clinical research in the above analysis were analyzed further using IMPAC II to determine if they were also coded as a Phase III clinical trial. If the grant had a Phase III clinical trial code during any 1 or more years of the project period, it was counted as Phase III for the purpose of this analysis.

- **Analysis of *Special Diabetes Program* Budget Supporting Clinical Research:** For clinical research consortia (T1DGC, TrialNet, TEDDY, SEARCH, ITN, CIT, CITR, DRCR.net, TRIGR, DirecNet, GoKinD, EDIC, and FIND), the entire research budget was included in the analysis. For non-consortia grants, grants coded as clinical research in the above analysis were further analyzed using IMPAC II to capture budget data by year. If a project year was coded as clinical research, the budget for that year was included in the budget total for clinical research. If a project year was coded as non-clinical research (codes 10 or E4), the budget for that year was not included in the analysis. Only funds from the *Special Diabetes Program* were included in the analysis; if grants received funds from regular NIH or CDC appropriations, those budgets were not included.

The total clinical research budget was then calculated by adding the budgets of the clinical research consortia with the budgets of clinical years of the non-consortia grants. The analysis included the entire grant portfolio analyzed by e-SPA, including R, U, K, T, DP2, and DP3 mechanism grants. It also included contracts, but excluded supplements to grants or centers.

The total budget over this time period was $1.29 billion. However, to calculate the percent clinical budget, the denominator was reduced by the budgets of the supplements that were excluded from the analysis. Thus, the FY 1998-2009 budget used in the denominator of this calculation was $1.27 billion.

RECRUITMENT AND SUPPORT OF DIABETES RESEARCHERS

A high priority of the *Special Diabetes Program* is the recruitment and retention of new investigators into diabetes-related research. Understanding the underlying causes of type 1 diabetes and finding new ways to prevent and cure this disease requires the concerted efforts of many investigators with diverse expertise. Relevant fields of scientific inquiry that can contribute to diabetes research include genetics, epidemiology, bioinformatics, genomics and proteomics, immunology, pathogen discovery, cell biology, bioengineering, transplantation surgery, neuroscience, cardiology, nephrology, ophthalmology, radiology, and others.

The *Special Diabetes Program* has used several mechanisms to attract new talent to type 1 diabetes research. Institutional clinical investigator training and career development programs for pediatric endocrinologists were established at seven medical institutions. Pilot and feasibility grants give new researchers the opportunity to test novel hypotheses that have conceptual promise. This type of award is also useful for established investigators who want to explore a new application or direction for their research. In addition, new research talent has been recruited through initiatives that pair established diabetes investigators with other scientists who can bring a new perspective or technology to the field. Finally, new research talent has been specifically recruited through an initiative directed to new investigators—the DP2 grant mechanism, also known as the Type 1 Diabetes Pathfinder Award. These mechanisms can be a magnet for drawing to diabetes research bright, capable investigators with creative research ideas to undertake innovative studies. Through these mechanisms, the *Special Diabetes Program* attracted investigators who had not previously received NIH funding, as well as scientists who were new to diabetes research.

In this evaluation, two approaches were considered to determine whether a grant supported by the *Special Diabetes Program* was submitted by a new investigator. First, grant applications in the NIH database IMPAC II have a "New Investigator" flag that denotes whether the grantee has had prior NIH funding. However, tracking of this parameter by the NIH began in 1999 and has been phased in over time. Therefore, it does not provide an accurate estimate of the number of new investigators for the date range of this evaluation. In a second approach, which was employed here, the investigator's earliest funded grant that disqualified him/her from being a new investigator was identified using IMPAC II. As currently defined by the NIH, an investigator can still be considered a "New Investigator" on a grant application if they previously held NIH subprojects or grants with the following activity codes: D43, G07, G08, G11, G13, G20, L30, L32, L40, L50, L60, R00, R03, R13, R15, R21, R25, R34, R36, R41, R43, R55, R56, R90, RL5, RL9, S10, S15, S21, S22, SC2, and SC3. In addition, previous F, K, and T grant mechanisms were not considered in the selection of an investigator's earliest grant application. NIH definition of a new investigator was accessed at: http://grants.nih.gov/grants/new_investigators/#definition in February 2010. The earliest funded grant application that disqualifies an investigator from "New Investigator" status was compared to the grant application funded by the *Special Diabetes Program*. A project was considered to have a "New Investigator" if the fiscal year of the *Special Diabetes Program* grant was the same as, or earlier than, the investigator's earliest disqualifying grant application. Data for the NIH-wide comparison group was collected using the same methodology.

From the inception of the program, FY 1998, through FY 2009, the *Special Diabetes Program* awarded 384 new research project grants (R01, R21, and DP2; this total does not include supplements to ongoing R01 grants). The analysis described above indicated that 147 (38 percent) of these were grants to new NIH investigators. These data are comparable with NIH-wide data for grant applications from new investigators (39 percent). The distribution of grants to new investigators by the *Special Diabetes Program* each year is summarized in Figure B6. Thus, the *Special Diabetes Program* is extending NIH's efforts to invest in human research capital by attracting and supporting new investigators.

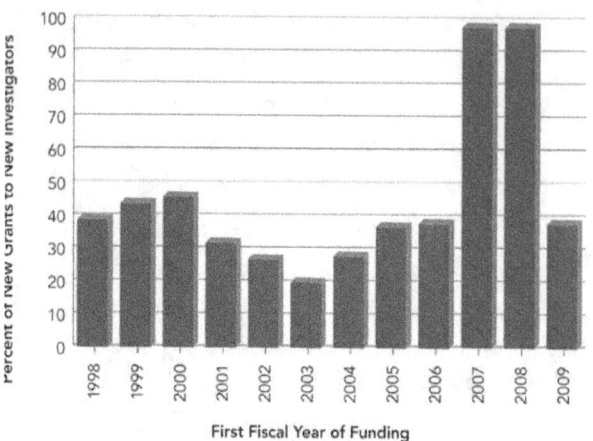

Figure B6: Recruitment of New Investigators
Data on *Special Diabetes Program*-funded investigators collected from NIH grant application database.

BROADLY CONSULTATIVE PLANNING PROCESS FOR PRIORITY SETTING AND RESOURCE DISTRIBUTION

The input of the diabetes research and voluntary communities in all aspects of planning, implementing, and evaluating the use of the *Special Diabetes Program* has been critical to its success. Leading scientific and lay experts with expertise relevant to type 1 diabetes and its complications have provided input on the priority-setting process for framing special type 1 diabetes initiatives, helped to evaluate the accomplishments of the *Program*, and identified new opportunities for future research that have emerged from the *Special Diabetes Program*.

External Evaluation Meetings

The NIH and CDC have convened a series of planning and evaluation meetings since the inception of the *Special Diabetes Program* to seek external scientific and lay input on ongoing and future research efforts. These meetings have constituted critical sources of input to program planning and management.

State-of-the-Science, 1997

In 1997, a trans-NIH conference entitled "Diabetes Mellitus: Challenges and Opportunities" met to discuss the state of research on diabetes and its complications. Symposium participants recommended that diabetes research be intensified in order to close research gaps, take advantage of new technologies, and capitalize on highly promising research leads and advances. The specific conclusions of this group were a critical source of input when the *Special Diabetes Program* was launched the next year. Moreover, the chairs of four relevant subpanels from the symposium reconvened in 1998 to provide input to NIH on the initial deployment of the funds under this *Program*.

Planning New Initiatives, 2000

In April 2000, scientific experts provided input on proposed research initiatives for the deployment of a portion of the funds of the *Special Diabetes Program* that became available after completion of short-term projects launched in FY 1998 and 1999. The input from this group were especially valuable for rapidly identifying high-priority initiatives when the *Special Diabetes Program* was expanded in duration and funding level in FY 2001.

Implementation, 2002

A similar panel of external experts met in May 2002 to review the use of the *Special Diabetes Program* at that time and to identify new research objectives and opportunities that arose from the expansion of research efforts on type 1 diabetes through the *Special Diabetes Program*. The input from this panel constituted a significant guide to NIH's research efforts on type 1 diabetes.

Mid-course Assessment, 2005

In January 2005, a third panel was convened for a 2-day meeting for a mid-course program assessment. The focus of the meeting was to evaluate the progress of 25 major research consortia, trial networks, and infrastructure-development initiatives. The panel also reviewed innovative research ideas proposed by the larger research community and discussed other emerging opportunities for research in type 1 diabetes that were enabled by the *Special Diabetes Program*.

Planning and Evaluation, 2008 and 2009

Conduct of *ad hoc* External Evaluation Meetings: In order to obtain external input on the progress and future directions of consortia supported by the *Special Diabetes Program*, NIDDK convened two recent ad hoc external evaluation meetings. These meetings were conducted similarly, as described below.

Panel members were identified by NIH and CDC for participation based on their scientific expertise. Panelists were asked to identify any potential conflicts of interest prior to the meeting and were dismissed for discussions that would qualify as a conflict of interest. Prior to the meeting panelists received a briefing binder prepared by NIH and CDC staff. This briefing binder contained introductory material about the *Special Diabetes Program*, instructions to the panel, and information on the consortia to be discussed. For each consortium to be discussed, the briefing binder contained:

- Administrative summary
- Description
- Goals
- Top five accomplishments

- Details of program management

- Details of resources provided to the scientific community

- Problems encountered

- Future directions if the *Special Diabetes Program* is extended

- Future directions if the *Special Diabetes Program* is not extended

- Most recent External Evaluation Committee report and/or report of the Data and Safety Monitoring Board

- List of publications generated

Panelists were informed prior to the meetings that the discussion was to serve as a means to obtain input on both current efforts and future directions on each consortium or network. The panel was asked to address the following questions:

- Does the consortium address a compelling scientific opportunity?

- How might scientific progress of each consortium be improved?

- Are processes in place to modify consortium plans in response to new scientific discoveries?

- Are there opportunities to better use resources generated by the consortium to advance type 1 diabetes research?

- Are there additional opportunities for coordination of consortia with each other and with other efforts?

The meetings were organized by consortium. Each session, which focused on a particular consortium, began with a presentation from a scientist participating in that consortium. The presentation provided an overview of the consortium, scientific accomplishments to date, current efforts, and future directions. The scientist then answered questions from the panel before leaving the room for the panel discussion. Non-federal attendees, other than the panelists, were asked to leave the room for the panel discussion. Individual panel members were designated as primary or secondary chairs for each discussion prior to the meeting based on their scientific field. The primary and secondary chairs for each session made introductory remarks and led the group discussion on each consortium or network. Following the introductory remarks, the chairs opened the floor to comments from the other panelists. Panelists provided individual input and opinions on the consortium and the discussion questions. At the end of the meeting, each panel member had an opportunity to provide input on future directions for research outside of the context of the ongoing programs.

Meeting on Clinical Research Supported by the *Special Statutory Funding Program for Type 1 Diabetes Research*, 2008: An external panel of 13 scientific experts with expertise in clinical trials, autoimmune diseases, immunology, transplantation, epidemiology, and biostatistics convened in Rockville, Maryland on April 29-30, 2008 (see Acknowledgments for a list of panelists). The goal of the 2-day planning and evaluation meeting was to perform a mid-course assessment of ongoing clinical research efforts supported by the *Special Statutory Funding Program for Type 1 Diabetes Research.*

The meeting was devoted to sessions to evaluate the following nine clinical research consortia supported by the *Special Diabetes Program*:

- Type 1 Diabetes TrialNet
- Immune Tolerance Network (ITN)
- Clinical Islet Transplantation (CIT) Consortium
- Collaborative Islet Transplant Registry (CITR)
- Diabetic Retinopathy Clinical Research Network (DRCR.net)
- The Environmental Determinants of Diabetes in the Young (TEDDY)
- Trial To Reduce IDDM in the Genetically at Risk (TRIGR)
- SEARCH for Diabetes in Youth (SEARCH)
- Diabetes Research in Children Network (DirecNet)

Much of the input provided by members of the expert panel cut across multiple research efforts. Cross-cutting input included:

- **Continue ongoing studies:** To capitalize on the investment made to date, it is important to continue all ongoing clinical research studies. All of the consortia have the potential to have a dramatic impact on the prevention and treatment of type 1 diabetes, and ending them prematurely would jeopardize the ability to acquire the extensive knowledge that can be gained through the studies.
- **Enhance collaboration among consortia:** The panel members acknowledged the efforts of the NIH, CDC, and the research consortia to coordinate their activities and noted that enhanced collaboration and coordination could propel research progress.

- **Develop a means to broadly advertise and distribute resources to the type 1 diabetes research community:** The consortia are collecting a significant number of biosamples and generating copious amounts of data that will be of benefit to the diabetes research community. It would be valuable for research consortia to develop a means to advertise the availability of biosamples and data and to ensure that policies and methods are in place to efficiently distribute these resources.
- **Encourage ancillary studies of ongoing clinical trials:** In order to maximize the investment in ongoing research programs, several panel members stressed the importance of engaging the scientific community in conducting ancillary studies of ongoing clinical trials.
- **Encourage mechanistic studies:** It is important that clinical trials be accompanied by mechanistic studies to understand why a particular therapy was or was not successful. These studies can also uncover new knowledge about mechanisms underlying type 1 diabetes disease onset and progression.

After reviewing the clinical consortia portfolio, the panel members commended NIH and CDC on the many accomplishments that have been achieved through the *Special Diabetes Program* in such a short period of time and noted that the research portfolio that has been established under the NIDDK's leadership has been a very wise investment of funding.

Meeting on Pre-Clinical Research Supported by the *Special Statutory Funding Program for Type 1 Diabetes Research*, 2009: An external panel of 14 scientific experts with expertise in beta cell biology, immunology, diabetes complications, and animal models convened in Rockville, Maryland on June 17-18, 2009 (see Acknowledgments for a list of panelists). The goal of the 2-day planning and evaluation meeting was to perform a mid-course assessment of ongoing pre-clinical research efforts supported by the *Special Statutory Funding Program for Type 1 Diabetes Research*.

The meeting was devoted to sessions to evaluate the following nine pre-clinical research consortia supported by the *Special Diabetes Program*:

- Type 1 Diabetes-Rapid Access to Intervention Development (T1D-RAID)

- Testing for Preclinical Efficacy in Prevention or Reversal of Type 1 Diabetes in Rodent Models (Type 1 Diabetes Preclinical Testing Program [T1D-PTP])

- Testing for Preclinical Efficacy in Prevention or Reversal of Diabetic Complications in Rodent Models (Type 1 Diabetes Preclinical Testing Program [T1D-PTP])

- Animal Models of Diabetic Complications Consortium (AMDCC)

- Type 1 Diabetes Mouse Resource (T1DR)

- Beta Cell Biology Consortium (BCBC)

- Cooperative Study Group for Autoimmune Disease Prevention

- Immunobiology of Xenotransplantation Cooperative Research Program (IXCRP)

- Non-Human Primate Transplantation Tolerance Cooperative Study Group (NHPCSG)

Cross-cutting input provided by the panel regarding pre-clinical research included:

- **Enhance utilization of resources:** Many of the pre-clinical consortia generate resources or provide services to assist research in this field. Suggestions from individual panelists included improving advertising of these resources, offering more flexible receipt dates for applications for services, and increasing the availability of biosamples generated by pre-clinical research consortia.

- **Enhance collaboration among consortia:** The panel members acknowledged the efforts of NIH, CDC, and the research consortia to coordinate their activities and noted that enhanced collaboration and coordination could propel research progress.

- **Improve animal models of human disease:** Many panel members felt that efforts to improve animal models of human disease so that they are more representative of disease are important research opportunities.

After reviewing the pre-clinical program portfolio, the panel members were enthusiastic about the progress and accomplishments of the pre-clinical consortia supported by the *Special Diabetes Program*. The NIDDK and NIAID were commended for their leadership of these consortia.

The input obtained at these evaluation meetings has been critically important for informing the government's program planning efforts for this time-limited appropriation. For example, at both meetings, panel members encouraged the government to enhance coordination across existing research consortia, to make the best use of existing resources and maximize research progress. One example of how coordination has been enhanced is through collaboration on a new clinical trial. Two research consortia—one with expertise in glucose monitoring technology and another with expertise in testing therapies for early treatment of type 1 diabetes—are collaborating on a clinical trial testing whether early and intensive blood glucose control at disease onset could preserve insulin production. In the trial, patients are placed on an inpatient closed-loop system and sent home with a sensor-augmented insulin pump. Thus, the combined expertise of the two consortia has been instrumental in enabling the conduct of this trial.

At the pre-clinical research meeting, the panel evaluated a consortium studying porcine to non-human primate models of xenotransplantation (solid organ, tissue, or cell transplantation between species). Panel members felt that the consortium's research was extremely valuable as an approach to relieve the shortage of solid organs for transplantation, but the research was less relevant to islet transplantation. Based on that feedback, the consortium is no longer supported by the *Special Diabetes Program*, but does continue to receive support from regularly appropriated funds for research on solid organ transplantation. Panel members at the clinical meeting felt that it was important to bolster research toward the development of an artificial pancreas. Based on this input, NIDDK developed new initiatives, with support from the *Special Diabetes Program*, to solicit research proposals from small businesses toward developing new technologies to inform development of an artificial pancreas. This example demonstrates how external evaluation led to a shift in use of the funds based on ongoing surveillance of scientific opportunities and how NIH has implemented input from the evaluation panels to enhance research supported by the *Special Diabetes Program*. The input received at these meetings continues to be invaluable as the government makes plans for future research directions.

Strategic Planning for Diabetes Research

The NIH utilizes strategic planning, with broad external input, to inform research directions, including research supported by the *Special Diabetes Program*. Strategic planning efforts that have informed program planning are described below.

1999 Diabetes Research Working Group Strategic Plan

In 1999, the independent, congressionally established Diabetes Research Working Group (DRWG) issued its strategic research plan for conquering diabetes, including both type 1 and type 2 diabetes. This panel of scientific experts engaged in a year-long, in-depth process to gather input from the diabetes research and voluntary communities. The DRWG's recommendations of relevance to type 1 diabetes have informed the planning and implementation of the *Special Diabetes Program*. These areas of DRWG emphasis include research opportunities identified in the areas of genetics; autoimmunity and the beta cell; clinical research and clinical trials; diabetic complications; special populations, including children; and resource needs. The Report can be accessed at: http://www2.niddk.nih.gov/NR/rdonlyres/95751201-0104-400D-AF6D-DC32E6BE74FE/0/DWG_1999_Report.pdf

2006 "Advances and Emerging Opportunities in Type 1 Diabetes Research: A Strategic Plan"

Responding to input from the January 2005 *ad hoc* mid-course assessment of the *Special Diabetes Program*, the Director, NIDDK, launched the development of a strategic plan for type 1 diabetes research under the auspices of the statutory Diabetes Mellitus Interagency Coordinating Committee (DMICC). The 18-month planning process involved creating five scientifically focused working groups to evaluate the state-of-the-science and to propose research objectives for type 1 diabetes research for the next 10 years. Each working group was composed of external scientific experts, members of the DMICC and other NIH officials, representatives from patient advocacy organizations, and lay members. The Type 1 Diabetes Research Strategic Plan can be accessed at: www.T1Diabetes.nih.gov/plan

2010 *"Advances and Emerging Opportunities in Diabetes Research: A Strategic Planning Report of the DMICC"*

In August 2008, the DMICC determined that the time was right to identify high-priority opportunities for diabetes research that can be accomplished in the next 5 to 10 years. As chair of the DMICC, NIDDK spearheaded the collaborative effort across federal agencies and with input from the external research and patient advocacy communities to develop a new Diabetes Research Strategic Plan. To formulate the Strategic Plan, working groups were convened to address each of 10 scientific areas of extraordinary opportunity in diabetes research. An additional working group composed of representatives from each of the other 10 groups addressed overarching needs for scientific expertise, tools, technologies, and shared resources. Each working group was chaired by a scientist external to NIH, and was comprised of external scientific experts—including basic scientists, clinicians, and engineers—as well as representatives of DMICC member organizations and diabetes voluntary organizations. This Plan will guide NIH, other federal agencies, and the investigative and lay communities in their pursuit of the goal of conquering diabetes. The Diabetes Research Strategic Plan can be accessed at: http://diabetesplan.niddk.nih.gov

Peer Review

Grants, cooperative agreements, and contracts supported by the *Special Diabetes Program* have been subject to peer-review mechanisms of NIH and CDC funding processes. This review system ensures that the funds are expended for scientifically- and technically-meritorious research that is responsive to the goals and priorities of the *Special Diabetes Program*. A limited number of administrative supplemental research awards were also made to existing projects.

Consortia External Evaluation Committees

For most large consortia supported by the *Special Diabetes Program*, NIH and CDC have established panels of scientists external to the consortia to provide ongoing oversight. These panels meet regularly to review progress and provide input on allocation of resources and future directions for the consortia.

Collaboration with the Diabetes Voluntary Community and Other Non-Federal Funding Sources

The major diabetes voluntary organizations—ADA and JDRF—have been committed and essential partners with HHS in providing critical input on the scientific goals and strategies of the *Special Diabetes Program*. Representatives of these groups have participated in the planning, assessment, and evaluation meetings that have aided in the formulation of a scientifically credible and productive plan for the *Special Diabetes Program*. Moreover, by co-sponsoring several of the special type 1 diabetes research initiatives, these organizations help HHS to maximize the resources available for achieving the goals of the *Special Diabetes Program*.

APPENDIX C

EVALUATION OF MAJOR RESEARCH CONSORTIA, NETWORKS, AND RESOURCES

This Appendix includes evaluation of the major research consortia, networks, and resources supported by the *Special Statutory Funding Program for Type 1 Diabetes Research* (*Special Diabetes Program* or *Program*). These sections were developed so that all the information on a single Consortium is found under that Consortium, rather than cross-referencing other sections of this Appendix. Therefore, information that is relevant to two different consortia will be repeated under each Consortium. This approach, although repetitive, was intentionally used so that complete information could be found in each Consortium's evaluation in a self-contained way. Consortium evaluations include the following sections:

- *Program Description*: The value added by the Consortium in the context of the overall research portfolio.

- *Highlights of Progress*: Examples of the progress achieved through spring 2010.

- *Anticipated Outcomes*: Description of anticipated future progress and the impact that the research effort could have on the health of people with type 1 diabetes.

- *Ongoing Evaluation*: Descriptions of regular oversight mechanisms, such as reviews by external evaluation panels.

- *Program Enhancements*: Descriptions of how the project has evolved over time to enhance research progress, based on input from external experts or from internal discussions within the program.

- *Coordination with Other Research Efforts*: Examples of how the research Consortium or network collaborates and coordinates its efforts with other research efforts to maximize and synergize progress.

- *Administrative History*: Programmatic details, including years of duration and agencies that support the Consortium.

In this Appendix, the consortia and networks are organized by Goal:[32]

Goal I: Identify the Genetic and Environmental Causes of Type 1 Diabetes

- o Type 1 Diabetes Genetics Consortium
- o The Environmental Determinants of Diabetes in the Young
- o SEARCH for Diabetes in Youth
- o Type 1 Diabetes Mouse Resource

Goal II: Prevent or Reverse Type 1 Diabetes

- o Type 1 Diabetes TrialNet
- o Immune Tolerance Network
- o Cooperative Study Group for Autoimmune Disease Prevention
- o Standardization Programs: Diabetes Autoantibody Standardization Program, C-peptide Standardization, and Improving the Clinical Measurement of Hemoglobin A1c
- o Trial To Reduce IDDM in the Genetically At-Risk
- o Type 1 Diabetes–Rapid Access to Intervention Development[33]

---

[32] Many consortia are relevant to Goal VI (Attract New Talent and Apply New Technologies to Research on Type 1 Diabetes), so there is not a separate section on Goal VI.

[33] Also relevant to Goal V.

Goal III: Develop Cell Replacement Therapy

o   Beta Cell Biology Consortium
o   Non-Human Primate Transplantation Tolerance Cooperative Study Group
o   Clinical Islet Transplantation Consortium
o   Islet Cell Resource Centers
o   Integrated Islet Distribution Program
o   Collaborative Islet Transplant Registry

Goal IV: Prevent or Reduce Hypoglycemia in Type 1 Diabetes

o   Diabetes Research in Children Network

Goal V: Prevent or Reduce the Complications of Type 1 Diabetes

o   Epidemiology of Diabetes Interventions and Complications Study
o   Animal Models of Diabetic Complications Consortium
o   Genetics of Diabetes Complications
o   Diabetic Retinopathy Clinical Research Network

Goal I: Identify the Genetic and Environmental Causes of Type 1 Diabetes

TYPE 1 DIABETES GENETICS CONSORTIUM (T1DGC)

The T1DGC is organizing and implementing international efforts to identify genes that determine an individual's risk of developing type 1 diabetes. Teasing apart the multiple gene combinations that predispose someone to this complex disease requires analysis of a very large dataset covering thousands of patients and closely related family members who may or may not have developed the disease. The goal of the monumental first phase of the project, completed in FY 2007, was to recruit families particularly those with multiple siblings with type 1 diabetes, to join the study and to collect DNA samples for analysis. Later on, the Consortium also initiated collection of trio families, and cases and controls from populations with a low prevalence of disease. A Consortium database containing clinical, genetic, and medical history information has been established to facilitate the search for susceptibility genes. The database and centralized DNA repository have and continue to serve as a resource accessible to genetics researchers both within and outside the T1DGC.

HIGHLIGHTS OF PROGRESS

- Completed enrollment of over 2,800 families who have two or more siblings with type 1 diabetes and performed genome scans on these families.

- Completed enrollment of 500 families who have one member with type 1 diabetes and their parents, and 600 cases and 700 controls.

- Performed genome scans on all the 2,800 families who have two or more siblings with type 1 diabetes.

- Identified, with its collaborators, more than 40 genes or gene regions that are involved in type 1 diabetes.

- Established a Major Histocompatibility Complex fine-mapping project to study genes in this region involved in susceptibility to type 1 diabetes.

- Established a Rapid Response project to study candidate genes that could contribute to type 1 diabetes.

- Distributed samples and data to several investigators.

- Stored data and samples in NIDDK Central Repositories. These are available to scientists worldwide for application of the latest genetic technology to study DNA from this large and well-characterized set of affected families.

Anticipated Outcomes

The T1DGC is a large-scale, well coordinated effort to identify numerous genes and gene combinations that are important in predicting an individual's risk of developing type 1 diabetes or related autoimmune diseases. The T1DGC is building on the work of the Human Genome Project that spelled out the contents of human genes and the International HapMap Project that identified the points at which gene sequences differ from person to person. The T1DGC is resolving which of these genetic differences are significant for type 1 diabetes. In 2003, just three type 1 diabetes genes were known. Today, the T1DGC and its collaborators have identified more than 40 genes or gene regions that are associated with the disease.

As science progresses to the age of personalized medicine, clinicians may soon be able to determine the optimal treatment strategy for an individual based on his or her genetic background. With new insights into the genetic factors that play a role in type 1 diabetes, researchers may be able to identify with great precision those individuals at risk for the disease, and to develop and test prevention-oriented strategies. It is possible, for example, that certain therapies to delay or reverse the development of type 1 diabetes may be more effective in individuals with specific genetic changes that predispose to type 1 diabetes. Such new genetic knowledge could point the way toward better screening of newborns or to widespread screening of the general population to identify individuals at risk of developing type 1 diabetes. This knowledge would facilitate the design of more specific clinical trials for testing interventions specifically tailored to patients with similar risk profiles. These

are just a few examples of the enormously important, predictive and preemptive strides that can be envisioned and possibly attained by further understanding the genetic underpinnings of disease development.

Ongoing Evaluation

To ensure ongoing evaluation of the study design and the progress of the T1DGC, NIDDK established an External Evaluation Committee (EEC). The EEC is composed of investigators with scientific expertise relevant to research conducted by the T1DGC, but who are not members of the Consortium. The EEC meets annually to:

- Review activities that affect the operational and methodological aspects of the study (*e.g.*, quality control procedures; performance of clinical networks, data coordinating center, and core laboratories).

- Review data to ensure its quality, provide input on procedures for analysis and data display, and provide input on interpretation and implication of results.

- Review proposed major modifications to the protocol or operations of the study for appropriateness, necessity, and impact on overall study objectives.

In addition, the T1DGC has been evaluated by an external panel of scientific and lay experts at an *ad hoc* evaluation meeting convened by NIDDK in January 2005. This meeting was an opportunity for external experts to evaluate progress and provide input on future research directions (for more information, see the Executive Summary and Appendix B). Through *ad hoc* evaluation meetings and regular meetings of the EEC, NIDDK continually seeks external input to inform current and future directions for the T1DGC.

Program Enhancements

Because of the evolving nature of science, consortia supported by the *Special Diabetes Program* have evolved over time and have undergone enhancements to take advantage of new technologies and research findings, and to accelerate progress. Some enhancements have been made in response to external input and others have been initiated by the consortium members. Examples of program enhancements for the T1DGC include:

- To increase coordination with the other human genetics consortia supported by the *Special Diabetes Program*, the T1DGC participated in a meeting with these consortia and developed new initiatives to coordinate future research efforts among these studies.

- The T1DGC also utilizes T1Dbase (http://T1DBase.org) as a Web-based tool to coordinate, manage, and interpret human, mouse, and rat genetics data. Use of T1Dbase has improved coordination of genetics research in mice and humans. Data on T1Dbase are open access and all software is open source in order to maximize its usage by the broad research community.

Coordination with Other Research Efforts

The T1DGC coordinates its efforts with multiple other type 1 diabetes research consortia and networks supported by the *Special Diabetes Program*. Collaboration, coordination, and resource sharing serve to synergize research efforts and accelerate research progress. Examples of coordination with other consortia are given below. For a summary of ongoing collaborative efforts, please see Appendix D.

Coordinating Patient Recruitment Efforts:

- All 14 Type 1 Diabetes TrialNet clinical centers and 4 SEARCH for Diabetes in Youth (SEARCH) study sites are participating as recruitment centers for the T1DGC North American Network.

- T1DGC assisted TrialNet in establishing international recruitment sites.

Enhancing Data Comparison Among Studies:

- T1DGC, TrialNet, SEARCH, and The Environmental Determinants of Diabetes in the Young (TEDDY) are sharing information and reagents so that they can assess allele and haplotype frequencies of the same sets of genes including *Human Leukocyte Antigen* and other diabetes-predisposing genes. This coordination will permit comparisons of genetics data across all four studies, effectively increasing the power of each in learning which genes play a role in disease onset.

- T1DGC, TrialNet, and TEDDY share the same North American laboratory for measurement of autoantibodies (markers used to predict an individual's risk for developing type 1 diabetes). This coordination will permit direct comparison of results obtained in each study.

- Researchers in the Diabetes Autoantibody Standardization Program (DASP) provide tools that T1DGC laboratories use to standardize autoantibody data. Data standardization provides confidence that results are independent of the laboratory performing the measurements.

Coordinating Studies of Type 1 Diabetes Genetics:

- The T1DGC coordinates its research efforts with the other genetics consortia supported by the *Special Diabetes Program* (Epidemiology of Diabetes Interventions and Complications, Family Investigation of Nephropathy and Diabetes, and Genetics of Kidneys in Diabetes Study).

Sharing Samples, Data, and Resources with the Research Community:

- The T1DGC has developed a comprehensive public Web site with information on samples, data, and resources that are available to the scientific research community (www.t1dgc.org).

- The T1DGC is repositing samples and data in all three NIDDK Central Repositories (Biosample, Genetics, and Data Repositories). The Repositories were established to expand the usefulness of NIDDK-supported studies by allowing a broader research community to access these materials beyond the end of the study.

T1DGC Administrative History	
Date Initiative Started	2002
Date *Special Diabetes Program* Funding Started	2002
Participating Components	NIDDK, NIAID, NHGRI, and JDRF
Web site	www.t1dgc.org
T1DGC consists of a coordinating center and four clinical recruitment networks in Asia-Pacific, Europe, North America, and the United Kingdom.	

THE ENVIRONMENTAL DETERMINANTS OF DIABETES IN THE YOUNG (TEDDY)

Scientists directing six independent studies of environmental triggers of type 1 diabetes in the United States and Europe joined forces to create this international consortium. TEDDY is providing a coordinated, multidisciplinary approach to understanding the infectious agents, dietary factors, or other environmental conditions that trigger type 1 diabetes in genetically susceptible individuals. TEDDY investigators have screened newborns in the general population, as well as those who have a first-degree relative with type 1 diabetes. In this large-scale, long-term epidemiological effort, in which patient follow-up is estimated to continue through 2023, high-risk infants will be followed until they are 15 years of age. The TEDDY study is making progress toward amassing the largest data set and samples on newborns at risk for autoimmunity and type 1 diabetes anywhere in the world. To maximize the return on the investment in TEDDY, samples from the study will be made widely available to researchers worldwide.

HIGHLIGHTS OF PROGRESS

- Completed screening of 418,671 newborns from the general population.

- Completed recruitment of 7,487 newborns from the general population.

- Completed screening of 6,412 newborns with a first-degree relative with type 1 diabetes.

- Completed recruitment of 894 newborns with a first-degree relative with type 1 diabetes.

- Mapped the frequencies of genes that increase susceptibility to type 1 diabetes in diverse populations.

- Completed food composition database harmonization.

- Discovered significant differences in infant feeding practices between the United States and Europe and explored variability in infant nutrition within the U.S. population.

- Identified risk factors for why families drop out of the study.

Anticipated Outcomes

Until researchers know what causes type 1 diabetes, it is difficult to develop strategies to prevent it. Previous studies suggested that certain factors, such as early exposure to cereal or cow's milk, might predispose to type 1 diabetes. However, these studies were too small and too short to achieve statistically significant results, and no definitive environmental trigger of the disease has yet been identified. Therefore, TEDDY is a crucially important effort to tease out the environmental factors triggering disease onset. While it is a substantial investment of time and resources to follow individuals for many years, it is only through a long-term, coordinated study such as TEDDY that researchers are likely to answer critically important questions about type 1 diabetes risk and onset.

Realization of study goals could have an enormously positive impact on public health efforts regarding disease prevention. For example, if a viral trigger is revealed, a vaccine could possibly be developed to prevent disease onset in genetically-susceptible individuals.

Alternatively, if a dietary component is found to be causative or protective, individuals at risk could take steps to either eliminate or add it to their diets. By pinpointing the constellation of type 1 diabetes disease genes (as is being done by the Type 1 Diabetes Genetics Consortium), environmental triggers (as is being done in TEDDY), and their cascading effects on the immune system (see Goal II), researchers may be able to entirely prevent or reverse disease onset. Combating the disease at the "front-end" is especially beneficial because early steps could preclude or arrest the development of disease complications—including kidney failure, blindness, lower limb amputations, heart attacks, and strokes. Research on the genetic and environmental causes of the disease thus offers the real hope of preventing type 1 diabetes.

Importantly, the studies of environmental factors that play a role in type 1 diabetes may also contribute to understanding the development of celiac disease, a digestive disorder caused by autoimmunity directed at gluten proteins in wheat and other grains. Celiac disease affects about 2 million Americans and like type 1 diabetes, rates of the disorder are rising. Some genes confer susceptibility to both celiac disease and type 1 diabetes, and many people have both diseases. Therefore, ongoing studies to identify environmental triggers of type 1 diabetes are also investigating development of celiac disease. These studies may uncover environmental factors initiating both disorders, benefiting not only people with type 1 diabetes, but also people suffering from celiac disease and other autoimmune diseases.

Ongoing Evaluation

To ensure ongoing evaluation of the study design and the progress of TEDDY, NIDDK established an External Evaluation Committee (EEC) composed of scientific experts who are not participating in TEDDY. The EEC meets annually, in person or by conference call, to:

- Review activities that affect the operational and methodological aspects of the study (*e.g.*, quality control procedures; performance of clinical centers, data coordinating center, and core laboratories);

- Review data to ensure its quality, provide input on procedures for analysis and data display, and provide input on interpretation and implications of results; and

- Review proposed major modifications to the protocol or operations of the study for safety, appropriateness, necessity, and impact on overall study objectives.

In addition, TEDDY has been evaluated by external panels of scientific and lay experts at *ad hoc* evaluation meetings convened by NIDDK in January 2005 and April 2008. These meetings were an opportunity for external experts to evaluate progress and provide input on future research directions (for more information, see the Executive Summary and Appendix B). Through *ad hoc* evaluation meetings and regular meetings of the EEC, NIDDK continually seeks external input to inform current and future directions for TEDDY.

Program Enhancements

Because of the evolving nature of science, consortia supported by the *Special Diabetes Program* have evolved over time and have undergone enhancements to take advantage of new technologies and research findings, and to accelerate progress. Some enhancements have been made in response to external input and others have been initiated by the consortium members. Examples of program enhancements for TEDDY include:

- Because measurements of islet autoantibodies were not standardized, it was difficult to compare results across different TEDDY sites. To address this barrier, TEDDY scientists fostered development of an NIDDK Islet Autoantibody Measurement Harmonization Project. This effort is helping to standardize protocols for measuring autoantibodies not just within TEDDY, but within all NIDDK studies, and is thus having a far-reaching impact.

- It was recognized that materials being developed by TEDDY would be of use to other scientists studying type 1 diabetes, so the consortium expanded its public Web site to include the study protocol, manual of operations, study forms, and other study materials (www.teddystudy.org).

- To take advantage of new and emerging technologies, TEDDY developed a program and explicit guidelines for ancillary studies to facilitate access to TEDDY materials by researchers who seek to expand and embrace new technologies for inclusion into the TEDDY study group. The NIDDK developed an initiative to support investigator-initiated ancillary studies to ongoing research efforts, including TEDDY.

- TEDDY enhanced coordination with other type 1 diabetes research consortia studying newborns, such as the Trial to Reduce IDDM in the Genetically at Risk (TRIGR) and TrialNet.

Coordination with Other Research Efforts

TEDDY coordinates its efforts with multiple other type 1 diabetes research consortia and networks supported by the *Special Diabetes Program*, particularly those studying newborns.

Collaboration, coordination, and resource sharing serve to synergize research efforts and accelerate research progress. Examples of coordination with other consortia are given below. For a summary of ongoing collaborative efforts, please see Appendix D.

Coordinating Research Studies Involving Newborns:

- TEDDY investigators have met with researchers participating in other type 1 diabetes research studies involving newborns (TRIGR and TrialNet) to discuss opportunities for enhancing coordination and collaboration.

- TEDDY has shared the following materials with TrialNet investigators who are studying newborns in the Nutritional Intervention to Prevent Diabetes Study: genetic-screening procedures, data forms, and parts of the Manual of Operations concerning follow-up of high-risk children.

- TEDDY and TRIGR share the same Data Coordinating Center. This coordination has resulted in implementation of similar standards in data collection, entry, management of quality control, and analyses for both studies.

- TEDDY, TrialNet, and TRIGR have coordinated patient recruitment efforts to ensure that they are not adversely competing for patient participants in their studies.

- TRIGR and TEDDY investigators are considering collaborative efforts on recruitment after TRIGR accrual ends. Both groups are also considering a follow-up intervention protocol.

Enhancing Data Comparison Among Studies:

- T1DGC, TrialNet, SEARCH for Diabetes in Youth, and TEDDY are sharing information and reagents so that they can assess allele and haplotype frequencies of the same sets of genes including *Human Leukocyte Antigen* (*HLA*) and other diabetes-predisposing genes. This coordination will permit comparisons of genetics data across all four studies, effectively increasing the power of each in learning which genes play a role in disease onset.

- TEDDY, T1DGC, and TrialNet share the same North American laboratory for measurement of autoantibodies. This coordination will permit direct comparison of results obtained in each study.

- TRIGR and TEDDY have implemented similar standards in data collection and entry. This coordination is permitting direct comparison between results obtained in each study relevant to nutrition and to diabetes-associated variants of certain immune system genes (*HLA* genes).

- TEDDY scientists have fostered development of the NIDDK Islet Autoantibody Measurement Harmonization Project. Common protocols have been developed optimizing the methods used to measure antibodies in TEDDY. Protocols and standards have been distributed to all laboratories measuring antibodies in NIDDK studies and these laboratories are using a standard protocol and common standards to measure study samples.

Sharing Samples, Data, and Resources with the Research Community:

- TEDDY is repositing biological samples and data into the NIDDK Central Repositories and will make the material available to the broad scientific community. The NIDDK has developed an initiative to support investigator-initiated ancillary studies to ongoing studies, including TEDDY.

TEDDY Administrative History	
Date Initiative Started	2002
Date *Special Diabetes Program* Funding Started	2002
Participating Components	NIDDK, NIAID, NICHD, NIEHS, CDC, and JDRF
Web site	www.teddystudy.org
TEDDY is a consortium of six Clinical Centers and one Data Coordinating Center in the United States, Finland, Sweden, and Germany.	

SEARCH FOR DIABETES IN YOUTH (SEARCH)

Major impediments to diabetes research and efforts to improve public health include lack of uniform national information on the rates of childhood diabetes, whether these are changing over time, and the clinical course and evolution of different forms of diabetes in children and youth. While substantial increases in the incidence of type 1 diabetes have been reported in Europe, reliable data on changes over time in the United States, or even how many children in the United States have diabetes, were lacking. The SEARCH multicenter epidemiological study is identifying cases of diabetes in children and youth less than 20 years of age in six geographically dispersed populations that encompass the ethnic diversity of the United States. The study aims to identify the number of children and youth under age 20 who have diabetes; learn how type 1 diabetes and type 2 diabetes differ, including how they differ by age and race/ethnicity; learn more about the risk for acute and chronic complications of diabetes in children and youth; investigate the different types of care and medical treatment that these children and youth receive; and learn more about how diabetes affects the daily lives of children and youth in the United States. Now that the first baseline assessment of diabetes rates in children nationwide has been completed, the study is poised to evaluate trends in diabetes incidence and progression of the disease over time.

HIGHLIGHTS OF PROGRESS

- The SEARCH prevalence data indicate that at least 154,000 children/youth (1.8 per 1,000) in the United States have diabetes. Diabetes prevalence varies across major racial/ethnic groups:

  - In children 0-9 years of age, non-Hispanic whites had the highest prevalence (about 1/1,000) and type 1 diabetes was the most common form of diabetes across all race/ethnic groups.

  - Among adolescents and young adults, African American and non-Hispanic white youth had the highest burden of diabetes (about 1/300) and Asian/Pacific Islanders had the lowest (about 1/750). Prevalence of type 1 diabetes was 2.3/1,000 and was the most common form of diabetes in all racial/ethnic groups except in American Indian youth.

- The SEARCH incidence data indicated that annually 15,000 youth are diagnosed with type 1 diabetes. Diabetes incidence also varies across major racial/ethnic groups:

  - In children less than 10 years of age, most diabetes cases are type 1, regardless of race/ethnicity, and the incidence of type 1 diabetes is highest in non-Hispanic whites.

  - In older youth (10-19 years), the highest incidence of type 1 diabetes is in non-Hispanic whites; American Indian and Asian/Pacific Islanders have the lowest.

- Since 2002, approximately 5.5 million children less than 20 years of age (approximately 6 percent of the under 20 years U.S. population) with wide racial/ethnic, socioeconomic, and geographic representation, have been under surveillance at the SEARCH research centers each year to estimate how many children develop diabetes (incidence cases) per year by age, sex, race/ethnicity, and diabetes type.

- Over 10,000 children/youth with diabetes, and their families, have been surveyed for SEARCH and over 6,000 have participated in SEARCH in-person visits. Nearly 3,000 stored DNA specimens from these participants are being used to extend the genetic component of SEARCH.

- The SEARCH data demonstrated that about four out of five youth with antibody positive diabetes have clinically significant amounts of residual beta cell function within the first year after diagnosis. This finding emphasizes the importance of clinical trials aimed at preserving residual beta cell function after diabetes onset.

- Results from SEARCH determined that 17 percent of youth with type 1 diabetes have hemoglobin A1c (HbA1c) levels reflecting poor blood glucose control. African American, American Indian, Hispanic, and Asian/Pacific Islander youth with type 1 diabetes are significantly more likely to have higher HbA1c levels compared with non-Hispanic white youth. This indicates the need for more effective treatment strategies, and better technologies and approaches to assist youth with diabetes in managing the disease, especially for those in minority groups.

- The SEARCH data revealed that young people with type 1 diabetes were more likely to be overweight, but not obese, compared to youth who did not have diabetes, highlighting the need to understand the role of excess weight in the development of diabetes and its impact on treatment.

- The SEARCH data showed that youth with type 1 diabetes and suboptimal control of their blood glucose levels had abnormal lipid (fat) profiles—indicators of heart disease risk—even after a short duration of disease. Effective blood glucose control may help protect against these abnormalities, which provides further impetus for people with type 1 diabetes to implement early and intensive blood glucose control.

- The large population-based cohort and collaborative infrastructure built by SEARCH has created new opportunities for additional research into childhood diabetes, resulting in five completed and six currently ongoing ancillary studies.

Anticipated Outcomes

Research supported through the SEARCH consortium has led to numerous insights and further understanding of the natural history, complications, and risk factors of diabetes onset in childhood and adolescence. SEARCH has generated estimates of diabetes prevalence and incidence by age, sex, race/ethnicity, and diabetes type, and continues to assess the impact of quality of diabetes care in youth on short- and long-term diabetes outcomes, including quality of life. Ongoing yearly case ascertainment will determine trends in incidence in the United States. Acquiring these data is important in order to ultimately design and implement public health efforts to prevent the disease once prevention strategies are identified. Furthermore, the data that are acquired in the SEARCH study regarding the natural history and risk factors of diabetes can inform the design of new prevention and treatment strategies. High prevalence of cardiovascular disease risk factors, including obesity, dyslipidemia, and hypertension, has been documented in youth with type 1 diabetes, as well as youth with type 2 or hybrid diabetes. The need for identifying effective approaches to improve dietary intake in youth with diabetes has been clearly documented. By building on SEARCH findings, researchers may be able to design interventions that can prevent or delay disease onset in at-risk individuals and, of equal importance, to design interventions to reduce risk for both acute and chronic complications of diabetes.

Ongoing Evaluation

The SEARCH Steering Committee (SC) comprises the Clinical Center and Coordinating Center principal investigators and one additional co-investigator from each center, designated scientists from the collaborating government agencies (CDC, NIH), and the central laboratory principal investigator. The SEARCH SC holds monthly conference calls and has overall responsibility for assuring the scientific integrity and progress of the study. It is also charged with assuring equity of data access and promoting career advancement of junior scientists working with SEARCH. The SEARCH Planning and Coordinating Committee, comprised of the Study Chair and Vice-Chair, the Coordinating Center principal investigator, and the Principal Scientists of the funding agencies, meets weekly by phone to facilitate study progress particularly regarding publications, and assure overall study coordination. SEARCH has seven standing committees (Typology; Publications and Presentations; Ancillary Studies; Protocol Oversight; Recruitment and Retention; Quality of Care; Epidemiology; Project Managers).

To ensure ongoing evaluation of the study design and the progress of SEARCH, CDC and NIDDK have established an External Scientific Evaluation Committee (ESEC). The ESEC is comprised of investigators with scientific expertise relevant to research conducted by SEARCH, but who are not members of the Consortium. The ESEC meets annually to:

- Review activities that affect the operational and methodological aspects of the study (*e.g.*, quality control procedures; performance of research centers, data coordinating center, and central laboratory);

- Review data to ensure its quality, advise on procedures for analysis and data display, and provide input on interpretation and implications of results; and

- Review proposed major modifications to the protocol or operations of the study for appropriateness, necessity, and impact on overall study objectives.

Program Enhancements

Because of the evolving nature of science, consortia supported by the *Special Diabetes Program* have evolved over time and have undergone enhancements to take advantage of new technologies and research findings, and to accelerate progress. Some enhancements have been made in response to external input and others have been initiated by the consortium members. Examples of program enhancements for SEARCH include:

- To manage challenges in the interpretation and implementation of the Health Insurance Portability and Accountability Act (HIPAA) Privacy Rule, SEARCH increased the efforts of study personnel working with the Institutional Review Boards, conducting case ascertainment, and recruiting volunteers. SEARCH presented data on the impact of the HIPAA law in conducting epidemiological research involving children at an ad hoc meeting organized by the Institute of Medicine of the National Academies in May 2007.

- As a result of diabetes autoantibodies (DA) measurement data generated by several NIH-funded studies, including SEARCH, discrepancies in DA measurements were observed and led NIDDK to form a harmonizing committee to standardize DA measurements. The SEARCH laboratory is one of the six laboratories participating in the DA standardization program. In addition, DA for all SEARCH samples, including those previously assayed, are being measured using the new harmonized protocols.

- To make samples and data available to the scientific community for ancillary studies, SEARCH has developed a comprehensive public Web site with information on samples, data, and resources that are currently available to the scientific community (www.searchfordiabetes.org). The SEARCH Ancillary Study Policy provides a process whereby outside investigators can access the SEARCH samples in a way that ensures scientific integrity and appropriate communication and coordination across projects. A subcommittee has been created to specifically monitor available stored samples, and to track funded and planned future usage in order to maximize and coordinate use of this important resource.

- To increase the retention rate of study participants, a subcommittee of the SEARCH Protocol Oversight Committee has been formed to regularly review recruitment and retention rates and to develop new approaches to enhance success in this arena. These retention efforts have resulted in close to 80 percent of SEARCH subjects participating in at least one follow-up visit.

- SEARCH investigators played a key role in organizing an international workshop on the classification of diabetes in children and young adults. Sponsored by NIDDK and CDC, the workshop brought together diabetes researchers to share data on prevalence, incidence and classification of diabetes in youth. The goal of the workshop was to share and disseminate the most up-to-date data and identify key gaps that need to be addressed with further research.

- SEARCH investigators are playing a key role in organizing an international workshop on surveillance methods for diabetes and its complications in children and adolescents. Sponsored by CDC and NIDDK, this workshop will explore approaches to the surveillance of diabetes in youth from registries and integrated data systems in several locations in the United States and other countries, and discuss their advantages and disadvantages. The goal of the workshop is to inform the development of a research agenda that specifically addresses epidemiology and surveillance of pediatric diabetes, and to foster the adoption and modification of national and international surveys.

Coordination with Other Research Efforts

SEARCH coordinates its efforts with multiple other type 1 diabetes research consortia and networks supported by the *Special Diabetes Program*. Collaboration, coordination, and resource sharing serve to synergize research efforts and accelerate research progress. Examples of coordination with other consortia are given below. For a summary of ongoing collaborative efforts, please see Appendix D.

Coordinating Patient Recruitment Efforts:

- Four SEARCH study sites are participating as recruitment centers for the Type 1 Diabetes Genetics Consortium (T1DGC) North American Network, and SEARCH is sharing its genetics samples with T1DGC.

- The Colorado, Cincinnati, Seattle, and South Carolina SEARCH sites are informing participants about Type 1 Diabetes TrialNet studies and referring them to the TrialNet coordinator for information on enrollment.

- Three SEARCH sites (Colorado, California, and Seattle) are assisting with recruitment from the Trial to Reduce IDDM in the Genetically at Risk (TRIGR) by providing brochures and other information about TRIGR to potential study participants.

Enhancing Data Comparison Among Studies:

- T1DGC, TrialNet, SEARCH, and The Environmental Determinants of Diabetes in the Young (TEDDY) are sharing information and reagents so that they can assess allele and haplotype frequencies of the same sets of genes including *Human Leukocyte Antigen* and other diabetes-predisposing genes. This coordination will permit comparisons of genetics data across all four studies, effectively increasing the power of each in learning which genes play a role in disease onset.

Coordinating Research Studies Involving Children:

- SEARCH, TrialNet, TEDDY, and T1DGC investigators directly collaborate.

SEARCH Administrative History	
Date Initiative Started	2000
Date *Special Diabetes Program* Funding Started	2001
Participating Components	CDC, NIDDK
Web site	www.searchfordiabetes.org
SEARCH consists of a coordinating center, a central laboratory, and six research centers in California, Colorado, Hawaii, Ohio, South Carolina, and Washington state.	

Type 1 Diabetes Mouse Resource (T1DR)

This research resource, located at The Jackson Laboratory, was established to expand existing repositories for genetically altered mice to accommodate the many different mouse models that are important for type 1 diabetes research. In its second phase, this project was expanded in scope to include activities supporting the Animal Models of Diabetic Complications Consortium (AMDCC; described later in this Appendix). Animal systems that appropriately model type 1 diabetes and its complications are critical tools for identifying and testing new therapeutic approaches, and for supporting the translational research required to move new treatments from the laboratory bench to patients' bedside. It is also important that the broad scientific community have ready access to these animal models to facilitate their research efforts. The repository is enhancing access and ensuring the continued availability of these mouse models to the entire research community.

HIGHLIGHTS OF PROGRESS

- Collected and preserved over 199 stocks of mice important to diabetes research that have been made available for distribution to the scientific community.

- Over 6,000 mice have been shipped from the T1DR to over 840 researchers.

- Performed genetic and phenotypic quality control that further enhances research utility of mice used for research on diabetes and its complications.

- Generated 19 new mouse strains that are sensitized to the development of diabetes complications for use by the research community.

Anticipated Outcomes

Animal models of type 1 diabetes can significantly facilitate the translation of laboratory research findings to clinical research. For example, techniques for gene discovery in small model organisms are much more powerful than in humans. Discovery of diabetes-causing genes in animal models will foster research on corresponding genes in human tissue samples and will thus help to uncover the pathways in which the genes function. Furthermore, animal models of the disease are important for testing promising therapeutic agents identified in the laboratory prior to testing in human clinical trials. Therefore, animal models are a crucial resource for translating laboratory results from the bench to the bedside. The research community is taking advantage of the T1DR, as demonstrated by the fact that over 6,000 mice have been distributed to 840 researchers. These mouse models continue to be critically important for conducting type 1 diabetes research and are being used by the broad diabetes research community.

Ongoing Evaluation

Activities and progress of the T1DR are monitored by an External Evaluation Committee (EEC) comprised of experts in mouse genetics, mouse husbandry, and rodent models of type 1 diabetes. Members of the EEC are not affiliated with the T1DR or with The Jackson Laboratory. The EEC meets annually to:

- Review status of importation and distribution of stocks, identify and make recommendations for new strains to be solicited, and provide input on procedures to advertise repository holdings.

- Review quality control of genetics data on repository strains, including genome scans, chromosome-of-interest studies, and incidence studies.

In addition, the T1DR was evaluated by an external panel of scientific and lay experts at an *ad hoc* evaluation meeting convened by NIDDK in June 2009. This meeting was an opportunity for external experts to evaluate progress and provide input on future research directions (for more information, see the Executive Summary and Appendix B). Through *ad hoc* evaluation meetings and regular meetings of the EEC, NIDDK continually seeks external input to inform current and future directions for the T1DR.

Program Enhancements

Because of the evolving nature of science, consortia supported by the *Special Diabetes Program* have evolved over time and have undergone enhancements to take advantage of new technologies and research findings, and to accelerate progress. Some enhancements have been made in response to external input and others have been initiated by the consortium members. Examples of program enhancements for T1DR include:

- In its second phase, the T1DR was expanded in scope to include activities supporting the AMDCC to facilitate the production, phenotyping, repositing and distribution of strains that are important for type 1 diabetes complications research.

- The T1DR has made enhancements to ensure that investigators are able to obtain animals for study at their research institution. A subset of the T1DR protocols involves development of mouse strains that may be physiologically brittle and difficult to ship to investigators for further study. In circumstances where it is determined that strains may not survive shipment as adults, younger cohorts are developed specifically for shipment. In the most severe cases where shipment of live animals may not be feasible, the T1DR has developed protocols to support shipment of embryos to investigators for expansion at the investigator's institution for further study.

Coordination with Other Research Efforts

In coordination with other NIH-sponsored mouse repositories, the T1DR serves as an archive for mouse models generated by all scientists engaged in research relevant to type 1 diabetes. In its second phase, the scope of the T1DR was expanded to include activities supporting the AMDCC, thus providing coordination of activities relating to animal models of diabetes complications. The T1DR also services many basic science consortia engaged in type 1 diabetes research, such as the Beta Cell Biology Consortium (BCBC). Mouse models distributed from these NIH-supported repositories support translational research relevant to pancreas development, autoimmunity, and transplantation. For a summary of ongoing collaborative efforts, please see Appendix D.

T1DR Administrative History	
Date Initiative Started	2001
Date *Special Diabetes Program* Funding Started	2001
Participating Components	NIDDK (NCRR also supported first project phase)
Web site	http://type1diabetes.jax.org/
T1DR is located at The Jackson Laboratory, Bar Harbor, ME.	

Goal II: Prevent or Reverse Type 1 Diabetes

Type 1 Diabetes TrialNet (TrialNet)

TrialNet is an international network of investigators, clinical centers, and core support facilities that recruits patients and conducts research to advance knowledge about type 1 diabetes, and to test strategies for its prevention and early treatment. TrialNet supports the development and implementation of clinical trials of agents aimed at preventing the disease in people at risk for type 1 diabetes and slowing the progression of disease in newly diagnosed patients. The network's Natural History Study will enhance understanding of how the disease develops in individuals at risk and will thus help in the formulation of future trials. Biological samples collected from study volunteers are being stored at the NIDDK Central Repositories, and these valuable resources are being made available to the broader scientific community for further research on type 1 diabetes.

HIGHLIGHTS OF PROGRESS

- Completed the Diabetes Prevention Trial Type-1 (DPT-1) clinical trial of insulin for the prevention of type 1 diabetes in individuals at moderate and high risk for disease development, which showed that oral or injected insulin administration did not delay or prevent the disease in relatives of people with type 1 diabetes. However, in a subset of the moderate-risk patients studied (those with high levels of insulin-reactive autoantibodies), protection may have been observed. Because this result was not definitive, TrialNet has launched a new trial to further evaluate the role of oral insulin in delaying or preventing type 1 diabetes in this subset of people (see below).

- Determined that rituximab slows progression of type 1 diabetes in newly diagnosed patients. Rituximab treatment temporarily depletes B cells of the immune system and has been approved by the U.S. Food and Drug Administration for treatment of B cell non-Hodgkin's lymphoma and some autoimmune disorders, such as rheumatoid arthritis. Scientists tested whether four separate infusions of rituximab shortly after diagnosis could slow disease progression. After 1 year, people who had received the drug produced more of their own insulin, had better control of their diabetes, and did not have to take as much exogenous insulin to control their blood glucose levels, compared to people receiving placebo. The finding will propel research to find drugs targeting the specific B cells involved in type 1 diabetes because drugs such as rituximab that broadly deplete B cells can increase the risk of infection.

- Launched an oral insulin prevention trial in relatives of people with type 1 diabetes. As described above, a subset of individuals in the DPT-1 with high levels of insulin-reactive autoantibodies may have been protected from type 1 diabetes development with oral insulin administration. This suggestive result is being rigorously tested in TrialNet to determine if oral insulin could prevent or delay development of type 1 diabetes in this group of people.

- Completed a pilot study to test the role of omega-3 fatty acids in preventing type 1 diabetes, called The Nutritional Intervention to Prevent (NIP) Diabetes Study. The study was based on observations from epidemiologic studies that children who have received more omega-3 fatty acid (such as from fish)—either in the womb or during the first year of life—have a lower risk of developing type 1 diabetes. The pilot study demonstrated that increasing omega-3-fatty acids in breast milk through maternal supplementation or directly in formula or foods significantly increased blood levels of this substance. While measurable differences in omega-3 fatty acids were achieved, there was no difference in the immune marker studied so a full trial will not be launched.

- In addition to launching the two prevention studies already mentioned (oral insulin and NIP Diabetes Study), TrialNet has planned two other prevention studies: (1) a study of an anti-CD3 monoclonal antibody; and (2) a study evaluating glutamic acid decarboxylase (GAD)-alum vaccine.

- TrialNet launched the Natural History Study, which was begun to identify risk factors associated with development of type 1 diabetes and to document disease characteristics and progression. The Natural History Study will also identify and maintain a pool of individuals who would be candidates for participation in clinical trials. The first phase of the Natural History Study involves identification of those at risk by using a blood test for the presence of diabetes-related autoantibodies to screen close relatives of people with the disease. Thus far, over 74,000 individuals have been screened. The study plans to screen people at a rate of about 20,000 individuals per year. Participants are being offered enrollment in diabetes prevention and early intervention studies as they become available.

- TrialNet has begun or approved eight studies in new-onset type 1 diabetes to evaluate the effect of distinct interventions targeting an array of mechanisms putatively involved in the development of type 1 diabetes, including immunosuppressive agents (mycophenolate mofetil [MMF] and daclizumab), therapies directed at B cells (rituximab, described above), therapies directed at co-stimulation (CTLA-4 Ig [abatacept]), antigen-specific therapy (GAD-alum vaccine), and therapies aimed at improving beta cell function and/or mass (a study evaluating early aggressive, meticulous glycemic control facilitated by use of a continuous glucose sensor augmented insulin pump). In addition to the ongoing or approved trials, TrialNet accepts new proposals throughout the year, and received 15 new protocol proposals for consideration in 2009. TrialNet centers also participate in new-onset trials led by the NIAID-led Immune Tolerance Network (ITN), including those testing anti-CD3 (teplizumab) and thymoglobulin, as well as a phase 1 study examining the combination of IL-2 and rapamycin.

- The network completed a clinical study to compare reliability of two tests for beta cell function—the Mixed Meal Tolerance Test (MMTT) and intravenous Glucagon Stimulation Test (GST). Residual beta cell function (insulin secretion) in people with type 1 diabetes is known to result in improved glycemic control, reduced hypoglycemia, and reduced risk for complications. In insulin treated patients with diabetes, beta cell function is currently best measured by determining levels of human C-peptide. C-peptide is useful as an outcome measure in clinical trials: for example, trials testing agents to preserve beta cell function in new-onset diabetes. There are different ways to stimulate insulin production and, concomitantly, C-peptide production, but it has not been clear which of these conditions is optimal for enabling C-peptide measurement. The MMTT/GST clinical trial compared the reliability and burden on patients of two test conditions for stimulating insulin/C-peptide: one, MMTT, is a liquid meal; the other, GST, is an injection of the hormone glucagon. Results of this study showed that the MMTT test is superior. This knowledge has helped to inform the design of future type 1 diabetes clinical trials to prevent or reverse type 1 diabetes in which C-peptide must be measured to determine if the intervention is successful.

• Completed a T cell Validation Study to learn which T cell assays are most reliable and reproducible in identifying differences between people with and without type 1 diabetes. The first study involved the evaluation of blinded samples from the same people by four T cell laboratories in North America and a parallel test of one of the assays in the United Kingdom. Samples were drawn on two occasions to compare reproducibility, sensitivity, and specificity. The first validation study demonstrated that several of the assays were able to distinguish people with type 1 diabetes from healthy control individuals. This study represents the first blinded evaluation of T cell assay reproducibility in a large multicenter network with ongoing external quality control of all assays, an essential component for multicenter clinical trials. TrialNet hopes to continue to use this process to assess new biomarkers of disease progression.

Anticipated Outcomes

TrialNet is an international clinical research network focused on individuals at risk for or newly diagnosed with type 1 diabetes. Its efforts span the time period from birth in those at high genetic risk to the development of signs of increased risk (for example, autoantibodies), when prevention strategies are particularly urgent, and on through the time soon after diagnosis, when residual beta cell function may afford a unique opportunity for interventions to mitigate disease severity. TrialNet hopes to identify agents that safely delay or prevent the onset of type 1 diabetes, sparing those at risk from developing this devastating disease. TrialNet is also hoping to identify agents that can modulate the immune system of recently diagnosed patients so as to preserve remaining beta cell function and thus make it easier for them to control glucose levels and reduce their burden of complications. In addition to providing direct benefit to newly diagnosed patients, new-onset trials are expected to identify agents that have low risk of serious side effects and have promise for preventing or delaying onset of type 1 diabetes in at-risk populations.

In addition to the conduct of clinical trials, TrialNet's extensive recruitment and frequent sampling and metabolic testing of individuals at risk for or with new-onset disease is facilitating research into biomarkers of disease progression. Other clinical studies conducted by TrialNet have improved the tests and strategies for future type 1 diabetes clinical trials, for example, showing that MMTT is superior to GST for stimulating insulin production. The infrastructure of TrialNet is also used to enhance other efforts supported by the *Special Diabetes Program*, such as aiding the Type 1 Diabetes Genetics

Consortium (T1DCG) with identification of families with two siblings affected with type 1 diabetes and collection of samples for genetic studies from these families.

There is a rigorous process for consideration of studies proposed for conduct through this coordinated clinical research infrastructure. This involves review by experts in diabetes, immunology, safety/ethics, clinical trials, study design and analysis. As new therapeutic agents are identified through additional studies supported by the *Special Diabetes Program*, TrialNet's standing infrastructure will be indispensable for the testing of these promising agents in patients. Furthermore, TrialNet makes resources available to the broader scientific community. For example, they make available serum, RNA, and peripheral blood mononuclear cell samples from people enrolled in the Natural History Study for validation of new biomarkers of type 1 diabetes. They also invite the broad community to submit proposals for ancillary studies as an adjunct to ongoing protocols. The knowledge gained from TrialNet's Natural History Study will help to spur the design of new prevention and treatment approaches. TrialNet's current position of strength is the result of years of effort in outreach to the diabetes care and research communities, intensive training in research procedures, including sample collection and storage for mechanistic assays (in collaboration with the ITN), and the establishment of close collaborative ties among clinical diabetes and immunology researchers. TrialNet scientists also take proactive roles in critically reviewing, identifying, and prioritizing promising candidates for trials, considering both clinical feasibility and scientific merit.

Ongoing Evaluation

TrialNet is led by an Executive Committee consisting of study leadership from the Chairman's Office, the Coordinating Center, NIDDK, and NIAID. This committee provides ongoing oversight, discusses issues related to trial conduct, and coordinates various Study Group activities. The TrialNet Steering Committee, comprised of the principal investigator and a co-investigator from each clinical center, principal investigator from the Coordinating Center and each major laboratory, and representatives from NIDDK, NIAID, NICHD, and JDRF, meets two times yearly to evaluate proposed and ongoing protocols and to reach consensus for TrialNet activities. A Data and Safety Monitoring Board (DSMB), appointed by NIDDK, NIAID, and NICHD, reviews diabetes protocols from TrialNet, the ITN, and the Autoimmunity Centers of Excellence. The DSMB meets at least four times per year to monitor protocol progress and reviews all safety issues. A TrialNet External Evaluation Committee (EEC), appointed by NIDDK, provides expert input and external review of overall TrialNet activities yearly.

TrialNet's intensive, streamlined protocol review process involves five separate committees: (1) Scientific Review Committee (with veto power), (2) Clinical Feasibility Committee, (3) Infectious Disease Safety Review Committee, (4) Ethics Committee, and (5) Intervention Strategies and Prioritization Committee (which meets last and considers reports of the other four committees). Several of these committees include outside experts. Protocols may be advanced from these committees for approval by the Steering Committee. Once a protocol is approved, associated mechanistic studies to improve understanding of pathophysiology underlying the disease are developed by a Mechanistic Studies Committee. Following Steering Committee approval, NIH seeks external input (from the DSMB and/or the EEC) to decide whether to move forward with protocol implementation.

In addition, TrialNet has been evaluated by external panels of scientific and lay experts at *ad hoc* evaluation meetings convened by NIDDK in January 2005 and April 2008. These meetings were an opportunity for external experts to evaluate progress and provide input on future research directions (for more information, see the Executive Summary and Appendix B). Through *ad hoc* evaluation meetings and regular meetings of the EEC, NIDDK continually seeks external input to inform current and future directions for TrialNet.

Program Enhancements

Because of the evolving nature of science, consortia supported by the *Special Diabetes Program* have evolved over time and have undergone enhancements to take advantage of new technologies and research findings, and to accelerate progress. Some enhancements have been made in response to external input and others have been initiated by the consortium members. Examples of program enhancements for TrialNet include:

- Shortly after TrialNet began, it was recognized that the international community had much to contribute to the network both intellectually and logistically. With the agreement of NIDDK, the JDRF solicited applications for international clinical centers to join TrialNet. Three European sites and one Australian site are fully represented on the Steering Committee. These sites have contributed to the screening of

people for the Natural History Study, enrollment of participants into the new-onset intervention studies and into the Oral Insulin Prevention Study, and in mechanistic studies.

- The initial protocol review process relied heavily on primary review at the level of the Steering Committee. After a few years, the protocol submission and review process was modified to facilitate thorough and rapid review and prioritization of protocols before coming to the Steering Committee for formal consideration.

- For those proposals approved for inclusion in TrialNet, initiating investigators have joined investigators with special expertise in the network to form a Protocol Development Team to expedite protocol development. This includes staff from the Chairman's Office, the Coordinating Center, and NIDDK. The Team was convened to lead the development of all protocols and to coordinate activities of the individual committees that oversee each protocol. A common template is used, and institutional review board (IRB) and regulatory issues are considered early in the process to expedite protocol development.

- At the end of the initial 7 year grant period, Clinical Center cooperative agreement PIs were asked to re-compete for funding and center status, and affiliated sites were invited to join the competition to become new centers. This competition led to the selection of 14 outstanding centers, 12 of which were continuations of prior cooperative agreements, and 2 new centers that were formerly TrialNet affiliates. All of the centers successfully competed by demonstrating exceptional recruiting ability and scientific knowledge and innovation that will improve TrialNet now and into the future.

- In addition to a re-competition of TrialNet centers, the TrialNet biostatistics and data coordinating center, which was formerly funded by a cooperative agreement, was converted to a contract and was competed in an open contract Request for Proposals issued in 2008. A new contract was awarded to the University of South Florida Data Coordinating Center, which offered strengths in operational efficiency and electronic database capabilities. The coordinating center transition was accomplished during the latter part of 2008 and 2009. The network looks forward to many more years of strong biostatistical capability and leadership, and efficient data and network coordination.

Coordination with Other Research Efforts

TrialNet coordinates its efforts with multiple other type 1 diabetes research consortia and networks supported by the *Special Diabetes Program*. Collaboration, coordination, and resource sharing serve to synergize research efforts and accelerate research progress. Examples of coordination with other consortia are given below. For a summary of ongoing collaborative efforts, please see Appendix D.

Coordinating Patient Recruitment Efforts:

- TrialNet and the ITN jointly introduced and advertised the TrialNet Natural History Study, the ITN Insulin B chain Vaccine Study, the ITN Anti-CD3 Study, the ITN Thymoglobulin Study and the ITN IL-2/Rapamycin Study.

- North American TrialNet centers participated as recruitment centers for the T1DGC North American Network. TrialNet investigators supplied the T1DGC with 74.8 percent of the affected sib-pair or trio families collected in North America.

- T1DGC assisted TrialNet in establishing international recruitment sites.

- TrialNet, The Environmental Determinants of Diabetes in the Young (TEDDY), and the Trial to Reduce IDDM in the Genetically At-Risk (TRIGR) have coordinated recruitment efforts to ensure that they are not adversely competing for patient participants in their studies.

Coordinating the Conduct of Clinical Trials:

- TrialNet and DirecNet are jointly performing the Metabolic Control Study, a study evaluating early aggressive meticulous glycemic control facilitated by use of a continuous glucose sensor-augmented insulin pump.

- TrialNet collaborates with the ITN to facilitate implementation of clinical trials designed by ITN. More than 90 percent of ITN type 1 diabetes study participants have been recruited and followed at TrialNet sites. Conversely, the ITN assists TrialNet with sample collection, RNA purification, PBMC isolation, sample tracking, storage, and analysis of mechanistic samples. A coordinating committee facilitates the TrialNet-ITN interactions and a common DSMB is used for type 1 diabetes studies. Representatives from the ITN serve as full members of the TrialNet Mechanistic Study Committee.

- Protocols potentially of interest to TrialNet and ITN are considered by both consortia to assess the possibility for joint sponsorship.

- TrialNet communicates regularly with the Clinical Islet Transplantation Consortium on clinical and mechanistic issues.

Enhancing Data Comparison Among Studies:

- TrialNet, TEDDY, and T1DGC share the same North American laboratory for measurement of autoantibodies. This coordination will permit direct comparison between results obtained in each study.

- TrialNet uses laboratories certified through the HbA1c Standardization Program.

- The C-peptide Standardization Program included the TrialNet C-peptide measurement laboratory in its international comparison and harmonization efforts, which will continue with the development of the reference standards needed to harmonize the assay into the future.

- TrialNet has been an active participant in an NIDDK-led program to standardize and harmonize autoantibody measurements in all NIDDK-sponsored research networks, as well as the CDC-led Diabetes Autoantibody Standardization Program (DASP).

- T1DGC, TrialNet, SEARCH for Diabetes in Youth, and TEDDY are sharing information and reagents so that they can assess allele and haplotype frequencies of the same sets of genes including *Human Leukocyte Antigen* and other diabetes-predisposing genes. This coordination will permit comparisons of genetics data across all four studies, effectively increasing the power of each in learning which genes play a role in disease onset.

Coordinating Research Studies Involving Newborns:

- TrialNet investigators meet with investigators participating in other type 1 diabetes research studies involving newborns (TEDDY and TRIGR) to discuss opportunities for enhancing coordination and collaboration.

- TEDDY has shared the following materials with TrialNet investigators who are studying newborns in the NIP Diabetes Study: genetics-screening procedures, data forms, and parts of the Manual of Operation concerning follow-up of high-risk children. Through concerted action to define exclusive study geographic areas, investigators in the two studies have also avoided direct competition for eligible study participants.

TrialNet Administrative History	
Date Initiative Started	2001
Date *Special Diabetes Program* Funding Started	2001
Participating Components	NIDDK, NIAID, NICHD, NCRR, NCCAM, JDRF, ADA
Web site	www.diabetestrialnet.org

TrialNet is conducting clinical trials with researchers from 18 Clinical Centers in the United States, Canada, Finland, United Kingdom, Italy, and Australia. In addition, more than 150 medical centers and physician offices participate in TrialNet.

Immune Tolerance Network (ITN)

The ITN is an international consortium of over 80 scientists and physicians dedicated to evaluating therapies to reduce autoimmunity and other adverse immune responses by inducing, maintaining, and monitoring "immunological tolerance" in humans for islet, kidney, and liver transplantation; autoimmune diseases; and allergy and asthma. The goal of immune tolerance research is to identify and evaluate strategies to "re-educate" the immune system in a highly specific manner to prevent graft rejection or disease-causing immune responses. Examples of autoimmune processes targeted by the ITN include those that destroy insulin-producing beta cells in type 1 diabetes, or the immune responses that destroy transplanted islets. It is important, however, that these strategies not dampen the body's normal infection-fighting immune mechanisms. Particular trials may be conceived by the ITN itself, or by scientists and physicians not initially affiliated with the ITN, but who are invited to submit clinical trial proposals. The ITN then assists investigators with study development, implementation, monitoring, and analysis; access to cutting-edge technologies; and a wide range of other expert scientific, regulatory, and technical support. Clinical trials are augmented by mechanistic studies designed to uncover basic biological features of immune tolerance which will, in turn, help guide the design of future clinical trials.

HIGHLIGHTS OF PROGRESS

- *Conducting the first multicenter trial of islet transplantation:* Nine sites in North America and Europe successfully replicated the "Edmonton protocol" for islet transplantation in the ITN's multicenter study from 2001-2006. The "Edmonton protocol" was a revolutionary new procedure developed in Canada that greatly improved the outcomes for islet transplantation in a relatively small single-site study. The ITN study showed that it was possible to replicate the Edmonton study at multiple islet transplantation research centers. While most people experienced a gradual loss of transplanted islet function over a period of years, even those individuals who retained only partial islet function and did not remain "insulin-free" benefited greatly from improved post-transplant glycemic control. The study played a critical role in defining the challenges, obstacles, and feasibility of moving islet transplantation into the therapeutic arena.

- *Determining that autoantibody titers may predict islet transplant success:* Among the aberrant immune processes that occur in type 1 diabetes is the production of "autoantibodies" that recognize beta cell components. Autoantibody levels were measured pre-transplant in patients enrolled in the ITN multicenter study of the "Edmonton protocol." Investigators found that pre-transplantation levels of autoantibodies to two beta cell proteins correlate indirectly with long-term graft survival and insulin-free status following the transplant. If confirmed, this result may lead to the development of predictive biomarkers of graft survival. It also underscores the need to abrogate both the immune reactivity to transplanted (foreign) donor cells and the ongoing autoimmune response.

- *Completing a pilot study testing novel vaccine for new-onset type 1 diabetes:* A pilot study tested an insulin-B chain peptide vaccine designed to preserve function of insulin-producing beta cells in newly diagnosed patients.

People who received the vaccine exhibited an increase in insulin autoantibody levels and developed T cell responses to the insulin B-chain peptide, clear indications of humoral and antigen-specific cellular responses to the vaccine. Evidence of the induction of antigen-specific regulatory T cells that might impede disease progression was also observed in treated patients.

- *Completing trials testing anti-T cell therapies for treating new-onset type 1 diabetes*: A number of promising anti-T cell therapies are being evaluated in type 1 diabetes, including the anti-CD3 monoclonal antibody, hOKT3gamma1(Ala-Ala). This antibody was shown to prolong the "honeymoon" phase for up to 2 years in a small study of recently diagnosed type 1 diabetes patients. The ITN is currently evaluating this agent in an expanded, multicenter phase II study of 83 people using a modified dose schedule designed to prolong beta cell preservation. In addition, the ITN is enrolling a 66 person, multicenter, placebo-controlled study of antithymocyte globulin which showed promising rates of insulin remission in a pilot study in Europe.

- *Launching a phase I trial using a novel cocktail to promote regulatory T cells*: Interleukin-2 (IL-2) and sirolimus have been used successfully to suppress autoimmune destruction of islets in non-obese diabetic (NOD) mice. The data suggest that the combination therapy promotes the development and survival of regulatory T cells known to suppress autoimmunity. This ITN trial is assessing the safety of this combination in order to provide a foundation for testing its effectiveness in individuals with recent-onset type 1 diabetes.

- *Demonstrating that a combination of assays detects type 1 diabetes with high sensitivity and specificity*: ITN investigators showed that no single assay (such as an autoantibody test or any of several other types of assays) distinguishes non-diabetic individuals from those with type 1 diabetes. However, the combination of an autoantibody test and two types of assays for T cells identified a high proportion of patients with type 1 diabetes with no false positives.

- *Supporting an active pipeline of new studies to assess immunomodulatory interventions for treating new-onset type 1 diabetes*: ITN will open a multicenter phase II study of Alpha-1 Antitrypsin (AAT) in 2010. AAT has shown promising results in NOD mice leading to a sustained reversion from hyperglycemia to normal glucose values in some animals. AAT, which is currently approved for use in patients with genetic deficiencies of AAT production, is believed to play a role in dampening inflammatory responses. Two additional studies are in earlier stages of clinical trial development and other projects are completing preclinical toxicology studies.

Anticipated Outcomes

The ITN is adding to knowledge of the autoimmune response in type 1 diabetes and testing strategies for blocking destruction of beta cells. ITN research on assays of the immune system to detect those at risk may help in the early identification of research participants and lead to improved outcomes via earlier intervention. Research on tolerance-inducing agents brings hope of arresting the autoimmune destruction of beta cells; while the overall goal is maintenance of residual function, preservation of at least some insulin producing cells would facilitate glucose control with less risk of hypoglycemia. For those who undergo islet transplantation, modulation of the immune system is necessary, not only to block the diabetes-specific autoimmune reactions that destroy beta cells, but to prevent the general immune rejection that can occur with any transplanted tissue. When donor cells or organs are transplanted, the patient's immune system recognizes these as foreign. Consequently, immunosuppressive drugs are necessary to prevent transplant rejection. However, long-term immunosuppression carries an increased risk of infections and certain types of cancer and many drugs that are effective in suppressing the immune system are also toxic to beta cells. As another potential treatment strategy, scientists are exploring whether beta cells can be coaxed to regenerate to levels that will restore insulin production. If effective, such a treatment would also require blocking of the autoimmune response. The ITN's research may lead to immunosuppression-free protocols or to drugs with narrower specificity to blunt unwanted immune responses. Thus, these efforts hold promise for improving the lives of people with type 1 diabetes and for those at risk.

Ongoing Evaluation

The ITN's principal decision-making body is the Network Steering Committee (NSC), a group of approximately 20 leaders in the field of immune tolerance, transplantation, asthma, allergy, autoimmunity, clinical trial design, and bioethics who evaluate clinical trial proposals, conduct annual strategic assessments, and oversee the ITN research portfolio and policies. NSC recommendations are subject to prioritization and final approval by the Network Executive Committee, which consists of ITN Directors, additional experts, and NIAID staff. Day-to-day management of ITN operations is carried out by the ITN Director and his deputies. In addition, the ITN

and NIAID leadership convene for periodic meetings to establish milestones, assess progress, and conduct long-range planning. Meetings are held with industry cosponsors and potential partners on an as-needed basis. The majority of ITN/industry collaborations are supported through Clinical Trial Agreements executed between pharmaceutical or biotechnology companies and NIAID.

Concepts for ITN clinical trials are promoted through one of two pathways: the ITN's open call for proposals to the research community or via NSC annual strategic assessments. Strategic Assessment groups, assembled for each of the ITN clinical emphasis areas, are composed of NSC members and external experts in the respective fields. They are tasked with reviewing the ITN portfolio in their area, and identifying promising strategies for discussion and prioritization by the NSC. Each year, several of these are selected for feasibility assessment and protocol development. Studies selected for implementation are developed by the principal investigator, in collaboration with the ITN Clinical Trials Group, the ITN Tolerance Assay Group, and industry partners. NIAID provides regulatory, medical affairs, and project management support. NIAID contractors provide clinical monitoring, statistical data management, and drug distribution services for ITN trials. Study Management Teams—consisting of study investigators, ITN clinical, assay, and operations staff, NIAID project managers, contractors, and industry representatives— oversee the implementation of the study and meet regularly over the course of the trial to review study progress in relation to predefined milestones. The ITN Clinical Trials Group provides operations staff in charge of clinical project management, while the ITN Tolerance Assay and Data Analysis Group ensures the integrity of the associated mechanistic studies. The ITN also provides data analysis services for mechanistic studies, data warehousing, study logistics, and patient recruitment support for all trials.

The ITN type 1 diabetes projects were evaluated by external panels of scientific and lay experts at *ad hoc* evaluation meetings convened by NIDDK in January 2005 and April 2008. These meetings provided an opportunity for external experts to evaluate progress and provide input on future research directions (for more information, see the Executive Summary and Appendix B). Through *ad hoc* evaluation meetings and regular meetings of Committees described above, NIAID continually seeks external input to inform current and future directions for the ITN.

Program Enhancements

The *Special Diabetes Program* has had a significant impact on ITN studies and has stimulated and enhanced the development and conduct of additional clinical trials in early onset type 1 diabetes. Without the support of the *Special Diabetes Program*, many of the studies that are currently planned or ongoing within the Network could not have been conducted.

These resources have enabled the ITN and other NIAID contractors (statisticians, and those responsible for data management, site monitoring, etc.) to dedicate staff to this mission.

Coordination with Other Research Efforts

The ITN coordinates its activities with multiple other type 1 diabetes research consortia and networks supported by the *Special Diabetes Program*. Collaboration, coordination, and resource sharing serve to synergize research efforts and accelerate research progress. Examples of coordination with other consortia are given below. For a summary of ongoing collaborative efforts, please see Appendix D.

Coordinating Patient Recruitment Efforts:

- The ITN and TrialNet jointly introduced and advertised the ITN Insulin B-chain Peptide Study and the TrialNet Natural History Study.

Collaborating To Enhance Islet Transplantation Efforts:

- Islet Cell Resource Centers isolated and supplied human islets to the ITN Multi-centered Islet Transplantation Trial clinical sites.

- The Collaborative Islet Transplant Registry archives trial results.

- The Clinical Islet Transplantation (CIT) Consortium and ITN are sharing expertise and coordinating efforts in the planning of immunologic assays in CIT trials. ITN core labs will perform selected assays in CIT trials.

- The CIT Consortium, the ITN, and the Non-Human Primate Transplantation Tolerance Cooperative Study Group (NHPCSG) are interested in using similar reagents for islet transplantation or as immune modulators for the treatment of type 1 diabetes.

- The ITN shares information about scientific priorities and pre-clinical research needs with the NHPCSG and both organizations benefit from shared information about study outcomes.

- ITN priorities for pre-clinical testing of new therapeutics are considered in evaluating NHPCSG Opportunities Pool applications. Several ITN high-priority strategies have been funded as pilot projects.

Sharing of Other Resources and Information:

- ITN collaborates with TrialNet to facilitate implementation of clinical trials designed by ITN. Many ITN type 1 diabetes study participants have been recruited and followed at TrialNet sites. A coordinating committee facilitates the TrialNet-ITN interactions and a single DSMB reviews many NIDDK and NIAID type 1 diabetes clinical trials. The TrialNet chairman is a member of the ITN Steering Committee.

- Protocols potentially of interest to ITN and TrialNet are considered by both consortia with the opportunities for joint sponsorship.

- ITN-supported investigators have used the Type 1 Diabetes-Rapid Access to Intervention Development program for production and pre-clinical testing of novel reagents.

- TRIGR and the ITN are coordinating their efforts in the area of T cell assays.

ITN Administrative History	
Date Initiative Started	1999
Date *Special Diabetes Program* Funding Started	2001
Participating Components	NIAID, NIDDK, and JDRF
Web site	www.immunetolerance.org
The ITN consists of over 80 world leaders in the clinical and basic sciences of immune tolerance from academic research institutions around the world.	

COOPERATIVE STUDY GROUP FOR AUTOIMMUNE DISEASE PREVENTION (PREVENTION CENTERS)

The Cooperative Study Group for Autoimmune Disease Prevention (Prevention Centers) is a collaborative program of investigators that supports research on the development of new prevention and treatment strategies for autoimmune diseases and evaluates these approaches in pilot and clinical studies. The Prevention Centers aim to create improved models of disease pathogenesis and therapy to better understand immune mechanisms. Ultimately, these models will provide opportunities to test new prevention strategies and validate new tools for human studies. The Centers also support projects, such as the development of surrogate markers for disease progression and/or regulation, designed to encourage rapid translation of discoveries from animal models to human clinical trials.

HIGHLIGHTS OF PROGRESS

- *Identifying insulin as a primary target for the autoimmune response in the non-obese diabetic (NOD) mouse model of diabetes:* Mice have two insulin genes, and generation of a NOD mouse lacking the insulin 1 gene revealed that it is required for development of insulitis and diabetes. Subsequent experiments showed that diabetes did not develop in NOD mice engineered to produce a slightly altered insulin molecule not recognized by the mouse's immune system. This research suggests that autoimmune reaction against insulin may be a critical initiator of the pathway toward beta cell destruction.

- *Launching the NOD Roadmap Project on the NOD mouse model of type 1 diabetes:* This study has generated a comprehensive time course of disease in the NOD mouse model of type 1 diabetes, cataloguing phenotypes, transcripts, and histochemistry through multi-institutional collaborations. Initial transcript data and analysis are posted on an open source Web site. Ongoing work on this project will refine this analysis by focusing on gene expression in small groups of cells in the pancreas. This project lays an extensive groundwork for future investigations into the mechanisms underlying the pathogenesis of type 1 diabetes in this model and the extension of these results to human diabetes.

- *Demonstrating the role of the Deaf1 gene in the development of type 1 diabetes:* As part of the NOD Roadmap project, scientists found that cells in the murine pancreatic lymph nodes make two forms of a gene called Deaf1. One form encodes full-length, functional Deaf1 protein, while the other encodes a shorter, nonfunctional variant. Additional experiments in mice suggested that the functional form of Deaf1 may control the production of molecules needed to eliminate immune cells that can destroy insulin-producing cells in the pancreas, thus preventing type 1 diabetes. Researchers also found that levels of the variant form of Deaf1 were higher in people with type 1 diabetes compared to levels in people without the disease. The research suggests that the development of type 1 diabetes may be due to increased levels of the Deaf1 variant protein in pancreatic lymph nodes, which may, in turn, lead to reduced production of molecules that are required to "educate" the immune system not to attack the body's own cells, including the insulin-producing cells of the pancreas.

- *Enhancing the autoimmune disease prevention research enterprise:* The Centers launched new autoimmune disease prevention projects through pilot projects. Over one-third (36 percent) of the innovative high-risk and pilot/feasibility projects awarded using the Prevention Centers' special opportunities funds have matured into NIH Research Project Grants. Notably, seven of these pilot projects were awarded to young investigators, who subsequently have converted them into self-supporting, career-establishing grants. In addition, several large programs and major initiatives were launched or initially supported through this pilot program.

- *Developing new tools to predict and monitor disease onset and progression:* Developed biological tools to identify certain types of T cells that can attack beta cells based on recognition of the beta cell protein GAD65. These tools are "MHC class II tetramers," which are constructed to contain a segment of the GAD65 protein. Researchers can use these tools to retrieve, quantify, and characterize GAD65-reactive T cells from patients and individuals at risk for the disease. Such T cells are a potential marker of early disease, and this research will increase understanding about the destructive autoimmune response that underlies type 1 diabetes. In addition, the Centers developed tools for using proteomics technology that can facilitate detection of autoantibodies and other markers of autoimmune disease.

- *Characterizing the functional properties of cells called "CD4+CD25+ regulatory T cells:"* These cells help protect against autoimmune disease by suppressing the activities of autoreactive T cells. Investigators also have identified functional defects in this T cell subset in humans with autoimmune disease.

- *Demonstrating the mechanisms by which blockade of a particular molecular interaction between immune cells can prevent or modulate the course of diabetes and other autoimmune diseases:* In these studies, scientists administered to mice an agent that blocked the interaction between two important molecules. One molecule, called CD154, exists on the surface of many T cells, and another molecule, called CD40, is present on other types of immune cells. One of their findings was that blocking the CD154-CD40 interaction resulted in induction of a novel type of cell that is able to prevent the onset of type 1 diabetes in mice.

Anticipated Outcomes

Autoimmune diseases are significant contributors to the burden of chronic illness. The ultimate goals of autoimmune disease research are to understand the body's aberrant immune responses and to "re-educate" the body to become tolerant to the antigens and tissues that are the targets of an attack without impairing the immune system's ability to fight infection. To this end, the Prevention Centers support a multidisciplinary program of investigators focused on understanding the immune mechanisms that underlie the process of autoimmunity, determining novel approaches to modulation of the immune system, and applying this knowledge to the prevention of autoimmune diseases.

In people with type 1 diabetes, the immune system attacks insulin-producing beta cells in the pancreas, prohibiting the body from absorbing glucose. Investigators funded by the Prevention Centers are working to identify and characterize cells of the immune system, such as certain types of T cells, which attack and destroy the body's beta cells causing type 1 diabetes. Another research focus is to define the beta cell molecules that are targeted for autoimmune attack. Prevention Centers investigators have discovered that insulin is a primary target of this process in a mouse model. Researchers funded by the Prevention Centers also are examining how other aspects of the immune system, or experimental manipulations that alter the immune system, may confer protection against autoimmunity. For example, their research in mice suggests that the functional form of Deaf1 plays a role in the production of molecules needed to eliminate immune cells that can destroy insulin-producing cells in the pancreas. This research is helping to identify new markers of disease susceptibility and progression and opportunities for novel treatment strategies.

Ongoing Evaluation

The Prevention Centers' progress and study design are monitored and evaluated on an ongoing basis through Steering Committee meetings, annual all-investigator meetings, and external evaluations. The Prevention Centers Steering Committee meets to discuss ongoing pilot projects and new pilot proposals as well as the overall progress of the group. External reviewers attended the 2005 all-investigator meeting to provide feedback on the accomplishments and direction of the program.

In addition, the Prevention Centers have been evaluated by external panels of scientific and lay experts at *ad hoc* evaluation meetings convened by NIDDK in January 2005 and June 2009. These meetings were an opportunity for external experts to evaluate the progress and provide input on future research directions (for more information, see the Executive Summary and Appendix B). Through *ad hoc* evaluation meetings and all-investigator meetings, NIAID continually seeks external input to inform current and future directions for the Prevention Centers.

Program Enhancements

Because of the evolving nature of science, consortia supported by the *Special Diabetes Program* have evolved over time and have undergone enhancements to take advantage of new technologies and research findings, and to accelerate progress. Some enhancements have been made in response to external input and others have been initiated by the consortium members.

Examples of program enhancements for the Prevention Centers to encourage applications from the most talented scientists as well as submissions by young investigators include:

- NIAID created a Web site for the Prevention Centers to advertise funding opportunities: http://www3. niaid.nih.gov/about/organization/dait/CSGADP.htm. After the Web site's implementation, the percentage of projects awarded to investigators new to the program rose from 58 percent of projects in the previous funding period (FY 2001-2005) to 73 percent in the current funding period (FY 2006-2009).

- The Steering Committee emphasizes young investigators when selecting innovative projects. For the current funding period (FY 2006-2009), 38 percent of innovative project awards were made to new investigators, compared to 21 percent during the previous period.

Prevention Centers Administrative History	
Date Initiative Started	2001
Date *Special Diabetes Program* Funding Started	2001
Participating Components	NIAID, NIDDK, JDRF
Web site	www.niaid.nih.gov/about/organization/dait/Pages/CSGADP.aspx
This Consortium consists of six centers in the United States.	

STANDARDIZATION PROGRAMS: DIABETES AUTOANTIBODY STANDARDIZATION PROGRAM (DASP); C-PEPTIDE STANDARDIZATION; AND IMPROVING THE CLINICAL MEASUREMENT OF HEMOGLOBIN A1c (HbA1c)

The purpose of these programs is to develop and implement standardization programs designed to improve the measurement of: (1) aberrant molecules called "autoantibodies," which are predictive of type 1 diabetes; (2) C-peptide as an indicator of insulin production; and (3) HbA1c as an indicator of glycemic control. Such improvements and standardization are greatly advancing both research and patient care.

DASP

DASP seeks to improve the measurement of autoantibodies in blood that are predictive of type 1 diabetes, and to decrease laboratory-to-laboratory variation. Autoantibody production reflects abnormal and destructive immune system functioning. A normal immune system is designed to fight infections; one part of this complex process is the production of antibodies that target infectious agents. The immune system of a person who has—or is developing—type 1 diabetes, however, also makes "autoantibodies" that recognize insulin and other beta cell-derived molecules. Autoantibodies are currently the best predictors of the onset of type 1 diabetes before the appearance of increased blood glucose and clinical symptoms. In combination with genetic screening, autoantibody tests are used to identify individuals at elevated risk of developing type 1 diabetes and to characterize autoimmunity. DASP sets of serum samples are used as standards to evaluate the performance of diabetes laboratories throughout the world and serve as reference materials for developing new methods and technologies. They also have been used for the NIDDK Islet Autoantibody Measurement Harmonization Project, which is helping all the major research consortia standardize protocols for measuring autoantibodies. DASP also provides training and information to guide other laboratories in improving their performance.

DASP standardized assays are critical for research on all forms of diabetes in children because they are helpful in distinguishing type 1 and type 2 diabetes.

C-peptide Standardization Program

This program aims to establish reliability in measurements of C-peptide, which is a byproduct of insulin production by beta cells and thus useful as a marker of beta cell function. In people taking insulin as therapy for diabetes, C-peptide is used to assess insulin production from the beta cell. In clinical trials of agents designed to prevent the disease in at-risk persons, or to preserve beta cell function in individuals with new onset type 1 diabetes, C-peptide is being used as the key outcome measure. Residual beta cell function is associated with better glycemic control, lower risk of hypoglycemia, and lower risk of long-term diabetic complications.

National Glycohemoglobin Standardization Program (NGSP; HbA1c Standardization Program)

The purpose of the NGSP is to achieve standardization and reliability in measurement of HbA1c, a component of blood that is a good surrogate measure of long-term blood glucose control and, as such, reflects risk of diabetic complications. Clinical guidelines for controlling blood glucose to reduce diabetes complications set targets for control of blood glucose as assessed by this key test based on results from two landmark clinical trials:

the Diabetes Control and Complications Trial (DCCT) for type 1 diabetes and the United Kingdom Prospective Diabetes Study for type 2 diabetes. By successfully standardizing HbA1c testing so that clinical laboratory results can be related directly to the results of the DCCT, this program is enabling health care providers and patients to accurately and meaningfully assess glycemic control and risks for complications. The standardization of HbA1c measures is essential to public health efforts, such as those of the National Diabetes Education Program (NDEP), to improve diabetes control nationwide so that the public can reap the benefits of clinical trials proving that complications can be delayed or prevented. This effort also allows researchers to better define diabetes control and evaluate risk for complications, as well as foster comparison of results across multiple studies worldwide. The NGSP consists of a Steering Committee and a Laboratory Network. The NGSP network interacts with manufacturers and laboratories to assist with calibration and to certify methods as traceable to the DCCT. The NGSP also works with the College of American Pathologists to assign HbA1c values to proficiency testing specimens for better evaluation of HbA1c results in clinical laboratories.

HIGHLIGHTS OF PROGRESS

- DASP conducted and presented workshop evaluations of key international diabetes laboratories in 2000, 2002, 2003, 2005, 2006, and 2009.

- DASP validated improvement of two different technologies for measuring autoantibodies.

- DASP documented improvement in performance of the insulin autoantibody assay for laboratories with consistent participation in the DASP Training Program.

- DASP created laboratory reference materials (blood samples) from type 1 diabetes patients and healthy people that are available to ensure assay quality and to support further technology development.

- DASP sets of serum samples have been used for the NIDDK Islet Autoantibody Measurement Harmonization Project. This effort is helping to standardize protocols for measuring autoantibodies within numerous research consortia, and is thus having a far-reaching impact.

- Accurate measurement of antibodies through DASP have allowed improved characterization of childhood diabetes in the SEARCH for Diabetes in Youth study (see Goal I) and an appreciation of the existence of hybrid forms of diabetes with characteristics of both type 1 and type 2. Accurate antibody measurement has also benefitted enrollment in the NIDDK's Treatment Options for Type 2 Diabetes in Youth (TODAY) clinical trial. More precise measures have allowed more patients to enroll into the trial because eligibility excluded those with autoimmunity, and previous assays were non-specifically falsely identifying some potential participants as having autoimmunity.

- DASP validated the fourth major diabetes autoantigen, zinc transporter 8 (ZnT8) in DASP 2007 and DASP 2009. DASP 2010 will evaluate polymorphic ZnT8 dimer and trimer constructs.

- A new non-radioactive assay format, the Luminescent Immunoprecipitation System (LIPS) demonstrated the potential for good performance in DASP 2009 and the availability of LIPS reagents will be expanded to additional laboratories in DASP 2010.

- The C-peptide program evaluated the stability of C-peptide and effects of common interferences. The program is coordinating international laboratory comparisons of C-peptide measurement to harmonize the measurement technologies and to improve precision and reliability of results. Results of two comparisons have been published in *Clinical Chemistry*, in 2007 and 2008. In the latest comparison trial, two isotope-dilution liquid chromatography–mass spectrometry was used as a reference method to assign values to serum-sample calibrators, which helped to reduce the imprecision among methods and laboratories. This research is crucial for optimizing measurement techniques and harmonizing methods, which will enable the use of C-peptide endpoints in large multicenter clinical trials, and potentially, for clinical monitoring.

- The HbA1c standardization program has improved the standardization and reliability in measures of HbA1c so that clinical laboratory results can be used by health care providers and patients to accurately and meaningfully assess blood glucose control and risks for complications. Building on this success, the American Diabetes Association (ADA) recently recommended HbA1c as a more convenient approach to diagnose type 2 diabetes.

- Standardization of the HbA1c test supported the development of a national education campaign on "knowing your HbA1c number." The campaign is sponsored by the NDEP, which is a partnership of NIDDK and CDC.

- Building on the success of the HbA1c standardization program, NIDDK was able to launch a new campaign highlighting the importance of using accurate methods to test HbA1c in people who have sickle cell trait or other inherited forms of hemoglobin. Results have been published in *Journal of Diabetes Science and Technology* in 2009 and in *Clinica Chimica Acta* in 2010.

- Standardized HbA1c is the key outcome measure in studies testing efficacy of new drugs for diabetes treatment and is the basis for U.S. Food and Drug Administration approval of new diabetes medications.

- The CDC HbA1c laboratory and the NGSP have participated in efforts of the International Federation of Clinical Chemistry and Laboratory Medicine (IFCC) to develop a "higher level" reference method for measuring HbA1c. This reference method was approved by the IFCC and is now the basis for uniform standardization of HbA1c assays worldwide. The IFCC Working Group also developed a mathematical equation to facilitate comparison among results obtained by this IFCC reference method and the NGSP, as well as with methods in Sweden and Japan.

- For HbA1c measurements, between 1996 and 2006, there was an increase in the number of methods and laboratories certified by the NGSP as traceable to the DCCT. Methods and laboratories are certified each year.

Anticipated Outcomes

The autoantibody, C-peptide, and HbA1c standardization programs are extensive efforts to improve laboratory measures of critical markers for type 1 diabetes risk and disease progression. While key to research, the importance of these efforts extends beyond research to diagnosis and treatment of all forms of diabetes. Standardized assays are required for the success of multicenter clinical studies as different participating laboratories must be able to obtain measurements that are comparable and can be meaningfully analyzed together. Research progress will also be enhanced when the results of different trials are based on standardized measures to facilitate comparison. Patients and their health care practitioners will be better able to ascertain what a given blood test means in terms of health risks and treatment plans when test results are sufficiently reliable for comparison with relevant research studies. As a result of research toward standardizing autoantibody testing and identifying new biomarkers for predictive assays, those at risk for type 1 diabetes may be diagnosed earlier, permitting earlier intervention to diminish disease severity. Improved measurement techniques for C-peptide will impact research on agents that can preserve beta cell function, particularly in those with new-onset diabetes. C-peptide measurements are increasingly used in both government-funded and industry trials, since FDA has recently accepted C-peptide preservation as an important outcome measure of benefit for new-onset clinical trials. Improvements in HbA1c

testing have enabled the ADA to recommend the test as a more convenient approach for diagnosing type 2 diabetes. Thus, the standardization programs are already having wide-reaching implications for researchers, clinicians, and patients.

Ongoing Evaluation

Ongoing evaluation of the research and progress of the Standardization Programs is carried out as described below.

DASP: DASP efforts are managed by the Immunology of Diabetes Society (IDS) Autoantibody Standardization Committee, CDC, and NIDDK. The activities and progress are reviewed by IDS participants at the workshop presentations at the IDS meetings, and additional input is periodically sought from the IDS president and other prominent scientists in the field.

C-peptide: The C-peptide standardization program has project oversight from CDC. In addition, a C-peptide Standardization Advisory Committee provides input on research studies and assists in evaluation of results.

HbA1c: The effort to improve and standardize the measurement of HbA1c is divided between CDC and the NGSP (with CDC support) at the University of Missouri. The CDC and the NGSP Laboratory also participate as members in the IFCC Reference Laboratory Network for HbA1c Measurement.

In addition, these programs were evaluated by an external panel of scientific and lay experts at an *ad hoc* evaluation meeting convened by NIDDK in January 2005. This meeting was an opportunity for external experts to evaluate progress and provide input on future research directions (for more information, see the Executive Summary and Appendix B). Through *ad hoc* evaluation meetings and regular meetings of the Committees described above, CDC and NIDDK continually seek external input to inform current and future directions for these standardization programs.

Program Enhancements

Because of the evolving nature of science, Standardization Programs supported by the *Special Diabetes Program* have evolved over time and have undergone enhancements to take advantage of new technologies and research findings, and to accelerate progress. Some enhancements have been made in response to external input and others have been initiated by the consortium members. Examples of program enhancements for the Standardization Programs include:

- DASP is standardizing new autoantibodies as they are identified.

- Plans for future enhancements to the C-peptide harmonization effort include the establishment of reference methods and materials endorsed by the Joint Committee for Traceability in Laboratory Medicine and the World Health Organization. These methods and materials can be used to establish surveillance of commercial laboratory performance and achieve traceability goals.

- The HbA1c test has been examined in diverse populations both with regard to ensuring that commercial laboratories use tests that are valid in people with hemoglobinopathies and to look for variation in HbA1c levels in different racial and ethnic groups in conjunction with the ADA decision to use HbA1c for diagnosis.

Coordination with Other Research Efforts

The Standardization Programs coordinate their efforts with multiple other type 1 diabetes research consortia and networks supported by the *Special Diabetes Program*. Collaboration, coordination, and resource sharing serve to synergize research efforts and accelerate research progress. Examples of coordination with other consortia are given below. For a summary of ongoing collaborative efforts, please see Appendix D.

Enhancing Quality and Standardization of Laboratory Measures in Multicenter Clinical Trials:

- DASP interacts with The Environmental Determinants of Diabetes in the Young, Type 1 Diabetes Genetics Consortium, Type 1 Diabetes TrialNet, and SEARCH for Diabetes in Youth autoantibody labs, by providing laboratory materials and proficiency testing to facilitate their autoantibody measurements.

- The C-peptide program included two laboratories from TrialNet in an international comparison effort, the results of which illustrated the need to identify and minimize the major sources of variation in C-peptide measurements in multicenter, multi-laboratory clinical studies.

- TrialNet, Epidemiology of Diabetes Interventions and Complications, and other clinical studies supported by the *Special Diabetes Program* use laboratories certified through the NGSP.

Improving and Developing Technology:

- Because of limitations associated with autoantibody testing, DASP is working with NIDDK-supported investigators studying proteomics and type 1 diabetes, and collaborating with the Pacific Northwest National Laboratory, to find new biomarkers to improve diagnosis of and prediction of risk for this disease. This collaborative project will use blood samples collected by DASP from newly diagnosed type 1 diabetes patients and healthy people. The samples will be analyzed with proteomic and metabolomic technologies: that is, large-scale profiling and characterization of the component proteins and small molecules, respectively. Differences identified between samples from patients and healthy individuals can be further investigated for potential predictive or diagnostic value.

DASP Administrative History	
Date Initiative Started	1998
Date *Special Diabetes Program* Funding Started	1998
Participating Components	CDC, NIDDK, and Immunology of Diabetes Society

C-peptide Standardization Program Administrative History	
Date Initiative Started	2002
Date *Special Diabetes Program* Funding Started	2003
Participating Components	CDC, NIDDK, C-peptide Standardization Advisory Committee, and University of Missouri

HbA1c Standardization Program Administrative History	
Date Initiative Started	1996
Date *Special Diabetes Program* Funding Started	1998
Participating Components	CDC, NIDDK, NGSP
Web site	www.ngsp.org

The HbA1c program is carried out at the CDC-supported NGSP, as well as the Reference Laboratory for HbA1c at CDC, both members of the IFCC Reference Laboratory Network for HbA1c; NIDDK also funds this effort.

Trial To Reduce IDDM in the Genetically At-Risk (TRIGR)

TRIGR is an international clinical trial to determine, for infants at risk for type 1 diabetes, whether weaning to extensively-hydrolyzed formula, as compared to standard cow's milk formula, will reduce the risk of developing diabetes-predictive autoantibodies and, ultimately, type 1 diabetes. Environmental factors, such as exposure during infancy to foreign proteins from food, may interfere with normal immune system development in genetically-susceptible individuals, and formula is usually the first foreign food given to infants as they are weaned from human breast milk. Standard cow's milk formula contains proteins that are intact and thus capable of inciting the immune system. Hydrolyzing proteins breaks them into very small pieces, which are much less likely to elicit an immune response, and prior research has suggested that weaning to hydrolyzed (versus intact-protein) formula may reduce risk of type 1 diabetes. The first phases of TRIGR are extensive, multi-national efforts to identify several thousand infants at risk for type 1 diabetes by recruiting pregnant women who have the disease, or an affected family member, and subsequent screening of the infants for diabetes-associated variants of certain immune system genes (*Human Leukocyte Antigen* genes). As part of the study, exclusive breastfeeding will be encouraged, but once this is no longer possible, babies will enter the intervention portion of the study by being randomly assigned to receive either standard or extensively-hydrolyzed formula (up to age 8 months). Follow-up monitoring will assess autoantibody development and diabetes incidence up to age 10 years.

HIGHLIGHTS OF PROGRESS

- Completed enrollment of 2,160 eligible newborns.

- Achieved 89 percent retention rate over the first 5 years of the study, which is greater than the planned retention rate of 80 percent.

- Achieved 94 percent study-wide protocol compliance (*e.g.*, measuring visits, questionnaires, and blood samples).

- Had a successful intervention phase, which ended in mid-2007. Compliance with the intervention resulted with all planning parameters being met or exceeded.

- Found differences in infant feeding patterns between Europe and North America. In Europe, the first foods to be introduced were typically fruits and vegetables, whereas in North America, gluten-free cereals were introduced first.

- Found that the proportion of mothers with or without type 1 diabetes who initially breastfed their infants did not differ significantly. However, the duration of both exclusive and total breastfeeding was shorter among mothers with type 1 diabetes.

- Discovered that, although differences in early growth patterns were observed in Europe versus North America, in Canada versus the United States, and by maternal type 1 diabetes status, parameters were similar by 24 months of age. Early childhood growth elevations are consistent with the higher incidence of type 1 diabetes in Europe and Canada compared to the United States, and a lower incidence in children of mothers with type 1 diabetes.

Anticipated Outcomes

TRIGR is a large-scale, well-coordinated clinical trial to test the effect of a dietary intervention during infancy on the development of type 1 diabetes in genetically-susceptible individuals. If the results of this trial show that weaning to hydrolyzed infant formula, as compared to standard formula, reduces incidence of type 1 diabetes, then it will have validated a practical way to alter the course of autoimmunity development and reduce type 1 diabetes incidence in young children.

TRIGR builds on prior research in animals and on a pilot study in humans that investigated the association of different infant formulas with autoantibody appearance. It has been hypothesized that diabetes-related autoimmunity may be triggered when the immature gut of an at-risk infant encounters foreign dietary proteins. The use of extensively hydrolyzed formula during weaning would delay the introduction of more complex, intact foreign proteins. Thus, TRIGR may also shed further light on the role of the gut and its immune system in the development of type 1 diabetes. The potential for a dietary modification in infancy to reduce type 1 diabetes—along with biological data on the very large number of genetically susceptible infants being studied—makes the TRIGR study enormously beneficial to families at risk.

Ongoing Evaluation

To ensure ongoing evaluation of the study design and the progress of TRIGR, NICHD has established an External Data Safety Monitoring Board/Advisory Panel for this trial. Additional critical entities include the trial's International Coordinating Center, which integrates operations for all regions of the TRIGR Study Group, maintains and validates documents related to the operations of TRIGR, and is in charge of developing study forms and the

Manual of Operations. A Data Management Unit is responsible for data management systems; monitoring the study for protocol compliance, adverse events, and other issues; and data analysis and reporting. There are also a number of working committees focused on such topics as nutritional intervention, ancillary studies, and internal safety monitoring, among others.

In addition, TRIGR has been evaluated by external panels of scientific and lay experts at *ad hoc* evaluation meetings convened by NIDDK in January 2005 and April 2008. These meetings were an opportunity for external experts to evaluate progress and provide input on future research directions (for more information, see the Executive Summary and Appendix B). Through *ad hoc* evaluation meetings and regular meetings of the External Data Safety Monitoring Board/Advisory Panel, NICHD continually seeks external input to inform current and future directions for TRIGR.

Program Enhancements

Because of the evolving nature of science, consortia supported by the *Special Diabetes Program* have evolved over time and have undergone enhancements to take advantage of new technologies and research findings, and to accelerate progress. Some enhancements have been made in response to external input and others have been initiated by the consortium members. Examples of program enhancements for TRIGR include:

- To take advantage of new and emerging technologies, TRIGR developed a program and explicit guidelines for ancillary studies to facilitate access to TRIGR materials by researchers who seek to expand and embrace new technologies for inclusion into the TRIGR study group.

- TRIGR enhanced coordination with other type 1 diabetes research consortia studying newborns, such as The Environmental Determinants of Diabetes in the Young (TEDDY) and Type 1 Diabetes TrialNet.

- Because measurements of islet autoantibodies were not standardized, it was difficult to compare results across different studies. To address this barrier, an NIDDK Islet Autoantibody Measurement Harmonization Project was undertaken. This effort is helping to standardize protocols for measuring autoantibodies within all NIDDK studies, and is thus having a far-reaching impact. TRIGR will also be using the harmonized assay at the end of the study so that comparisons can be made.

Coordination with Other Research Efforts

TRIGR coordinates its efforts with multiple other type 1 diabetes research consortia and networks supported by the *Special Diabetes Program*. Collaboration, coordination, and resource sharing serve to synergize research efforts and accelerate research progress. Examples of coordination with other consortia are given below. For a summary of ongoing collaborative efforts, please see Appendix D.

Coordinating Research Studies Involving Newborns:

- TRIGR investigators have met with investigators participating in other type 1 diabetes research studies involving newborns (TEDDY and TrialNet) to discuss opportunities for enhancing coordination and collaboration.

- TEDDY and TRIGR share the same Data Coordinating Center. This coordination has resulted in implementation of similar standards in data collection, entry, management of quality control, and analyses for both studies.

- With the closure of the TRIGR accrual, two TRIGR sites began collaborative efforts on recruitment for TEDDY. Both groups are also considering a combined follow-up intervention protocol.

Coordinating Patient Recruitment Efforts:

- Two SEARCH for Diabetes in Youth sites assisted with TRIGR recruitment by providing brochures and other information about TRIGR.

- TRIGR, TrialNet, and TEDDY have coordinated recruitment efforts to ensure that they are not adversely competing for patient participants in their studies.

Enhancing Data Comparison Among Studies:

- TRIGR and TEDDY have implemented similar standards in data collection and entry.

- TRIGR and the Immune Tolerance Network are coordinating their efforts in the area of T cell assays.

TRIGR Administrative History	
Date Initiative Started	2001
Date *Special Diabetes Program* Funding Started	2001
Participating Components	NICHD, Canadian Institutes of Health Research, European Foundation for the Study of Diabetes, European Union, JDRF, Netherlands Diabetes Foundation, and Mead Johnson
Web site	www.trigr.org
TRIGR is taking place at 77 sites in 15 countries including the United States, 12 European countries, Canada, and Australia.	

TYPE 1 DIABETES–RAPID ACCESS TO INTERVENTION DEVELOPMENT (T1D-RAID)[34]

Promising ideas for novel therapeutic interventions can encounter roadblocks in movement from bench to bedside testing. Many investigators who have discovered a promising therapeutic agent in the laboratory do not have the resources or the background knowledge, for example, to "scale up" production of the agent for use in clinical trials. The T1D-RAID program was established to help overcome this major barrier to development of potential new therapeutics for type 1 diabetes and its complications. The program provides resources for pre-clinical development of drugs, natural products, and biologics that will be tested in clinical trials. The goal of T1D-RAID is to facilitate translation from the lab to the clinic of novel, scientifically meritorious therapeutic interventions for type 1 diabetes and its complications. T1D-RAID is not a grant mechanism and it does not sponsor clinical trials. Rather, it sponsors the work needed to get ready to do clinical trials. The program is assisting investigators by providing pre-clinical development steps, the absence of which may impede clinical translation.

HIGHLIGHTS OF PROGRESS

- Prepared lisofylline to meet product specifications for use in clinical trials. Lisofylline is now being tested in a clinical trial supported by the Clinical Islet Transplantation (CIT) Consortium (see Goal III) to determine if it can help to prevent recurrent autoimmunity after islet transplantation in humans.

- Established two master cell banks for manufacturing of a novel drug regimen (IL-2-Fc agonist and mut-IL 15-Fc antagonist) for a planned Immune Tolerance Network (ITN) (see Goal II) clinical study. Researchers in the Non-Human Primate Transplantation Tolerance Cooperative Study Group (NHPCSG) (see Goal III) demonstrated long-term survival of islets after transplantation when the animals were given the novel mixture of medicines that target the immune system. Based on these findings, the ITN approved a clinical trial to test this therapy in people with newly diagnosed type 1 diabetes to determine if the medicines can slow progression of disease.

- Stimulated the need for resources to do pre-clinical efficacy studies in type 1 diabetes and its complications. This resulted in the establishment of two contracts to provide preliminary and confirmation efficacy data in animal models (the T1D-Preclinical Testing Program [T1D-PTP]).

- Promptly terminated one project for a therapeutic for diabetic neuropathy after studies performed though the T1D-PTP failed to provide confirmation of efficacy previously provided by the principal investigator.

- Reviewed and referred six new potential projects to the T1D-PTP to conduct efficacy studies in animals to obtain stronger pre-clinical evidence prior to T1D-RAID investment.

---

[34] This program is also relevant to Goal V because it provides resources for therapies related to the complications of type 1 diabetes.

Anticipated Outcomes

Because clinical trials of agents to prevent, reverse, or treat type 1 diabetes and its complications are so important to realizing real improvements in the health and quality of life of patients, it is crucial to have a research continuum from the laboratory, where therapeutic agents are identified and initially tested, to the clinic, where agents are tested in patients. T1D-RAID provides a necessary resource that permits researchers to overcome the major barrier to moving promising agents from bench to bedside. T1D-RAID is already manufacturing agents for testing in type 1 diabetes clinical trials and is expected to produce several more. As more knowledge is gained about the underlying mechanisms of disease development, including genes and environmental factors that cause disease (see Goal I), as well as key immune system players (see Goal II), researchers could use this information to develop additional targets for disease prevention and treatment. Therefore, having the T1D-RAID resource in place will help to translate these new discoveries from the laboratory to the clinic, thereby accelerating the pace at which therapeutic agents can be used to prevent or treat type 1 diabetes.

Ongoing Evaluation

To determine which submitted requests are scientifically and technically meritorious, NIDDK specially convenes a T1D-RAID Review Panel consisting of outside experts from academia and industry who make recommendations to the Institute regarding whether a project should receive support. Final prioritization of the projects is made by NIDDK and takes into consideration the importance of the project to the NIH research agenda, portfolio diversity, and contract capacity. Investigators whose projects are supported are invited to present their project to a joint NIDDK/NCI T1D-RAID team, at which time questions can be asked. The Project Development Team, consisting of NIDDK T1D-RAID program directors, NCI staff experts, the principal investigator, and other Institute staff as necessary, decide on the necessary tasks and exact next steps. The NCI identifies and assigns available contractors for the tasks based on their expertise, capacity, and the time frame. The contractors then perform the T1D-RAID-approved tasks under the direction of NIDDK and NCI staff.

Milestones for progression of the project are then set by the Project Development Team. Monthly meetings of the NIDDK/NCI T1D-RAID team review the progress and roadblocks on each project to ensure that projects are progressing and that information is widely shared among all members of the principal investigator's team and the NIDDK and NCI staff managing the T1D-RAID program. In the event that a T1D-RAID project is encountering problems or overrunning its project budget in a way that will not readily lead to a desired data endpoint, a status review group will be convened to consider the likelihood that further work in the project area will be fruitful. The investigator and NIDDK staff will present progress to date to extramural scientists knowledgeable in the area. Following the presentations, the review group will meet in closed session to determine whether T1D-RAID efforts should continue with new project milestones or the project should be concluded.

In addition, T1D-RAID has been evaluated by external panels of scientific and lay experts at *ad hoc* evaluation meetings convened by NIDDK in January 2005 and June 2009. These meetings were an opportunity for external experts to evaluate progress and provide input on future research directions (for more information, see the Executive Summary and Appendix B). Through *ad hoc* evaluation meetings and other meetings described above, NIDDK continually seeks external input to inform current and future directions for T1D-RAID.

Program Enhancements

During the course of any long-term research project, adjustments need to be made to respond to a changing scientific landscape, which can include new and emerging areas of science and new discoveries that can inform future research directions. Because of the evolving nature of science, consortia supported by the *Special Diabetes Program* have also evolved over time and have undergone enhancements to take advantage of new technologies and overcome barriers to progress. Some enhancements have been made in response to gaps or opportunities identified by external input or by consortium members. Examples of program enhancements for T1D-RAID include:

- The inability to confirm the efficacy data provided in the original proposal submitted by an investigator was a concern of NIDDK and its reviewers and was resolved by the establishment of contracts by NIDDK to conduct animal efficacy studies.

- NIDDK program staff have worked closely with NIDDK's Technology Transfer Office to ensure that Material Transfer Agreements clearly establish ownership. NIDDK works with the principal investigator to ensure close communication in circumstances in which ownership of a project might change. This procedural change was established to ensure freedom for T1D-RAID to conduct pre-clinical development activities if ownership of the project changes. It is possible, as a project progresses, that ownership of the project may change from one entity to another (*e.g.*, a company transfers ownership of the material).

Coordination with Other Research Efforts

T1D-RAID is supporting the pre-clinical development of therapeutic agents that will be tested in clinical trials supported by the *Special Diabetes Program*. Therefore, this resource has been critically important in facilitating the translation of agents from bench to bedside, where they will be tested in people with type 1 diabetes. For a summary of ongoing collaborative efforts, please see Appendix D.

Facilitating Type 1 Diabetes Clinical Trials:

- T1D-RAID supported the manufacture of lisofylline, which is being tested in the CIT Consortium to determine if it can help reduce islet autoimmune destruction after islet transplantation.

- T1D-RAID is assisting in the manufacture and toxicology studies of a novel drug regimen (IL-2-Fc agonist and mut-IL 15-Fc antagonist), which will be tested in an ITN clinical trial. Researchers in NHPCSG demonstrated long-term survival of islets after transplantation when the animals were given this novel mixture of medicines.

T1D-RAID Administrative History

Date Initiative Started	2003
Date *Special Diabetes Program* Funding Started	2004
Participating Components	NIDDK, NCI
Web site	www.T1Diabetes.nih.gov/T1D-RAID/index.shtml

The T1D-RAID program was modeled after the NCI's RAID program and is a collaboration between NIDDK and NCI. The sponsors of approved requests to T1D-RAID gain access to the pre-clinical drug development contract resources of NCI's Developmental Therapeutics Program.

Goal III: Develop Cell Replacement Therapy

Beta Cell Biology Consortium (BCBC)

The BCBC is an international Consortium of investigators pursuing key challenges of enormous relevance to the development of therapies for type 1 diabetes by: (1) understanding how endogenous beta cells are made through the study of pancreatic development, with the hope of making pancreatic cells in culture; (2) exploring the potential of animal and/or human stem cells (embryonic[35] or adult) as a source of making pancreatic islets; and (3) determining the basic mechanisms underlying beta cell regeneration in the adult as a basis for producing new cellular therapies for diabetes. The BCBC is responsible for collaboratively generating necessary reagents, mouse strains, antibodies, assays, protocols, and technologies that are beyond the scope of any single research effort and that would facilitate research on the development of novel cellular therapies for diabetes.

HIGHLIGHTS OF PROGRESS

- Increased understanding of the events that occur during development that lead to the formation of pancreatic beta cells. This type of knowledge is being used in the development of strategies to generate beta cells from embryonic stem cells and/or other stem/progenitor cell populations, such as induced pluripotent stem cells.

- Identified progenitor cells in the adult mouse pancreas that form insulin-producing beta cells.

- Reprogrammed adult mouse exocrine cells into insulin-producing beta cells.

- Demonstrated spontaneous conversion of adult alpha cells into insulin-producing cells in beta cell-depleted mice.

- Developed a new mouse model for studying beta cell regeneration.

- Discovered a new marker for pre-clinical type 1 diabetes called ZnT8.

- Generated and/or listed on its Web site over 300 unique and useful resources of which 70 percent are publically available (those that are not remain in development and are released after validation and/or publication).

- Generated and/or validated more than 110 antibodies against markers expressed at different stages of stem cell to beta cell maturation and distributed more than 700 orders, to BCBC and non-BCBC investigators, since its inception. In a major development, a subset of these antibodies now allow researchers to obtain, for the first time, highly-purified fractions of the various endocrine cell types present in islets coming from human donors, including insulin-producing beta cells and glucagon-producing alpha cells.

- Created, for distribution to the scientific community, four PancChips (microarrays) that enable researchers to study genes expressed in the pancreas/islets of both humans and mice, as well as over 36,000 gene promoter regions in mice. Between 2002 and 2007, the core manufactured approximately 4,000 units of three different arrays, including over 2,300 that were shipped to investigators in 19 different countries.

---

[35] The NIH supports research using human embryonic stem cells within the NIH Guidelines for Human Stem Cell Research.

- Generated more than 50 new lines of genetically engineered mice or mouse embryonic stem cells to enable researchers to study pancreatic/islet cell development in animal systems. These mouse resources are available to the broad scientific community through a BCBC Web-based mouse database.

- Initiated http://genomics.betacell.org, previously known as EPConDB, a searchable database that provides sophisticated search tools for genes, their transcripts, and their profiles in expression studies. In addition, over 50 microarray studies related to the beta cell, and an additional 20, were extensively annotated and made available.

- Attracted new talent to beta cell biology through the Pilot and Feasibility (P&F) Program, funding seven new investigators.

- Attracted new talent to beta cell biology through the Seeding Collaborative Research in Beta Cell Biology (SCRBCB) Program. This mechanism permitted investigators outside the BCBC to collect preliminary data and form collaborative research teams prior to applying for full-scale grants during the BCBC re-competition.

- Stimulated productive collaborations among investigators with the Collaborative Bridging Project (CBP) which to date has supported 21 different short-term (1-3 years) projects. This program has yielded novel reagents and new methods, brought new skills and knowledge into the BCBC, and increased the number of formal collaborative interactions between BCBC participants by nearly 50 percent.

Anticipated Outcomes

The successful BCBC has made numerous scientific discoveries in the field of beta cell biology and accelerated progress toward the development of cell-based therapies for the treatment of type 1 diabetes. BCBC research has increased understanding of the developmental pathways required to produce a fully functioning pancreatic islet; the nature of stem/progenitor cells during normal pancreatic development and in the adult pancreatic islet; and the mechanisms of beta cell regeneration in the adult animal and human islet. With these insights and recent developments, the BCBC is shifting its efforts to take advantage of new emerging opportunities and increasing its focus on translational outcomes and scientific issues that stand in the way of developing new cell-based and regenerative therapies. First, the BCBC is working to reconstruct human type 1

diabetes in the mouse to produce a better animal model in which to study this disease. The model has two components: (1) type 1 diabetes patient-specific induced pluripotent stem cells that will differentiate into beta cells, blood stem cells, and cells of the immune system; and (2) a mouse recipient for the cells with genetic components of a human immune system. With these components, scientists expect the mouse to recapitulate the early events in the autoimmune destruction of human beta cells. This will allow them to study these events and test strategies to intervene in this process.

In addition, the BCBC will place a greater emphasis on studies of human cells and tissues to move new discoveries forward as quickly as possible. Efforts will be increased to generate beta cells from human embryonic stem cells,[36] to increase the human beta cell mass, and to uncover the mechanism to reprogram human

---

[36] The NIH supports research using human embryonic stem cells within the NIH Guidelines for Human Stem Cell Research.

adult cells into beta cells. Furthering basic research on beta cells will enhance efforts to produce an abundant supply of beta cells for transplantation and/or efforts to promote the generation of new beta cells within the body. The potential outcomes of BCBC research could permit scientists to grow islets in the laboratory for use in future research or clinical efforts. This knowledge could help scientists recreate an environment in the transplant patient that would optimize the success of the grafted islets, as well as make the treatment more widely available. Additionally, new knowledge could lead to the development of strategies to increase a person's beta cell mass *in vivo*, without the need for transplantation and immunosuppressive drugs.

The BCBC provides an infrastructure that is conducive to tackling these critical issues that can revolutionize type 1 diabetes research and, ultimately, the treatment of type 1 diabetes patients. BCBC researchers work collaboratively and are encouraged to share data and information on a regular basis through a coordinating center that organizes retreats, meetings, conference calls, and a comprehensive Web site. This rapid and efficient communication ensures that all members are aware of the "latest" research findings, and that they can tailor their own research endeavors to build upon that knowledge. Furthermore, research through this Consortium and in the broader scientific community is also accelerated by having core facilities that produce key laboratory reagents (*e.g.*, mouse models, antibodies, microarrays). This easy access to resources means that more time is spent performing real experiments, rather than preparing reagents to do the experiments. The *Special Diabetes Program* has facilitated the establishment of this multifaceted, interdisciplinary, collaborative, team-science approach to bring together leading experts in beta cell

biology to address fundamental questions about this important area of science, which is key to combating type 1 diabetes.

Ongoing Evaluation

The Executive Committee (EC), consisting of four NIDDK staff members and three BCBC investigators, is the principal governing body of the BCBC and actively guides the development of the BCBC. The EC is chaired by the leader of the Coordinating Center. An agenda is distributed in advance of every meeting, and minutes/action items are posted on the Web site. The EC meets regularly by teleconference to exchange information and build consensus in order to quickly and effectively resolve operational issues. In addition to the EC, a Steering Committee (SC) composed of all BCBC investigators and NIDDK program staff meets twice a year during the semiannual BCBC retreats. During this formal discussion, operational issues of potential interest to everyone are discussed. This provides a time during which strategic visions can be presented and discussed, and for any concerns that may have arisen to be openly discussed. An External Evaluation Committee (EEC), composed of 10 highly-regarded scientists, contributes to the scientific review of various projects (CBPs, P&F Program, and SCRBCB Program) and is often asked for input and advice on ongoing BCBC activities and future directions.

In addition, the BCBC has been evaluated by external panels of scientific and lay experts at *ad hoc* evaluation meetings convened by NIDDK in January 2005 and June 2009. These meetings were an opportunity for external experts to evaluate progress and provide input on future research directions (for more information, see the Executive Summary and Appendix B). Through *ad hoc* evaluation meetings and regular meetings of the EEC,

NIDDK continually seeks external input to inform current and future directions for the BCBC.

Program Enhancements

Because of the evolving nature of science, consortia supported by the *Special Diabetes Program* have evolved over time and have undergone enhancements to take advantage of new technologies and research findings, and to accelerate progress. Some enhancements have been made in response to external input and others have been initiated by the consortium members. Examples of program enhancements for the BCBC include:

- During the first funding cycle, the BCBC received critical scientific feedback, via a formal review process that involved the SC, the EEC, and a committee convened at the *ad hoc* planning and evaluation meeting in January 2005, that there was insufficient synergy among BCBC scientists. As a result, the CBP Program was created to support collaboration among various BCBC members and between the BCBC and other scientists. This highly flexible program has supported 21 different short-term (1-3 years) collaborative projects to date.

- Data sharing is critical to the success of the BCBC, however significant issues to protect the confidentiality of unpublished results and to avoid conflict of interest issues generated a barrier to this activity. Two actions were taken to ensure confidentiality to promote the sharing of preliminary research information and reagents. First, the Sharing Agreement that all BCBC members are required to sign was revised to make it more explicit and easier to understand. Second, access to resource information on the BCBC Web site was restructured to enable a high degree of access control. This assures that BCBC investigators can access all information that they have privileges to see, while maintaining confidentiality of unpublished results and avoiding conflict of interest issues.

- To increase the number of resources described on the BCBC Web site and assure that they become readily and publicly accessible, the BCBC took a multifaceted approach. First, the data collection process was simplified and, when possible, data standards were minimized. Second, descriptions of new reagents were sent to the Coordinating Center by NIDDK staff so that they could be correlated with database entries and released more quickly to the public. Third, the Coordinating Center hired scientists with experience in the fields of genetics, cell and development biology, and molecular biology to help oversee data entry and curation efforts. Finally, incentives were developed to stimulate students and post-doctoral fellows in member laboratories to enter this information into the databases.

Coordination with Other Research Efforts

The BCBC coordinates its efforts with multiple other type 1 diabetes research consortia and networks supported by the *Special Diabetes Program*. Collaboration, coordination, and resource sharing serve to synergize research efforts and accelerate research progress. Examples of coordination with other consortia are given below. For a summary of ongoing collaborative efforts, please see Appendix D.

Sharing Samples, Data, and Resources with the Research Community:

- The BCBC developed a comprehensive Web site (www.betacell.org) with information on mouse models, antibodies, microarrays, and data available to the scientific community.

- Collections of data and bioinformatics analytical tools developed by the BCBC are made available through the EPConDB database (http://genomics.betacell.org). This database has been linked to other relevant databases, such as the NIDDK-supported Diabetes Genome Anatomy Project database and the JDRF-sponsored T1Dbase.

Coordinating Research Efforts on Human Islets:

- BCBC investigators obtain human islets through the Islet Cell Resource Centers (ICR) for use in basic science research.

- Data collected from BCBC investigators using ICR samples are collected within the informatics coordination center of the ICR Consortium.

Collaboration Among Mouse Resources:

- Mouse strains developed by BCBC investigators are available through mouse repositories (Type 1 Diabetes Mouse Resource [T1DR] and Mutant Mouse Regional Resource Centers [MMRRC]), which provide greater access to the scientific community to these resources.

- The BCBC mouse database was designed to directly interface with T1DR and MMRRC to foster data sharing.

BCBC Administrative History	
Date Initiative Started	2001
Date *Special Diabetes Program* Funding Started	2001
Participating Components	NIDDK
Web site	www.betacell.org

The BCBC is comprised of a diverse group of 29 laboratories in the United States, Europe, and Israel. The BCBC Coordinating Center at Vanderbilt University oversees all collaborative scientific endeavors of the BCBC, including scientific cores, reagent databases, Steering Committee meetings, investigator retreats, the P&F Program, the SCRBCB Program, and the CBPs.

NON-HUMAN PRIMATE TRANSPLANTATION TOLERANCE COOPERATIVE STUDY GROUP (NHPCSG)

The NHPCSG is a multi-institution Consortium collaboratively developing and evaluating the safety and efficacy of novel therapies to induce immune tolerance in non-human primate (NHP) models of islet, kidney, heart, and lung transplantation. The program also supports fundamental research into the molecular mechanisms of immune tolerance and graft rejection; the identification of surrogate markers for graft rejection; and the induction, maintenance, and loss of tolerance. Two NIAID-funded specific pathogen-free NHP breeding colonies provide high-quality NHPs for these research studies. An Opportunities Pool supports innovative pilot projects, emerging research opportunities, and sharing of resources to further the goals of the NHPCSG. Pre-clinical research conducted by the NHPCSG provides critical information required to move promising therapeutic agents from the laboratory into clinical trials.

HIGHLIGHTS OF PROGRESS

- *Demonstrating long-term and sustained pancreatic islet beta cell function without continuous immunosuppressive therapy following islet transplantation in a drug-induced diabetic NHP model:* The researchers discontinued immunosuppressive treatments 14 days after the transplant. The 14-day tolerance induction protocol, which consisted of anti-CD3 conjugated with immunotoxin (to deplete T cells) and 15-deoxyspergualin (to arrest pro-inflammatory cytokine production and maturation of dendritic cells), was sufficient to protect the transplanted islets from immune rejection and loss of functional islet mass. More than half of the NHPs treated with this regimen remained insulin-free for more than 6 years without the need for pharmacologic immune suppression. Toxicity of immunosuppressive drugs is a major barrier in human islet transplantation. Therefore, if follow-on studies in humans achieve similar outcomes, then islet transplantation may be an option for more individuals with type 1 diabetes.

- *Demonstrating, in a steroid-free immunosuppressive protocol, an immune cell costimulatory blocking protein known as belatacept (LEA29Y) prolonged islet survival in a primate model:* This promising study provided the basis for a phase II kidney transplantation clinical trial. The trial has demonstrated promising results and has led to the development of a pilot study currently being conducted by the NIH Clinical Islet Transplantation (CIT) Consortium. An additional kidney transplantation clinical trial using LEA29Y in a steroid-free protocol is being conducted by the Immune Tolerance Network (ITN) (see Goal II).

- *Prolonging transplanted islet cell survival using a combination of IL-2/IL-15 fusion proteins with a steroid-free protocol:* A clinical trial in patients with new-onset type 1 diabetes is approved for development by the ITN once good manufacturing practice (GMP) grade reagents are available. The Type 1 Diabetes-Rapid Access to Intervention Development (see Goal II) program is undertaking production of reagents for pharmokinetic and toxicology studies before initiating a clinical trial.

- *Providing basis for a new ITN clinical trial for patients with new-onset type 1 diabetes:* The results of NHPCSG islet transplantation studies of an anti-inflammatory, alpha 1 anti-trypsin molecule provided support for an ITN clinical trial.

- *Demonstrating that a fusion protein, alefacept (lymphocyte function-associated antigen-3-Ig; LFA-3-Ig), selectively eliminated memory T cells and, when combined with abatacept (CTLA-4-Ig), prevented renal allograft rejection and alloantibody formation in NHPs:* These results are promising for the development of future clinical trials in islet transplantation.

- *Demonstrating that elevation of cytotoxic lymphocyte (CL) gene expression preceded the rejection of transplanted islets in NHPs:* These findings also extended to clinical studies in humans in which increased CL gene expression preceded clinical evidence of graft rejection. These results may help identify early stages of islet graft rejection and lead to clinically useful biomarkers that signal the need for early graft-saving interventions.

- Evaluating over 15 different protocols to establish immune tolerance and/or islet graft acceptance.

- Establishing two specific pathogen-free NHP breeding colonies to provide high-quality primates for type 1 diabetes research studies.

- *Performing pedigree analysis and histocompatability gene typing of key primate colony breeders and offspring to enable establishment of selective breeding groups:* Understanding the degree of Major Histocompatibility Complex (MHC) disparity between the transplant donor and recipient is crucial for interpretation of transplant outcomes. This gene typing program will greatly enhance the value of the colony for future transplantation studies.

Anticipated Outcomes

Model systems in which to study autoimmune disorders and organ transplantation are essential for translation of basic research into clinical practice. The NHPCSG uses primate models for the study of islet, kidney, heart, and lung transplantation since the NHP immune system and physiology most closely approximates those of humans. These studies are critical for the design of scientifically sound and ethically acceptable clinical trials to induce transplantation tolerance. However, there are also limitations in the use of NHP models. Because these animals do not spontaneously develop islet autoimmunity and type 1 diabetes, they lack the complication, seen in humans, of recurrent autoimmunity following transplantation. The latter is a major barrier to success of islet transplantation efforts in humans. Nonetheless, NHPCSG studies have led to clinically relevant discoveries. Most notably, researchers have demonstrated the ability of transplanted islets to survive in NHPs without the requirement for long-term immunosuppression. Through consortium building, sharing reagents, developing novel protocols, and directing the primate colony breeding program, researchers have made significant contributions to the field of islet transplantation; many of these advances are already being translated to clinical trials. In particular, two agents, a modified costimulatory blocking protein known as LEA29Y and a combination of IL-2/IL-15 fusion proteins, tested in NHPCSG studies demonstrated the safety and feasibility necessary to progress to human clinical trials. Future NHP studies using novel therapeutic agents may enable control of the immune response in humans, resulting in long-term islet cell graft survival, with limited requirements for short-term immunosuppressive therapy. These primate models serve the crucial role of bridging the gap between basic research and clinical advances in type 1 diabetes research.

Ongoing Evaluation

The NHPCSG Steering Committee (SC) serves as the governing body and is composed of the Principal Investigators (PIs) for each grant and an additional PI from multi-project grants. Program Directors of NIAID and NIDDK serve as non-voting members of the SC. Investigators report on progress and issues that arise in their research at annual meetings. In addition, research agendas, collaborations, and plans for resource development/sharing are established and implemented by the SC. The NHPCSG SC also directs the program's efforts to coordinate research agendas with NIAID and NIDDK clinical trial networks. The NIAID Program Officer coordinates activities of several subcommittees of the SC that maximize resources and promote group collaborations. The NIAID and NIDDK program officers also conduct annual evaluations of individual grants to ensure that appropriate progress has been made prior to the release of funds. The SC establishes guidelines for the identification of appropriate research milestones, and conducts peer review of proposals for support from the NHPCSG Opportunities Pool. Finally, the SC provides recommendations and guidance for the development and content of a secure NHPCSG Web site.

The NHPCSG chair of the SC provided an update of progress to the NIAID Advisory Council (NIAID Division of Allergy, Immunology, and Transplantation Subcommittee) during the open session of the January 30, 2006, meeting. Council members concurred that the NHPCSG has made excellent progress and has made many valuable contributions to transplantation immune tolerance research.

In addition, the NHPCSG was evaluated by external panels of scientific and lay experts at *ad hoc* evaluation meetings convened by NIDDK in January 2005 and June 2009. These meetings were an opportunity for external experts to evaluate progress and provide input on future research directions (for more information, see the Executive Summary and Appendix B). Through these and other meetings described above, NIDDK and NIAID continually seek external input to inform current and future directions for the NHPCSG.

Program Enhancements

Because of the evolving nature of science, consortia supported by the *Special Diabetes Program* have evolved over time and have undergone enhancements to take advantage of new technologies and research findings, and to accelerate progress. Some enhancements have been made in response to external input and others have been initiated by the Consortium members. Examples of program enhancements for the NHPCSG include:

- A longstanding obstacle to NHP transplantation research is the lack of high-quality, specific pathogen-free animals with well characterized histocompatibility genes. NIAID addressed this need by establishing dedicated breeding colonies and selecting progeny based on MHC haplotypes. Other NIAID-sponsored contract programs support NHP MHC gene/allele discovery and the discovery and development of novel methods to type for these alleles.

- Another major impediment is the lack of reagents that will work, or that work optimally in the NHP model, both for monitoring the immune responses and as immunotherapeutics. NIAID contract support for the NIH NHP Reagent Resource was established to address these needs. This program is producing monoclonal antibodies and other biological reagents when the corresponding biologics licensed, or under investigation, for human use are less than optimally active in NHP.

- To promote and enhance new interactions, training, and collaborations within the NHPCSG, the Consortium holds meetings of the NHPCSG SC 1-2 times per year. The meetings provide a venue for sharing ideas and solutions to specific research problems, evaluating progress, and enhancing ongoing collaborations. Subcommittees of the SC also have periodic conference calls and meetings. For example, a subcommittee for the rhesus macaque colony provides recommendations to NIAID regarding breeding strategies that enhance the utility of the colony.

- The NHPCSG has also engaged the scientific community to develop the highly specialized skills, standardized reagents, assays, and techniques needed for NHP transplantation studies. The NHPCSG has held three NHP Transplantation Techniques Workshops that included NHP transplantation researchers outside of the NHPCSG, and experts on NHP genomics and NHP diseases and disease models. These workshops also engaged many graduate students and fellows to

promote future growth of an experienced cadre of investigators in this highly specialized field. A direct outcome of these workshops is a web-based initiative that shares hundreds of protocols and standard operating procedures both within and outside the Consortium. In addition, Consortium investigators have established collaborations with experts in NHP microarray, genomics, and genetics as a result of these workshops.

- Progress in transplantation biology has been hampered by a lack of resources to validate or exclude immunosuppressive strategies showing promise in rodent models. The establishment of the NHPCSG Opportunities Pool has helped to address this need. An Opportunities Pool funding program within the Consortium provides additional support for collaborations within and outside the NHPCSG with an emphasis on cutting edge research studies. The NHPCSG Opportunities Pool has funded 16 projects, including five that were awarded to non-PI or junior investigators, and at least two outside collaborators were involved in the studies.

Coordination with Other Research Efforts

The NHPCSG coordinates its efforts with multiple other type 1 diabetes research consortia and networks supported by the *Special Diabetes Program*. Collaboration, coordination, and resource sharing provide synergy to research efforts and accelerate research progress. Examples of coordination with other consortia are given below. For a summary of ongoing collaborative efforts, please see Appendix D.

Coordinating Research Studies:

- Cross-representation of investigators between the NHPCSG and the CIT Consortium facilitates collaborative design of pre-clinical testing of novel therapeutics in NHPs.

- ITN priorities for pre-clinical testing of new therapeutics are considered in evaluating NHPCSG Opportunities Pool applications. Several ITN high-priority strategies are currently funded as pilot projects.

- The CIT Consortium, ITN, and NHPCSG are analyzing similar reagents and approaches for the treatment and prevention of type 1 diabetes or for islet transplantation.

- The NHPCSG and the ITN share information about scientific priorities and interests for research planning.

NHPCSG Administrative History	
Date Initiative Started (Islet and Kidney Models)	1999
Date *Special Diabetes Program* Funding Started	2002
Date NHPCSG Expanded to Include Heart and Lung Transplantation Models	2005
Participating Components	NIAID, NIDDK
The NHPCSG is a multi-institution Consortium consisting of 9 research cooperative agreements, including 3 multi-project awards.	

CLINICAL ISLET TRANSPLANTATION (CIT) CONSORTIUM

The CIT Consortium is a network of clinical centers that conducts clinical and mechanistic studies in islet transplantation, with or without accompanying kidney transplantation, for the treatment of type 1 diabetes. Consortium investigations focus on improving the isolation of islets, determining why donor islets fail, reducing the complications of islet transplantation, and limiting the side effects of immunosuppression.

HIGHLIGHTS OF PROGRESS

- *Launching seven clinical trials, with associated immunologic, metabolic, and mechanistic studies, of islet transplantation in individuals with normal kidney function and type 1 diabetes with severe hypoglycemic events despite intensive medical management:* In collaboration with the U.S. Food and Drug Administration (FDA), CIT investigators are conducting a Phase III multicenter clinical trial that may support future FDA licensure of an islet product. Five pilot trials will test new, innovative islet transplantation approaches. The seven trials will use comparable inclusion criteria and manufacturing specifications to ensure the comparability of study results.

- *Conducting a phase III, multicenter clinical trial that includes Medicare beneficiaries, as mandated by the Medicare Prescription Drug Improvement and Modernization Act of 2003 (Public Law 108-173):* The target population consists of individuals with type 1 diabetes who have previously undergone kidney transplantation for diabetic nephropathy and are thus already receiving immunosuppressive therapy to prevent rejection of the donor kidney. This trial has required close collaboration among NIDDK, NIAID, and the Centers for Medicare & Medicaid Services.

- *Developing an FDA licensure pathway for an islet product based primarily upon the two phase III trials described above:* These trials will use "standard" anti-rejection regimens for both islet-alone and islet-after-kidney transplant protocols. A key FDA requirement for consideration of islet licensure was the development and implementation of a common isolation process with standardized documentation at all sites. The CIT Consortium met these requirements by developing a master production batch record for islet isolation.

Anticipated Outcomes

Islet transplantation is a promising therapy that can yield long-lasting, beneficial results for individuals with difficult-to-manage type 1 diabetes including those with kidney failure. Much has been learned about islet cell biology and the processes leading to rejection of transplanted islets and loss of islet function. In addition, pre-clinical studies are evaluating new approaches to immunomodulation in conjunction with islet transplantation in animal models. Challenges remain, however, in improving the safety and long-term outcomes of islet transplantation in people with type 1 diabetes. To address these issues, CIT investigators hope to minimize the toxic effects of anti-rejection drugs and identify potential methods to prevent graft rejection without the need for global immunosuppression. Other Consortium research is aimed at abolishing life-threatening hypoglycemic events and achieving long-lasting control of blood glucose with only a single islet transplant. Ultimately, the knowledge gained from these and other CIT investigations can enable the greater use of islet transplantation in individuals with type 1 diabetes.

Ongoing Evaluation

The CIT Consortium is managed jointly by the NIDDK and the NIAID. NIAID assumes principal leadership for regulatory affairs. The Consortium's clinical protocols are reviewed by the NIDDK Islet Transplantation Data and Safety Monitoring Board, which is composed of outside experts in diabetes, clinical trial design, ethics, transplantation, and biostatistics. The Steering Committee is responsible for the overall Consortium governance and is composed of the chair, the PIs of the six awarded clinical centers and the data coordinating center, the chair of the Mechanistic Studies Subcommittee, and representatives from NIDDK and NIAID.

To inform the CIT Consortium's current and future research directions, NIDDK and NIAID seek external expert review. Through an External Evaluation Committee, input on the design of the CIT Consortium's Islet After Kidney trial was sought. In addition, the Consortium has been evaluated by external panels of scientific and lay experts at *ad hoc* evaluation meetings convened by NIDDK in January 2005 and April 2008. These meetings were an opportunity for external experts to evaluate the progress and provide input on future research directions (for more information, see the Executive Summary and Appendix B).

Program Enhancements

Because of the evolving nature of science, consortia supported by the *Special Diabetes Program* have evolved over time and have undergone enhancements to take advantage of new technologies and research findings, and to accelerate progress. Some enhancements have been made in response to external input and others have been initiated by the Consortium members. Examples of program enhancements for the CIT Consortium include:

- Establishing a collaboration between the CIT Consortium, the IIDP (Integrated Islet Distribution Program), and Collaborative Islet Transplant Registry (CITR) to harmonize data dictionaries of the three programs, reduce the time involved in data entry, increase data accuracy, and facilitate data sharing.

- Developing and implementing new adverse event reporting, and standard operating and reagent manufacturing procedures to meet FDA requirements for the conduct of a multicenter cellular therapy phase III trial to license an islet product.

- Expanding the Statistical and Data Coordinating Center of the CIT Consortium to increase clinical site monitoring and specimen tracking functions of protocols. In addition, an advisory group to the Coordinating Center has been established.

Coordination with Other Research Efforts

The CIT Consortium coordinates its efforts with multiple other type 1 diabetes research consortia and networks supported by the *Special Diabetes Program*. Collaboration, coordination, and resource sharing serve to synergize research efforts and accelerate research progress. Examples of coordination with other consortia are given below. For a summary of ongoing collaborative efforts, please see Appendix D.

Sharing Data Among Consortia Studying Islet Transplantation:

- Data sharing agreements have been developed among the CIT Consortium, CITR, and the IIDP.

These agreements include use of shared data dictionaries and source verification of data by CIT clinical site monitors, with corrections transmitted to all participants. Monthly teleconferences ensure communication about maintaining up-to-date information. This effort will minimize redundancy in data collection and enhance data dissemination.

- The CITR will list all active islet transplantation protocols on its Web site. The Consortium will use this information as part of its informed consent process for clinical trial participants.

Coordinating Research Studies:

- Cross-representation of investigators between the Non-Human Primate Transplantation Tolerance Cooperative Study Group (NHPCSG) and the CIT Consortium will facilitate collaborative design of pre-clinical studies and pre-clinical testing of therapeutics in non-human primates.

- The CIT Consortium, ITN, and NHPCSG are interested in analyzing similar reagents to be used as immune modulators for the treatment of type 1 diabetes or for islet transplantation.

- The CIT Consortium and ITN are sharing expertise and coordinating efforts in the planning of immunologic assays in CIT trials. ITN core labs will be used for selected assays in CIT trials.

- The Type 1 Diabetes-Rapid Access to Intervention Development program is supporting the manufacture of reagents for use in CIT trials.

CIT Consortium Administrative History	
Date Initiative Started	2004
Date *Special Diabetes Program* Funding Started	2004
Participating Components	NIDDK, NIAID
Web site	www.citisletstudy.org
The CIT Consortium is composed of 11 clinical centers in the United States, Canada, Sweden and Norway, and one data coordinating center.	

Islet Cell Resource Centers (ICRs)

The notable advances made in understanding human islet function and improving the efficacy and safety of islet transplantation have been facilitated by making human islets available to researchers. Importantly, isolation of human islets from the pancreas is a complex technology mastered by few investigators and facilities. The ICRs were a consortium of the most experienced academic centers that provided human islets for research and helped establish the efficacy and safety of islet transplantation as a treatment for type 1 diabetes. The initial mission of the ICRs was three-fold: (1) to purify clinical-grade pancreatic islets from whole pancreata and distribute them for clinical transplantation; (2) to provide pancreatic islets for basic research studies; and (3) to perform research and development to improve isolation techniques, islet quality, the shipping and storage of islets, and assays for characterizing purified islets.

Islet transplantation research requires multidisciplinary isolation laboratories that meet or exceed FDA guidelines for good manufacturing practice (GMP). The staff must include experts in clinical research and basic science and have specific expertise in the preparation of islets from cadaver pancreata. Over 92 million human islets were produced by the ICRs from 2004-2009. Some clinical-grade human islets were distributed throughout the United States to transplant centers that enrolled patients in approved clinical protocols. Islets were also distributed to approved investigators who used them in basic research protocols. The ICR program was facilitated by a coordinating center at the City of Hope (Duarte, CA) that provided infrastructure support to both the islet production facilities and the research community. The ICR consortium was the first and largest cooperative effort in the world to provide human islet preparations for research while simultaneously addressing the need to improve isolation and transplantation technologies.

HIGHLIGHTS OF PROGRESS[37]

- Provided more than 92 million islet equivalents for transplantation in 78 patients.

- Distributed more than 201 million islet equivalents for research to 273 investigators. The number of islet equivalents distributed for basic research grew steadily from 1.3 million in 2004 to 22.3 million in 2008. Similarly, the number of approved institutions and research studies steadily increased from 16 institutions and 19 studies in 2004 to 105 institutions and 156 studies in 2008.

- Of the total 1,076 documented pancreata, 202 (19 percent) were used in clinical islet transplantation and 809 (75 percent) were used for basic research studies. Sixty-five (6 percent) pancreata were not used because consent for research was not obtained or islet quantity or quality did not meet clinical criteria.

- Demonstrated that the oxygen-carrier, perfluorocarbon, stabilizes cadaver pancreata during transportation.

- Optimized the use of shipment materials for transport of purified islets to improve islet viability and quality. An immediate electronic notification mechanism simplified the distribution process and contributed to broadening the availability of pancreatic islets for clinical studies or research.

---

[37] This section includes progress through July 2009 because the ICRs concluded in July 2009 and were replaced, in part, by the Integrated Islet Distribution Program (see this Goal).

Outcomes

The regional ICRs were successful in the support of national demands for clinical islets and distributed approximately 300 million islet equivalents in 8 years. Using a centrally located, objectively monitored priority list, the centers distributed islets throughout the United States. As a result, institutional access to islets for transplantation and basic research increased since the ICRs were created. This fostered a growing appreciation of the uniqueness of human islet biology as compared to rodent counterparts and accelerated the pace of discovery. Furthermore, the ICRs created a collaborative infrastructure that fostered refinement of preservation and cell culture solutions, optimization of shipping devices for both pancreas and islets, and advances in laboratory technologies to isolate islets. The collaborations helped to meet the challenges inherent in the provision of viable islets with an optimal chance for survival after transplantation. During pancreatic transport and islet purification, preservation, and shipping, the islets are at risk of suffering irreversible damage that reduces their viability and effectiveness as transplanted tissue. ICR research demonstrated that perfluorocarbon stabilized cadaver pancreata during transportation and led to the development of specialized containers for the shipment of purified islets. These achievements improved islet viability, quality, and availability for transplantation and basic research.

Research designed to enable durable islet viability and survival is expected to improve diabetes control after transplant, with a consequent improvement in the recipient's quality of life and health status. However, cadaver islets are foreign tissues for the recipients. Thus, immunosuppressive therapy is required to sustain transplant survival, in addition to optimally prepared donor islets. Further refinements in laboratory assessment of islet potency and viability, purification procedures, and detection of viable islets within the recipient using noninvasive methods are critical. Durable islet survival could lower the number of islets required per patient for successful transplantation, reduce from two to one the number of transplants currently required, reduce the risks and costs associated with transplantation, and extend the availability of islet transplant to a greater number of people with diabetes.

Evaluation

The ICR Steering Committee (SC), composed of the PIs of each ICR, the Administrative and Bioinformatics Coordinating Center (ABCC, City of Hope), NCRR, NIDDK, JDRF, and FDA, as well as a select group of experts and administrators, provided continuous evaluation, oversight, and guidance to the ICRs. In addition, the SC included members of transplantation centers from Canada, the Nordic Network (Sweden), and the Australian Transplant Consortium. Inclusion of non-U.S. experts in islet preparation was intended to extend the breadth of the group's experience and provide objective, cutting-edge analysis of the ICRs' progress in islet purification, stabilization, and transport. They reviewed procedures and outcomes, adverse events, protocols for scientific studies, and policy matters. The ABCC also received feedback concerning islet quality from users of the pancreatic islets supplied by the ICRs. Finally, the ICRs were evaluated by an external panel of scientific and lay experts at an *ad hoc* evaluation meeting convened by NIDDK in January 2005. This meeting was an opportunity for external experts to evaluate progress and provide input on future research directions.

Program Enhancements

Because of the evolving nature of science, consortia supported by the *Special Diabetes Program* have evolved over time and have undergone enhancements to take advantage of new technologies and research findings, and to accelerate progress. Some enhancements have been made in response to external input and others have been initiated by the consortium members. Examples of program enhancements for the ICRs include:

- To improve further the quality of islets for islet transplantation, the ICRs studied islet shipping procedures and conditions. Efforts were developed to evaluate three islet shipping containers that were designed by ICR scientists and one small business. Two Small Business Innovation Research (SBIR) grants supported applied research in this area and the beta prototypes were tested in conjunction with ICR investigators.

- An *ad hoc* evaluation committee established milestones for ICR participation. Based on their input, three ICR centers failed to demonstrate the required activity and proficiency in their transplant programs and were discontinued.

- Utilizing islets of the highest-quality possible is critical to conducting research. To foster research targeted towards islet quality improvement, a competitive Opportunities funding program was established in 2006 within the Consortium. This mechanism provided additional opportunities for collaborations within and outside the ICRs and allowed for timely research studies in response to the emergence of promising new technologies. In addition, the ICRs shared new developments with the community through their comprehensive Web site, review of clinical and basic science research proposals, and frequent relevant publications.

Coordination with Other Research Efforts

The ICRs coordinated efforts with multiple other type 1 diabetes research consortia and networks supported by the *Special Diabetes Program*. Collaboration, coordination, and resource sharing served to synergize research efforts and accelerate research progress. Examples of coordination with other consortia are given below. For a summary of ongoing collaborative efforts, please see Appendix D.

Enabling Clinical and Basic Research Studies:

- The ICRs provided clinical grade islets for trials conducted within the Clinical Islet Transplantation (CIT) Consortium.

- The ICRs provided islets for multicenter clinical studies using the "Edmonton protocol" in the Immune Tolerance Network (ITN).

- Type 1 Diabetes–Rapid Access to Intervention Development supported the manufacture of reagents that were tested for their effects on improving the survival and function of islets in culture.

- Investigators from the following consortia received islets used for clinical assays and for basic research through the ICR basic science human islet distribution program:

  o SEARCH for Diabetes in Youth study;

  o ITN;

  o Autoimmune Disease Prevention Centers;

  o Genetics of Kidneys in Diabetes Study; and

  o Beta Cell Biology Consortium (BCBC).

Sharing Data Across Multiple Research Consortia Studying Islets:

- Investigators who used ICR resources agreed to place their clinical study data in the Collaborative Islet Transplant Registry (CITR).

- The CITR performs on-site data review of transplantation centers and electronically shared the results with the ICRs. The data included determination of islet quality and collection of transplant outcome information.

- The CIT Consortium, CITR, and ICRs developed data sharing agreements. These agreements included use of shared data dictionaries and source verification of data by CIT clinical site monitors with corrections transmitted to all participants. Monthly teleconferences ensured communication about maintaining up-to-date information. This effort minimized redundancy in data collection and enhanced its dissemination.

- Data from BCBC investigators who used ICR samples were collected within the informatics coordination center of the ICR Consortium.

Improving Characterization of Islet Quality:

- ICR and BCBC investigators shared reagents and expertise to develop improved methods of characterizing islet quality and viability.

ICRs Administrative History	
Date ICRs Started	2001
Date ICRs Ended	2009
Date *Special Diabetes Program* Funding Started	2001
Participating Components	NIDDK, NCRR, JDRF
Web site	http://icr.coh.org

A total of 14 different ICRs participated from 2001-2009, with eight ICRs in operation at the close of the program. The ABCC coordinated the activities of the ICRs and the SC, including the administrative, supervisory, and collaborative achievements required to achieve the goals of the program.

Integrated Islet Distribution Program (IIDP)

The availability of human islets as a resource for research is critical to advancing islet transplantation and other cell-based therapies as treatment for type 1 diabetes. Importantly, human islets differ from rodent models with respect to the regulatory and metabolic milieu affecting their function, susceptibility to injury, and their adaptive responses for replication. Recognition of these differences underscores the need for human islet investigations. The IIDP is a new program, launched in July 2009, to process and distribute high-quality human cadaveric islets to the diabetes research community for basic research. This new program builds upon the experience of the Islet Cell Resource Centers program that was operative from 2001-2009.

Anticipated Outcomes

The IIDP consists of a single coordinating center (City of Hope, Duarte, CA) that subcontracts with 11 carefully selected islet isolation facilities to process and distribute human cadaveric islets. The coordinating center responsibilities include:

- Maintenance of investigator database

- Monitoring islet production centers

- Implementation and maintenance of notification algorithm

- Financial management of program

- Shipment and tracking of islet tissues

- Performance site and user satisfaction analyses

- Assessment of human islet resource value

- Interaction with the External Evaluation Committee (EEC)

- Completion of reporting requirements

Because pancreas procurement, processing, and testing procedures are expensive, cost sharing by the investigator is required, but with considerable subsidization from NIDDK through the *Special Diabetes Program*. Therefore, the IIDP fulfills the existing need for affordable human islet resourcing for investigators. The IIDP is fully operative and is distributing these precious resources that will ultimately advance human islet biology and assure the clinical relevance of basic research.

Ongoing Evaluation

The IIDP consists of project officers from NIDDK and JDRF, an EEC, and the Coordinating Center at City of Hope. The EEC currently has five non-Federal members and convenes through regular teleconferences and an annual meeting. The EEC is charged with providing guidance to and assessment of the performance of the Coordinating Center. EEC functions include, but are not limited to:

- Development of criteria required for competitively derived subcontract awards.

- Development of equitable compensation fee schedules for islet production facilities and cost sharing fee schedules for islet recipient investigators.

- Peer review of new investigator proposals that do not have extramural NIH, JDRF, or ADA funding.

- Development of governance policies concerning equitable systems of islet allocation per investigator and project. Implementing policies that enable ongoing progress reviews and criteria for expanding, curtailing, or discontinuing approved studies.

- Review of subcontract performance with evaluation criteria emphasizing maintenance of certification records, lot release data, human islet production and shipment activity, islet quality assessments from users, shipment compliance, compliance for correcting recognized deficiencies, and technological innovation.

- Development of islet viability standards necessary for lot release.

- Monitoring performance of the Coordinating Center with respect to implementation of procedures and policies and providing input on modifications where necessary.

Coordination with Other Research Efforts

The IIDP coordinates its efforts with multiple other type 1 diabetes research consortia and networks supported by the *Special Diabetes Program*. Collaboration, coordination, and resource sharing serve to synergize research efforts and accelerate research progress. Examples of coordination with other consortia are given below. For a summary of ongoing collaborative efforts, please see Appendix D.

Enabling Clinical and Basic Research Studies:

- Investigators from the following consortia receive islets used for clinical assays and for basic research through the IIDP:

  - o   SEARCH for Diabetes in Youth study;
  - o   Immune Tolerance Network;
  - o   Autoimmune Disease Prevention Centers;
  - o   Genetics of Kidneys in Diabetes Study; and
  - o   Beta Cell Biology Consortium (BCBC).

Sharing Data Across Multiple Research Consortia Studying Islets:

- The Clinical Islet Transplantation (CIT) Consortium, Collaborative Islet Transplant Registry, and IIDP developed data sharing agreements. These agreements include use of shared data dictionaries and source verification of data by CIT clinical site monitors with corrections transmitted to all participants.

- Data from BCBC investigators who use IIDP samples are collected within the informatics coordination center of the IIDP.

Improving Characterization of Islet Quality:

- IIDP and BCBC investigators share reagents and expertise to develop improved methods of characterizing islet quality and viability.

IIDP Administrative History	
Date IIDP Started	2009
Date *Special Diabetes Program* Funding Started	2009
Participating Components	NIDDK, JDRF
Web site	http://iidp.coh.org

The IIDP consists of a single coordinating center that subcontracts with carefully selected islet isolation facilities to process and distribute human cadaveric islets.

Collaborative Islet Transplant Registry (CITR)

The CITR expedites progress and promotes safety in islet transplantation through the collection, analysis, and communication of comprehensive and current data on all islet transplants performed in North America. Through additional support from the JDRF, CITR has begun collection of data from selected European and Australian sites. The CITR collects both retrospective and prospective data from participating islet transplant programs. All islet transplants performed since January 1, 1999, are expected to be captured by the CITR, as well as future islet transplants performed through 2013. The CITR prepares an annual report with data on recipient and donor characteristics; pancreas procurement and islet processing; immunosuppressive medications; function of the donated islets; patients' lab results with confidential information removed; and adverse events. This information is widely disseminated throughout the islet transplant and diabetes communities, and also made available to the general public. The data collected and analyzed by the CITR will help to define the overall risks and benefits of islet transplantation as a treatment option for people with type 1 diabetes, and identify the most optimal maintenance therapy. To date, only human-to-human cadaveric islet transplantation has been reported to the CITR.

HIGHLIGHTS OF PROGRESS

- Publication of six annual reports for 2004-2009 with over 200 pieces of data analysis.

- Results from the Annual Report have provided the basis for publications and communications at international transplantation meetings; information for the Islet Investigators Brochure used for recruitment for the Clinical Islet Transplantation (CIT) Consortium; and data to fine-tune eligibility requirements for CIT Consortium trials.

- Determined that episodes of dangerously low blood glucose (hypoglycemia), encountered in most patients prior to transplantation, were nearly absent after islet transplantation. The data were obtained from an analysis of 138 poorly controlled type 1 diabetes patients who had the procedure at 19 medical centers in the United States and Canada.

- Reported that, 1 year after the last islet infusion, 58 percent of recipients no longer had to inject insulin to maintain normal glucose levels, a successful clinical outcome.

- Reported that, for islet-alone recipients, 72 percent achieved insulin independence at least once. Of those who achieved insulin independence, 70 percent retained this status 1 year after achieving it and 55 percent remained insulin independent after 2 years.

- Reported that, 1 year after islet infusion, those individuals still requiring insulin injections had a 69 percent reduction in insulin requirements.

- Current North American database includes information on 339 allogeneic islet recipients (80 percent of all those known done in North America), 658 allogeneic infusion procedures, 722 donor pancreata, 213 autograft recipients and their islets, from 28 centers ever active since 1999 (some have closed). Each transplant center in CITR received inspection, training, software integration, and quality assurance visits.

Anticipated Outcomes

Important components of clinical studies are careful monitoring and reporting of findings. The CITR collects data on patients who have undergone islet transplantation procedures and produces reports that document study parameters and clinical outcomes. This monitoring system enables researchers to track the progress of successful patients as well as to follow patients who experienced graft failure. Importantly, long-term data regarding islet transplantation outcomes are collected for analyses. CITR has reported that 72 percent of islet alone recipients achieved insulin independence at least once and identified factors that are associated with the achievement of insulin independence. The Registry also reported that 1 year after islet infusion, individuals still requiring insulin injections had a 69 percent reduction in their insulin requirements. However, some patients require additional islet transplants, and successful outcomes are not uniformly observed. Tracking these patients is essential to determine the factors that contribute not only to graft function and longevity, but to graft failure. These analyses will also provide the comparative basis needed for determining long-term benefits of induction and maintenance therapies that are most successful. Because islet transplantation is a complex, multifaceted process, and because it is conducted at numerous centers with funding from NIH, voluntary organizations, and local institutions, the CITR is needed as a structure for making valuable assessments that will guide continued improvements.

Ongoing Evaluation

To ensure ongoing evaluation of the CITR's data collection process and procedures, the CITR is both peer reviewed and reviewed at least annually by a Scientific Advisory Committee (SAC). The SAC was established by the Coordinating Center, in consultation with NIDDK. Current voting members include representatives from University of Miami, United Network for Organ Sharing (UNOS), VA Puget Sound Health Care Systems, UCLA Immunogenetics Center, and the Nordic Network (Sweden). *Ad hoc* members include representatives from the U.S. Food and Drug Administration, Centers for Medicare & Medicaid Services, Health Resources and Services Administration, JDRF, NCRR, NIAID, and NIDDK. In addition, yearly investigator meetings are held, including contributors from the international islet transplantation community. These meetings serve to review the annual activities of the registry and provide guidance for the evolving challenges. Finally, monthly teleconferences including the Scientific Advisor, Program Officer, and CITR investigators provide a forum for discussion of time sensitive issues. Participating investigators and transplant coordinators/data managers serve on the following CITR Committees that review its functions, procedures, and status on a minimum quarterly basis:

- The Compliance Committee monitors participant and islet transplant program compliance, identifies barriers to consistent compliance with participant registration and follow-up, and suggests mechanisms to improve compliance. The Committee also reviews the results of each onsite data audit and recommends appropriate action based on the results of the audit.

- The Data Elements Committee is responsible for monitoring changes in the standard practice of islet transplantation (which includes islet isolation, purification, transplant technique, immunosuppression medications, and metabolic tests) and recommending appropriate modifications to the CITR data definitions and collection tools.

- The Transplant Coordinators/Data Managers Committee provides logistical information to the SAC regarding the working of the CITR from the Coordinators' perspective.

- The Publications and Presentations Committee is responsible for reviewing all proposals, manuscripts, abstracts, and presentations for primary and secondary analysis of the data and dissemination of results.

In addition, the CITR has been evaluated by external panels of scientific and lay experts at *ad hoc* evaluation meetings convened by NIDDK in January 2005 and April 2008. These meetings were an opportunity for external experts to evaluate progress and provide input on future research directions (for more information, see the Executive Summary and Appendix B). Through *ad hoc* evaluation meetings and regular meetings of the SAC, NIDDK continually seeks external input to inform current and future directions for the CITR.

Program Enhancements

Because of the evolving nature of science, consortia supported by the *Special Diabetes Program* have evolved over time and have undergone enhancements to take advantage of new technologies and research findings, and to accelerate progress. Some enhancements have been made in response to external input and others have been initiated by the consortium members. Examples of program enhancements for the CITR include:

- An active collaboration between the CIT Consortium, the Islet Cell Resource Centers (ICR), and CITR was established. One important accomplishment of this collaboration was the successful harmonization of the data dictionaries for

the databases of the three programs to reduce the time involved in data entry at the participating sites, and to facilitate data sharing.

- To respond to general data reporting and storage needs, CITR developed a unified islet module designed to capture detailed procurement, processing, and performance characteristics information on all islet preparations whether used for clinical transplantation or not. The preparations used for clinical transplantation are linked to the recipient and donor information for full analysis.

- To attain and maintain currency in islet transplantation, CITR has recruited all but two centers within North America who have conducted islet transplants since 1999, and is collecting current and historical islet transplant data from these centers. CITR has also launched new electronic data forms for pancreatic islet autograft patients and is collecting these data as well for 1999-2013.

Coordination with Other Research Efforts

The CITR coordinates its efforts with multiple other type 1 diabetes research consortia and networks supported by the *Special Diabetes Program*. Collaboration, coordination, and resource sharing serve to synergize research efforts and accelerate research progress. Examples of coordination with other consortia are given below. For a summary of ongoing collaborative efforts, please see Appendix D.

Sharing Data Across Multiple Consortia Studying Islets:

- The CITR provides all data collection forms, data dictionaries, and code lists to all type 1 diabetes consortia and networks studying islets and islet transplantation.

- Data sharing agreements have been developed among the CIT Consortium, CITR, the UNOS, and the ICRs. These agreements include use of shared data dictionaries and source verification of data by CIT clinical site monitors, with corrections transmitted to all participants. Monthly teleconferences ensure communication about maintaining up-to-date information. This effort will minimize redundancy in data collection and will enhance its dissemination. The CITR is implementing separate data sharing agreements with each of the islet processing centers (former ICR sites) to continue collecting the islet data for transplanted islets.

- Investigators who use CIT resources must agree to place their clinical study data in the CITR, with recipients' consent.

- On-site data review of transplantation centers is performed by the CITR and is provided to the CIT Consortium. Data include determination of islet quality and collection of transplant outcome information.

- Meeting minutes of special interest committees such as the CITR Metabolic Monitoring Committee and the Health Related Quality of Life Committee are shared with all type 1 diabetes consortia and networks studying islets. Members from these groups are invited to participate on these committees.

- The CITR is planning to list all active islet transplantation protocols on their Web site. The CIT Consortium will be using this information as part of its informed consent process for enrollees.

- The CITR archives data from the Immune Tolerance Network islet transplantation trials.

CITR Administrative History	
Date Initiative Started	2001
Date *Special Diabetes Program* Funding Started	2001
Participating Components	NIDDK, JDRF
Web site	www.citregistry.org
The CITR currently consists of one Coordinating Center (The EMMES Corporation, Rockville, MD) and 28 CITR North American centers. Three European and two Australian CITR sites are supported by the JDRF.	

Goal IV: Prevent or Reduce Hypoglycemia in Type 1 Diabetes

DIABETES RESEARCH IN CHILDREN NETWORK (DIRECNET)

DirecNet is a multicenter clinical research network investigating the use of technology advances in the management of type 1 diabetes in children and adolescents. DirecNet is also developing a better understanding of hypoglycemia, the dangerous drop in blood glucose that can lead to seizures, loss of consciousness and, in extreme cases, coma or death. Specific goals for DirecNet have been to: (1) assess the accuracy, efficacy, and effectiveness of devices that continuously monitor blood glucose levels in children with type 1 diabetes, the population of patients at highest risk for consequences of hypoglycemia; (2) determine the optimal utilization of continuous glucose monitors (CGMs) in the management of diabetes in children; (3) determine the extent to which exercise contributes to the risk of hypoglycemia; (4) assess the impact of continuous glucose monitoring on quality of life for the child and family; (5) develop tools to incorporate CGMs into diabetes self-management; (6) evaluate and develop distinct, age-appropriate treatment approaches to type 1 diabetes in children; (7) characterize the daily blood sugar profile of nondiabetic children with continuous monitoring; and (8) develop statistical methods for the analysis of continuous glucose monitoring data.

After the completion of the first phase of DirecNet, and in response to a competitive renewal process, DirecNet continued into a second phase in 2007. The goals of DirecNet were to continue trials related to continuous glucose monitoring technologies in children utilizing the information obtained during the first phase of DirecNet. In addition, new specific goals were added to include: (1) evaluating interventions to reduce hypoglycemia in children and young adults with diabetes; (2) studying the pathophysiology of protection against and recognition of hypoglycemia in children; (3) determining the effects of hypoglycemia on brain structure and function using state-of-the-art neuroimaging methodologies and neurocognitive evaluations; (4) determining whether intensive therapy including initial closed loop control followed by pump and continuous glucose monitoring therapy can preserve islet cell function; and (5) expanding the understanding of the effects of exercise on blood glucose control, especially the risk of hypoglycemia.

HIGHLIGHTS OF PROGRESS

- Successful completion of nine protocols on children with or without type 1 diabetes, with five more in progress.

- Showed that the risk of nocturnal hypoglycemia increased nearly two-fold on nights following exercise.

- Showed that the risk of hypoglycemia can be markedly reduced in patients treated with insulin pumps by suspending the basal insulin infusion during exercise.

- Demonstrated that counterregulatory hormone responses to spontaneous nocturnal hypoglycemia are blunted throughout the nighttime period with or without antecedent exercise.

- Demonstrated that most pediatric patients with well-controlled type 1 diabetes fail to release epinephrine, a specific counterregulatory hormone, until blood glucose levels are approaching values that indicate a shortage of glucose in the brain.

- Showed that levels of adiponectin, a protein secreted by fat cells, are stable from day to day, not affected by acute exercise or metabolic control, and vary inversely with obesity in children with type 1 diabetes. Increased levels of adiponectin appear to be associated with a decrease in hypoglycemia risk.

- Showed that both low-fat and high-fat bedtime snacks provide equal protection against nocturnal hypoglycemia. This study also highlighted the feasibility of web-based research in the patients' home environment.

- Demonstrated that continuous glucose monitoring is a better method compared with 8-point glucose profiles as an outcome measure to assess glucose variability in diabetes clinical trials.

- Developed and tested new treatment satisfaction and adherence measures for use in clinical trials of continuous monitoring systems.

- Developed standard algorithms for patients and clinicians to use to adjust basal and bolus insulin doses based on continuous glucose monitoring data.

- Determined sensor accuracy, sensitivity, specificity, and reliability of first generation continuous glucose monitors in detecting hypoglycemia.

- Developed and implemented pilot studies to assess two bedtime interventions (terbutaline and glutamine) in the prevention or reduction of nocturnal hypoglycemia. One of these (terbutaline) proved difficult to recruit for and the other (glutamine) appeared ineffective. Neither was pursued by the study group for a long-term clinical trial.

- Developed and implemented a randomized, controlled trial of continuous glucose monitoring in children 4 to less than 10 years old. This trial is currently under way with 100 patients enrolled and is due for completion in late summer 2011.

- Developed and implemented a pilot and feasibility study of CGM use in children with type 1 diabetes less than 4 years old. This study is ongoing with 28 patients enrolled and is due for completion in early 2011.

- Developed and implemented a protocol designed to assess the relationship of beta cell reserve and glucagon (and epinephrine) response to hypoglycemia in children and adolescents with recent-onset (less than 1 year) type 1 diabetes. Mixed meal tolerance tests and hypoglycemic clamp tests have been performed in 20 patients.

- Developed and implemented a randomized trial, in collaboration with Type 1 Diabetes TrialNet, evaluating whether intensive glycemic control from the time of diagnosis of type 1 diabetes with initial closed loop therapy followed by pump-CGM therapy can preserve islet cell function.

- Developed a protocol to assess the relationship between hypoglycemia and brain structure and function using state-of-the-art magnetic resonance imaging technology and neurocognitive testing in young children with type 1 diabetes. Recruitment for this study will start in summer 2010.

- Developed a pilot protocol to inform the design of a clinical trial to develop and evaluate algorithms to minimize hypoglycemia during and after exercise in active adolescents with type 1 diabetes.

Anticipated Outcomes

In the absence of a functioning endocrine pancreas, people with diabetes are unable to respond to changes in blood glucose levels with insulin release. Over the past 80 years, improvements in technology have allowed patients to measure glucose levels and calculate the amount and variant of insulin to inject. These technological advances have saved many lives, but are far from perfect. The static measurement of glucose levels does not account for changes in diet or activity; there is a lag time between injecting insulin and its effect on the body; and too much injected insulin or inappropriately timed insulin action can lead to dangerous hypoglycemic episodes. The fear and danger of hypoglycemic episodes impede patients from achieving optimal control of blood glucose levels despite definitive evidence from the Diabetes Control and Complications Trial and the Epidemiology of Diabetes Interventions and Complications study that rigorous control can prevent diabetes complications. To address these issues, DirecNet has been testing the next generation of technologies: sensors that continuously monitor glucose levels and sound an alarm if levels cross certain thresholds; measurements that are sensitive to the rate of glucose change, not just the absolute amount of glucose; and insulin pumps that control insulin delivery under the skin. The ultimate goal of the network is to "close the loop" between automatic glucose level measurements and appropriate insulin delivery responses. The ideal artificial pancreas would relieve the patient of the burden of constantly testing glucose levels and adjusting insulin doses and dietary intake. The role of DirecNet is to determine if the new technologies are safe and effective, particularly for use in children.

DirecNet is a prime example of the interface between industry, academia, health care, and government-sponsored research. DirecNet has carried out independent and scientifically rigorous studies to determine the true benefit of new monitoring technologies. Without the commitment of DirecNet to perform these studies, it could have been many years before the manufacturers of these devices were willing to conduct studies in the pediatric population. The DirecNet group is well positioned to assess new devices for their accuracy, as well as their clinical usefulness in the home environment.

Ongoing Evaluation

The overall decision making body of DirecNet is the Steering Committee (SC) which consists of the principal investigator, one co-investigator, and one coordinator from each clinical center; representatives of the Coordinating Center; and representatives from NICHD and NIDDK. For each protocol being considered, a Protocol Development Group is formed. This group develops a concept document outlining the planned protocol for discussion and approval by the SC and then the Protocol Review Committee, an NIH-appointed, external review committee. Once the Protocol Review Committee approves the concept document, the Protocol Development Group develops a complete protocol which requires approval by the SC, the Protocol Review Committee, and the Data Safety and Monitoring Board (DSMB).

The DirecNet DSMB is an independent group of experts who meet at least 2 times each year or more frequently if needed to review clinical research protocols in the Network. The primary responsibilities of the DSMB are to: (1) periodically review and evaluate the accumulated study data for participant safety, study conduct and progress, and, when appropriate, efficacy; and (2) make recommendations to the SC concerning the continuation, modification, or termination of the trial. The DSMB considers study-specific data, as well as relevant background knowledge about the disease, technology, or patient population under study. Open session meetings involve DSMB members as well as DirecNet investigators who are chairpersons for specific protocols, the DirecNet SC Chair, Coordinating Center staff, and NIH representatives. The open sessions are followed by closed sessions involving only DSMB members and NIH representatives.

In addition, DirecNet has been evaluated by external panels of scientific and lay experts at *ad hoc* evaluation meetings convened by NIH in January 2005 and April 2008. These meetings were an opportunity for external experts to evaluate progress and provide input on future research directions (for more information, see the Executive Summary and Appendix B). Through *ad hoc* evaluation meetings and other meetings described above, NICHD continually seeks external input to inform current and future directions for DirecNet.

Program Enhancements

Because of the evolving nature of science, consortia supported by the *Special Diabetes Program* have evolved over time and have undergone enhancements to take advantage of new technologies and research findings, and to accelerate progress. Some enhancements have been made in response to external input and others have been initiated by the consortium members. Examples of program enhancements for DirecNet include:

- In order to continually advance progress, DirecNet worked to maintain a steady stream of protocols in the development phase while one or more studies were being implemented. This allowed new studies to be implemented rapidly once resources were available.

- The scope of DirecNet was broadened in 2007 by soliciting competitive proposals in response to a new Request for Applications (RFA). In addition, NIH convened a panel of scientists with hypoglycemia expertise to obtain input on the 2007 research solicitation and to encourage the participation of such experts.

- As DirecNet adds neuroscience and neuroimaging measures to studies of hypoglycemia, NIDDK and NICHD sought the participation of NINDS to further assist in the effort.

Coordination with Other Research Efforts

The DirecNet coordinates its efforts with other type 1 diabetes research consortia and networks supported by the *Special Diabetes Program*. Collaboration, coordination, and resource sharing serve to synergize research efforts and accelerate research progress. Examples of coordination with other consortia are given below. For a summary of ongoing collaborative efforts, please see Appendix D.

Coordinating Research Studies:

- Coordination with TrialNet on Effect of Metabolic Control at Onset of Diabetes on Progression of Type 1 Diabetes Trial: This trial is testing the impact of intensive metabolic control from the onset of diabetes on the preservation of beta cell function. The therapy consists of a short inpatient course of sub-cutaneous closed-loop diabetic control at the onset of diabetes followed by real-time continuous glucose monitoring associated with continuous subcutaneous insulin infusion.

DirecNet Administrative History	
Date Initiative Started	2001
Date *Special Diabetes Program* Funding Started	2001
Participating Components	NICHD, NIDDK
Web site	http://public.direc.net
DirecNet consists of a Coordinating Center, five pediatric diabetes centers, and a central laboratory.	

Goal V: Prevent or Reduce the Complications of Type 1 Diabetes

EPIDEMIOLOGY OF DIABETES INTERVENTIONS AND COMPLICATIONS (EDIC)

The aim of EDIC is to study the clinical course and risk factors associated with the long-term complications of type 1 diabetes, using the cohort of 1,441 patients who participated in the landmark Diabetes Control and Complications Trial (DCCT). Completed in 1993, the DCCT revolutionized diabetes management by demonstrating the benefit of intensively controlling blood glucose levels with frequent monitoring and insulin injection for preventing or delaying the early complications of the disease. Both the "conventional" and "intensive" treatment groups from DCCT are being followed observationally, but all participants are now recommended to follow the intensive therapy guidelines. DCCT/EDIC is a prospective study: one of its major strengths is the well-studied cohort of patients in which disease progression has been followed for over 25 years before most complications developed. The *Special Diabetes Program*'s support has been pivotal to the success of EDIC. Major findings highlighted below derive from studies to measure the onset and progression of cardiovascular disease (CVD), diseases of the urinary tract (uropathy), and diseases of the nerves that communicate with the internal organs such as the bladder, bowel, and sexual organs (autonomic neuropathy) and with the hands and feet (peripheral neuropathy). A separate genetics component is described in the section entitled "Genetics of Diabetic Complications."

HIGHLIGHTS OF PROGRESS

- Results show that after 30 years of diabetes, DCCT participants randomly assigned to intensive glucose control had lower rates of eye damage, kidney damage, and cardiovascular events than the conventional group. The phenomenon of long-lasting effects of a period of intensive or nonintensive glucose control has been termed "metabolic memory," and suggests that implementing intensive glucose control as early in the course of diabetes as possible could help people avoid life-threatening complications.

- Metabolic memory may wane over time, based on reduction in risk of retinopathy in participants assigned to intensive glucose control.

- Results show that intensive control of blood glucose levels cut the number of CVD events (heart attacks, strokes, or death) in half relative to the control group in the DCCT. This is the first demonstration of the long-term beneficial effects of intensive diabetes therapy on macrovascular complications in type 1 diabetes patients.

- Evaluation of DCCT patients 12 years after the conclusion of the study, using the same neuropsychological tests administered during the DCCT trial, revealed no link between multiple severe hypoglycemic reactions and impaired cognitive function in people with type 1 diabetes in the study. This result means that people with type 1 diabetes do not have to worry that acute episodes of hypoglycemia will damage their mental abilities and impair their long-term abilities to perceive, reason, and remember.

- Results of carotid ultrasonography show significant thickening in arteries of EDIC diabetes patients relative to non-diabetic controls and significantly less progression in the DCCT intensively treated group compared to the conventionally-treated group.

- Results also show that the DCCT intensively treated group has reduced coronary calcification (a subclinical progression of CVD).

- Occurrence of cardiac autonomic neuropathy was significantly lower in the former DCCT intensively treated EDIC cohort compared to the conventionally treated.

- Prevalence of urinary incontinence (urge and stress incontinence) was found to be significantly higher in women in the EDIC cohort than in women in the general U.S. population. Urinary tract infections, however, were not more prevalent in EDIC women, compared to the general population.

- Sexual dysfunction in both men and women in the EDIC cohort were common.

- DDCT/EDIC data and biosamples have been made available to the scientific community through multiple means, including the NIDDK Central Repositories.

Anticipated Outcomes

The dramatic results of the DCCT/EDIC demonstrate the benefits of a long-term prospective study. The DCCT proved conclusively that intensive diabetes therapy reduces the risk and progression of eye disease (retinopathy) by 47 to 76 percent, of kidney damage (nephropathy) by 39 to 54 percent, and of nerve damage (neuropathy) by 60 percent. The EDIC study continues to follow participants in the DCCT study to determine the long-term benefit of intensive blood glucose control and recently reported additional striking results. After 30 years of diabetes, DCCT participants randomly assigned to intensive glucose control had about half the rate of eye damage compared to those assigned to conventional glucose control (21 percent versus 50 percent). They also had lower rates of kidney damage (9 percent versus 25 percent) and cardiovascular events (9 percent versus 14 percent) compared to those receiving conventional glucose control.

Only in the long-term follow-up EDIC study (average 17 years of follow-up) have the benefits for CVD become apparent as well: intensive diabetes therapy reduces non-fatal CVD events by 57 percent. Heart disease is a chronic condition, developing over decades. It is difficult to prospectively study a population continuously from a young age before the onset of symptoms through CVD events, such as heart attacks and strokes. Yet as shown in EDIC, therapy early in the course of disease has profound consequences decades later. Because pharmaceutical companies and the biotechnology industry have a limited willingness to develop products that require years of testing before their clinical effects can be realized, it is therefore important to develop and validate subclinical biomarkers that the U.S. Food and Drug Administration (FDA) will accept as a basis for approval of new drugs for diabetes complications. For example, the DCCT demonstrated that the level of hemoglobin A1c (HbA1c)—a modified form of hemoglobin that circulates in the blood and correlates to the average blood glucose levels over a 3-month period—can be used as a surrogate endpoint for therapies that seek to reduce complications of diabetes. This test has subsequently become an important outcome measure for future clinical trials of both type 1 and type 2 diabetes. The use of HbA1c as an outcome measure was the basis for FDA approval of improved forms of insulin, as well as many other new drugs for type 2 diabetes.

Comprehensive and meticulous data collection in the DCCT/EDIC cohort for more than 25 years, with participation rates of about 95 percent, has created an unparalleled resource of individuals with type 1 diabetes that is ideal for future study of the clinical course of diabetes and its complications and for the validation of surrogate endpoints that can facilitate future drug development. These include assessment of subclinical markers such as testing new imaging techniques to measure the clogging, narrowing, and hardening of major arteries (atherosclerosis), heart muscle function, and other signs of CVD. EDIC has pioneered the use of new noninvasive diagnostic tools such as using ultrasound to measure the thickness of the carotid artery, or use of a "heart scan" (electron beam computed tomography) and multi-detector scanning to determine the extent of coronary calcification, and most recently using cardiac magnetic resonance imaging (MRI) to assess the structure and function of the heart allowing detection of silent heart attacks and congestive heart failure. By validating new analytical tools for early detection of CVD complications before events occur, the results of EDIC are paving the way for future trials that are smaller, shorter in duration, and less expensive to conduct.

Longitudinal assessment of the cohort allows analysis of the rate-of-change of complications over time, including the interactions among complications and co-occurrence of complications, as well as further evaluation of the longer-term effects of original DCCT interventions on advanced complications. This study is also leading to an examination of the longevity of the metabolic memory phenomenon and whether it applies to all diabetic complications, as was mentioned earlier with the waning of metabolic memory found with retinopathy. Important insights will be gained regarding the disease-causing mechanisms that underlie the development and progression of diabetic complications.

Ongoing Evaluation

To ensure ongoing evaluation of the study design and progress of the EDIC, NIDDK has established an External Evaluation Committee (EEC). The EEC is composed of investigators with scientific expertise relevant to research conducted by the EDIC, but who are not members of the Consortium. The EEC meets annually to:

- Review activities that affect the operational and methodological aspects of the study (e.g., quality control procedures and performance of clinical centers, data and clinical coordinating centers, central laboratories, and reading centers);

- Review data to ensure its quality, provide input on procedures for analysis and data display, and provide input on interpretation and implications of results; and

- Review proposed major modifications to the protocol or operations of the study for appropriateness, necessity, and impact on overall study objectives.

In addition, *ad hoc* groups have been assembled to review new initiatives being proposed in EDIC and to review progress once initiatives have been implemented. Examples of these groups have included an *ad hoc* group for genetics studies, review groups for proposals to obtain EDIC nonrenewable biologic samples, and groups recommending specific measures to be obtained for assessing CVD and autonomic and peripheral neuropathy.

Finally, EDIC has been evaluated by an external panel of scientific and lay experts at an *ad hoc* evaluation meeting convened by NIDDK in January 2005. This meeting was an opportunity for external experts to evaluate progress and provide input on future research directions (for more information, see the Executive Summary and Appendix B). Through *ad hoc* evaluation meetings and regular meetings of the EEC, NIDDK continually seeks external input to inform current and future directions for the EDIC.

Program Enhancements

Because of the evolving nature of science, consortia supported by the *Special Diabetes Program* have evolved over time and have undergone enhancements to take advantage of new technologies and research findings, and to accelerate progress. Some enhancements have been made in response to external input and others have been initiated by the consortium members. Examples of program enhancements for EDIC include:

- To capitalize on the long-term investment in resources in this select cohort of patients and because this cohort provided a good opportunity to examine subclinical CVD markers (e.g., carotid intima-medial thickness, coronary calcification, myocardial function), EDIC developed additional cardiovascular studies. A total of three

measurements of carotid intima-medial thickness have been taken so that changes in atherosclerosis can be measured over time. The cohort is currently undergoing a cardiac MRI procedure to assess the structure and function of the heart, allowing detection of silent heart attacks and congestive heart failure.

Coordination with Other Research Efforts

EDIC coordinates its efforts with multiple other type 1 diabetes research consortia and networks supported by the *Special Diabetes Program*. Collaboration, coordination, and resource sharing serve to synergize research efforts and accelerate research progress. Examples of coordination with other consortia are given below. For a summary of ongoing collaborative efforts, please see Appendix D.

Enhancing Data Comparison Among Studies:

- The National Glycohemoglobin Standardization Program certifies clinical laboratories to use the standard set by DCCT/EDIC for measurements of HbA1c. Nearly all commercial laboratories providing this clinical test in the United States are now certified though this program supported by the *Special Diabetes Program*. This has allowed the National Diabetes Education Program to promulgate a nationwide public health campaign to achieve targeted HbA1c values based on the DCCT/EDIC and led the American Diabetes Association to recently recommend HbA1c as a more convenient approach to diagnose type 2 diabetes.

EDIC Administrative History

Date Initiative Started	1994
Date *Special Diabetes Program* Funding Started	1998
Participating Component	NIDDK
Web site	http://www2.bsc.gwu.edu/bsc/oneproj.php?pkey=10

EDIC is a long-term follow-up study to the DCCT of 1,441 patients with type 1 diabetes conducted between 1983 and 1993.

Animal Models of Diabetic Complications Consortium (AMDCC)

The AMDCC is an interdisciplinary Consortium designed to develop animal models that closely mimic the human complications of diabetes for the purpose of studying disease pathogenesis, prevention, and treatment. In addition to creating animal models, the goals of the AMDCC include defining standards to validate each diabetic complication for its similarity to the human disease, testing the role of candidate genes or chromosomal regions that emerge from genetic studies of human diabetic complications, and facilitating the sharing of animals, reagents, and expertise between members of the Consortium and the greater scientific community via its bioinformatics and data coordinating center. In its second funding cycle, the AMDCC formed a close partnership with the Type 1 Diabetes Mouse Resource (T1DR, described earlier in this Appendix) and the Mouse Metabolic Phenotyping Centers (MMPCs).

HIGHLIGHTS OF PROGRESS

- Generated about 40 animal models of type 1 diabetes that closely mimic various aspects of the human complications of diabetes.

- Published over 180 scientific publications in highly respected peer-reviewed journals.

- Published about 60 laboratory protocols on the AMDCC public Web site (www.amdcc.org) for use by the research community.

Anticipated Outcomes

Animal models are an important scientific resource because they enable researchers to investigate underlying disease processes that cannot be studied in humans. For example, the demonstration of the key role of immune cells in the destruction of beta cells in type 1 diabetes would not have been possible without animal models. These models also permit assessment of novel therapeutic interventions before they are tested in people. The creation of the non-obese diabetic (NOD) mouse provided investigators with a critical tool for pre-clinical testing of new drugs for type 1 diabetes. Just like people with type 1 diabetes, the NOD mouse has genetic susceptibility due to molecules regulating the immune response; the disease is influenced by environmental encounters; the animal produces autoantibodies against beta cell proteins; and the white blood cells infiltrate the pancreatic islets. In the animal model, beta cell destruction can be attenuated through application of agents capable of influencing the immune response. Following this successful approach, the AMDCC is creating better animal models of diabetes complications. Because the Consortium has invested in infrastructure to share its resources with the larger scientific community, the impact of its efforts on drug discovery is enormous. Animal models also provide an opportunity to identify surrogate markers for diabetic complications. Diagnosing intermediate stages of disease progression is a major challenge inhibiting clinical translation because disease progression is long-term. With about 40 new animal models and 180 peer-reviewed scientific publications, the AMDCC has played a critical role in propelling research progress by developing, validating, and distributing animal models with greater fidelity to human type 1 diabetes and its complications.

Ongoing Evaluation

The AMDCC is jointly managed by NIDDK and NHLBI, with input from NINDS, NEI, and JDRF staff. NIH staff and AMDCC investigators participate in monthly conference calls to discuss business and science. An External Evaluation Committee (EEC) meets with the AMDCC investigators annually. This meeting usually lasts 2 days and includes an open session where the investigators present their work and a closed session where NIH staff and the EEC evaluate progress and discuss future directions. The EEC prepares a written report of their deliberations, to which the investigators must respond in writing. AMDCC investigators also prepare an annual progress report. This document provides a written summary of yearly progress, an appraisal of the interactions between the ongoing projects at each site, and a description of the existing and planned collaborations with other members of the Consortium. All annual progress reports are available to the public at www.amdcc.org. A representative from the JDRF often participates in the monthly conference calls and always participates in AMDCC face-to-face meetings.

In addition, AMDCC has been evaluated by external panels of scientific and lay experts at *ad hoc* evaluation meetings convened by NIDDK in January 2005 and June 2009. These meetings were an opportunity for external experts to evaluate progress and provide input on future research directions (for more information, see the Executive Summary and Appendix B). Through *ad hoc* evaluation meetings and regular meetings of the EEC, NIDDK continually seeks external input to inform current and future directions for the AMDCC.

Program Enhancements

Because of the evolving nature of science, consortia supported by the *Special Diabetes Program* have evolved over time and have undergone enhancements to take advantage of new technologies and research findings, and to accelerate progress. Some enhancements have been made in response to external input and others have been initiated by the consortium members. Examples of program enhancements for AMDCC include:

- In its second funding cycle, the AMDCC formed a close partnership with the T1DR and the MMPCs to ensure that all interesting models are screened across multiple complications.

- Recognizing the need to bolster research efforts for both diabetic retinopathy and neuropathy, the AMDCC worked closely with the MMPCs to organize a workshop entitled "Advances Toward Measuring Diabetic Retinopathy and Neuropathy" in April 2007. The meeting provided a forum for identifying needs and research opportunities for the AMDCC and MMPC Pilot & Feasibility (P&F) programs. Two P&F awardees targeted by this workshop presented their exciting work at the AMDCC meeting in June 2008: one discussed a novel technique for measuring intraretinal ion activity and retinal thickness in diabetic mice using manganese-enhanced magnetic resonance imaging and another presented data on the use of "hyperspectral" imaging for diabetic peripheral neuropathy and wound healing.

- The AMDCC has been working with the broader neuropathy community to enhance pre-clinical studies. The AMDCC and JDRF supported a planning meeting in late 2007 to set the agenda for a 2-day meeting in 2008 entitled "Consensus meeting on experimental models of diabetic neuropathy" to establish a definition of diabetic neuropathy in experimental rodent models. A distinguished group of basic and clinical researchers from around the world produced a definition including assessments of functional, sensory, behavioral, and anatomical measures.

Coordination with Other Research Efforts

The AMDCC coordinates its efforts with other type 1 diabetes research consortia and networks supported by the *Special Diabetes Program*. Collaboration, coordination, and resource sharing serve to synergize research efforts and accelerate research progress. Examples of coordination with other consortia are given below. For a summary of ongoing collaborative efforts, please see Appendix D.

Synergism with Consortia Studying Animal Models:

- The AMDCC collaborates with the T1DR to enhance model development and phenotype characterization under controlled husbandry conditions. One example of this collaborative partnership is an ongoing investigation to examine the significant variation seen in the susceptibility of inbred mouse strains to the development of diabetic nephropathy. Consortial studies have characterized the differential responses of mouse strains to the development of hyperglycemia. They have also delineated mouse strains that are most and least susceptible to development of albuminuria and renal histopathologic changes in response to diabetes. These findings have been widely disseminated in the research community and have had a profound and fundamental impact on the design of studies of experimental diabetic nephropathy.

- The AMDCC also supports the MMPCs to enhance phenotyping of mouse models of diabetic complications. The MMPCs are charged with providing the scientific community with standardized, high-quality metabolic and physiologic phenotyping services for the mouse. The MMPCs provide state-of-the-art technologies to investigators for a fee, and with AMDCC support, the MMPCs have expanded their services to include a wide range of tests for diabetic nephropathy, retinopathy, and cardiovascular disease. The MMPCs also support a P&F program to develop new technologies for phenotyping animal models, and with the input of the AMDCC have provided focused solicitations in the areas of diabetic complications.

- The AMDCC has partnered with the Type 1 Diabetes-Rapid Access to Intervention Development (T1D-RAID) project, in which the T1D-RAID contractor acts as a histology and phenotyping resource for diabetic neuropathy. Tissue specimens received from The Jackson Laboratories as part of ongoing AMDCC projects are processed to blocks, analyzed, and stored. Stored tissues are available to all interested members of the research community.

AMDCC Administrative History

Date Initiative Started	2001
Date *Special Diabetes Program* Funding Started	2001
Participating Components	NIDDK, NHLBI, NINDS, NEI, and JDRF
Web site	www.amdcc.org

The AMDCC is comprised of thirteen "pathobiology sites" that study complications such as diabetic nephropathy, uropathy, neuropathy, cardiomyopathy, and vascular disease. The Consortium also supports and has formed a close partnership with the T1DR and the MMPCs. All data and resources from the consortium and its partners are freely available through a joint AMDCC-MMPC Coordinating and Bioinformatics Unit.

Genetics of Diabetes Complications

The following three consortia were grouped because they all address genetic factors that predispose people with diabetes to, or protect them from, developing complications in various organs. Each has unique attributes that make it highly valuable for genetic studies: the Epidemiology of Diabetes Interventions and Complications' strength is the careful characterization of the cohort over 25 years of follow-up; the Family Investigation of Nephropathy and Diabetes has a very large collection of families in which two or more siblings have diabetes; and the Genetics of Kidneys in Diabetes Study matches people with type 1 diabetes, with and without kidney complications, and collects information from their parents.

Epidemiology of Diabetes Interventions and Complications (EDIC)

The aim of EDIC is to study the clinical course and risk factors associated with the long-term complications of type 1 diabetes, using the cohort of 1,441 patients who participated in the landmark Diabetes Control and Complications Trial (DCCT), which showed that intensive glucose control can prevent or delay microvascular (eye, kidney, and nerve) disease complications. To capitalize on the long-term investment in the select EDIC cohort, the *Special Diabetes Program* supports a study on the genetics underlying diabetes complications in these patients. The study is analyzing expanded data regarding the progression of complications in EDIC participants and their affected and non-affected family members to identify DNA sequence differences that influence susceptibility to diabetic complications.

Family Investigation of Nephropathy and Diabetes (FIND)

The FIND Consortium is carrying out studies to elucidate the genetic susceptibility to kidney disease (nephropathy) in people, especially those with diabetes, as well as genetic susceptibility to eye disease (retinopathy) in people with diabetes. Five to ten percent of the people in FIND have type 1 diabetes. FIND is primarily supported by regularly appropriated NIH funds; however, support from the *Special Diabetes Program* permitted expansion of FIND by initiation of a study of the genetic determinants of diabetic retinopathy in persons enrolled in the FIND family study. This component of the study seeks to identify genes that may influence the development and severity of diabetic eye disease. FIND has also created a resource of genetic samples and data for use by investigators outside the FIND study group, for ancillary or follow-up studies. FIND represents the first large-scale study of the genetic determinants of retinopathy.

Genetics of Kidneys in Diabetes Study (GoKinD)

People with type 1 diabetes have a high risk of developing kidney disease. The fundamental aim of GoKinD was to facilitate investigator-driven research into the genetic basis of diabetic nephropathy by creating a resource of genetic samples from people who have both type 1 diabetes and renal disease, and "control" patients who have type 1 diabetes but no renal disease. With this design, the genes that confer risk for renal disease can be distinguished from those that are primarily risk factors for type 1 diabetes. The GoKinD study was concluded in 2007. Any researcher can apply for access to this collection of samples and data to investigate the role of specific genes.

HIGHLIGHTS OF PROGRESS

- Genome-wide association studies (GWAS) examine genetic variation across the entire human genome to try and identify genetic differences that are associated with a particular disease. GWAS have been completed for cohorts of patients with type 1 diabetes in the GoKinD Study and the EDIC Study. The data are being shared through the NIH's Database of Genotypes and Phenotypes (dbGAP). In 2009, samples from the FIND study were tested using GWAS; analysis of these data is ongoing. The resulting data from DCCT/EDIC and GoKinD have been used by numerous investigators in various genetic analyses to identify genetic regions associated with a disease, to replicate promising findings from other studies, or to refine analytic methods. Some of these studies are highlighted below.

- Using GWAS data from the DCCT/EDIC cohort, researchers identified a gene region, which is near the *SORCS1* gene, associated with hemoglobin A1c (HbA1c) levels. Other genetic regions were also found to be associated with HbA1c levels, and some of the regions were also associated with low blood glucose levels and eye complications of diabetes. The association with the *SORCS1* gene region was replicated in the GoKinD study control group.

- The GoKinD GWAS data was used to identify two genes/genetic regions associated with diabetic nephropathy: *FRMD3* and *CARS*. The results from the genotyping were confirmed by comparison to the GWAS data from the DCCT/EDIC study.

- Using GWAS data from the GoKinD collection, scientists determined that *ELMO1* is associated with diabetic nephropathy, thereby further establishing the gene's role in the susceptibility of this disease.

- Studying three European-American cohorts, including GoKinD participants, researchers identified a gene associated with risk of kidney and eye complications of diabetes. They compared 11 genes in people with type 2 diabetes who either had or did not have proliferative diabetic retinopathy (PDR; a serious form of diabetic eye disease) and end-stage renal disease (ESRD). The researchers found that variation in a region of DNA near the erythropoietin gene was associated with PDR and ESRD. They also analyzed genes of people with type 1 diabetes and found the same result, suggesting even more strongly a link between this genetic variation and diabetic eye and kidney disease in people of European American ancestry.

- *HLA DRB1*04* alleles have been associated with protection from some of the injurious hyperglycemic effects related to diabetic nephropathy in the GoKinD study population.

- A region upstream of the *PLEKHH2* gene on chromosome 2p21 that is exclusively expressed in the glomerulus has been associated with diabetic nephropathy by transmission to trio probands, and as a risk factor for diabetic nephropathy in the independent case/control population of the GoKinD study. This region was found by a GWAS of *human leukocyte antigen*-matched GoKinD case and control samples that minimized the problem of population stratification.

- FIND investigators studied 2,368 people with diabetes from 767 families enrolled in the FIND-Eye study. They determined that the overall prevalence of diabetic retinopathy was high: 33.4 percent had proliferative diabetic retinopathy; 7.5, 22.8, and 9.5 percent had severe, moderate, and mild nonproliferative diabetic retinopathy, respectively; 26.6 percent had no diabetic retinopathy. They also found that the severity of diabetic retinopathy was significantly associated with severity of diabetic kidney disease.

- Using genome-wide scans of samples collected from over 1,200 people with diabetes-related kidney disease and their relatives, FIND researchers identified four regions on chromosomes 7, 10, 14, and 18 where subtle variations correlated with an increased risk of diabetic kidney disease. Similar scans identified three regions on chromosomes 2 and 15 and a different part of chromosome 7 associated with elevated protein in the urine. The strength of the linkages varied with the ethnic background of participants. These findings confirm earlier studies implicating regions of chromosomes 7, 10, and 18 in increased risk of diabetic kidney disease, and identify a new region of interest on chromosome 14.

Anticipated Outcomes

Through these research efforts, many new insights into the genetic underpinnings of diabetes complications have emerged. With more complete knowledge of the genetic factors that contribute to different complications, the patient's doctor may be able to personalize therapy and intervene early to prevent or delay specific complications. For example, a patient genetically predisposed to diabetic nephropathy could employ clinical strategies such as carefully controlling blood pressure and taking angiotensin-converting enzyme (ACE) inhibitors or angiotensin receptor blockers, which lower protein in the urine and are thought to directly prevent injury to the kidney's blood vessels. In another example, understanding the genetic factors that contribute to patients' control of HbA1c levels may provide insights as to why people on similar treatment regimens have different HbA1c values and inform personalized therapies to achieve similar levels.

Although these genetic findings are extremely exciting in and of themselves, they represent just the beginning of new knowledge that is expected to emerge as research is setting the stage for even more scientific breakthroughs. For example, a newly associated gene may produce a protein that interacts with numerous other proteins. Therefore, discovering the disease association not only implicates that protein in the disease, but also the proteins with which it interacts. This knowledge could illuminate several new therapeutic targets for disease prevention or treatment. Studying genes that were not thought to be involved in a disease can lead to brand new avenues for research that would likely not have been pursued otherwise. Identifying the functions of genes may not only enhance understanding of molecular mechanisms that underlie disease, but may also reveal new targets for therapy.

In addition to the genes and genetic associations with diabetes complications that have been discovered and are still emerging from EDIC, FIND, and GoKinD, each of these consortia also serves as a resource for ongoing and future efforts: tissue, genetic samples, data, and analytic methods from each study are stored in a repository or database. The large and diverse sample and data collections—with families, cases, and controls—

are a widely-used resource for genetic studies of susceptibility to diabetic complications. The availability of immortalized cell lines for each participant provides a renewable source of DNA, allowing investigators to explore novel hypotheses or analytical approaches.

Ongoing Evaluation

To ensure ongoing evaluation of the study design and the progress of FIND and EDIC, NIH has established External Evaluation Committees (EEC). Each EEC is composed of investigators with scientific expertise relevant to research conducted by the Consortium, but who are not members of the Consortium. Please see a description of the EDIC EEC in the EDIC section of this Appendix. The FIND EEC meets periodically to review the progress of the study. The experts comment specifically on activities that affect the operational and methodological aspects of the study (*e.g.*, quality control procedures and performance of clinical centers, data and clinical coordinating centers, and central laboratories and reading centers), review data to ensure its quality, provide input on procedures for analysis, and review proposed significant modifications to the protocol or operations of the study for appropriateness, necessity, and impact on overall study objectives. The GoKinD Executive Committee oversaw the day-to-day operation of the study and consisted of representatives from academia, government, and voluntary organizations. An external Steering Committee consisting of scientific and lay reviewers met once a year to review the study and make recommendations. The GoKinD study was concluded in 2007.

In addition, these programs were evaluated by an external panel of scientific and lay experts at an *ad hoc* evaluation meeting convened by NIDDK in January 2005. This meeting was an opportunity for external experts to evaluate progress and provide input on future research directions (for more information, see the Executive Summary and Appendix B). Through *ad hoc* evaluation meetings and regular meetings of the EECs, NIDDK and CDC continually seek external input to inform current and future directions for these research programs.

Program Enhancements

Because of the evolving nature of science, consortia supported by the *Special Diabetes Program* have evolved over time and have undergone enhancements to take advantage of new technologies and research findings, and to accelerate progress. Some enhancements have been made in response to external input and others have been initiated by the consortium members. Examples of program enhancements for FIND, GoKinD, and EDIC include:

- Since the inception of these research programs, new and emerging genetics technologies have become available. The FIND and GoKinD studies were designed and launched at a time when genetic analyses focused on sibling pairs and only low resolution methods were available for gene hunting. Over time, the two consortia responded to the emergence of novel methodologies by changing their genotyping strategies to use GWAS. The robust design of each consortium's recruitment allowed them this flexibility: both relatives and unrelated individuals were recruited in enough numbers to permit the older and newer analytic methods to be used. The EDIC study also changed its strategies from examining familial clustering of diabetic complications (in siblings and parents of EDIC probands), to examining candidate genes, to using GWAS in conjunction with FIND and GoKinD.

- Resources for sharing samples and data have also changed these projects significantly. The NIDDK

Central Repositories, created in 2001, facilitate rapid and efficient sharing of samples and data. In addition, the NIH's dbGAP database and associated mandated GWAS data sharing policies ensure maximum rapid access to GWAS data. These two changes, external to the consortia, made some of the organizational and administrative functions of the consortia redundant, and they were reduced accordingly.

Coordination with Other Research Efforts

The consortia studying the genetics of complications coordinate their efforts with each other and with multiple other type 1 diabetes research consortia and networks supported by the *Special Diabetes Program.* Collaboration, coordination, and resource sharing serve to synergize research efforts and accelerate research progress. Examples of coordination with other consortia are given below. For a summary of ongoing collaborative efforts, please see Appendix D.

Coordinating Studies of Genetics in Type 1 Diabetes:

- EDIC, FIND, and GoKinD participated in a coordination meeting with the T1DGC.

- Key personnel from the FIND study served in official advisory capacities for GoKinD.

Developing Interoperable Databases for Data Sharing:

- A series of database coordination meetings between FIND, EDIC, and GoKinD helped standardize vocabularies, allowing investigators to search data across databases.

- The NIDDK is supporting the development of tools at the NIDDK Central Repositories to allow searching across the stored data from major clinical studies, which include EDIC, GoKinD, and FIND.

- The uniformity of GWAS data allows results from EDIC, GoKinD, and FIND to be housed in a single location (dbGAP), and still be accessed by investigators through the NIDDK Central Repositories. dbGAP works cooperatively with the NIDDK Central Repositories to provide easy, interoperable access to all three datasets.

EDIC Administrative History

Date Initiative Started	1994
Date *Special Diabetes Program* Funding Started	1998
Participating Components	NIDDK
Web site	http://www2.bsc.gwu.edu/bsc/oneproj.php?pkey=10

EDIC is a long-term follow-up study to the DCCT of 1,441 people with type 1 diabetes conducted between 1983 and 1993.

FIND Administrative History

Date Initiative Started	1999
Date *Special Diabetes Program* Funding Started	2001
Participating Components	NIDDK, NEI, NCMHD

Ten percent of the people in the FIND family study have type 1 diabetes. Funds from the *Special Diabetes Program* permitted expansion of FIND to support ancillary studies searching for determinants of diabetic retinopathy.

GoKinD Administrative History

Date Initiative Started	1998
Date *Special Diabetes Program* Funding Started	1998
Participating Components	CDC, JDRF
Web site	www.jdrf.org/gokind
Concluded	2007

Saved DNA, blood plasma, blood serum, and urine samples as well as data are being stored in the NIDDK Central Repositories for use by any investigators in the diabetes research community based on a review process.

Diabetic Retinopathy Clinical Research Network (DRCR.net)

The DRCR.net is a collaborative, nationwide network of eye doctors and investigators conducting clinical research of diabetes-induced retinal disorders (diabetic retinopathy, diabetic macular edema, and associated conditions). The DRCR.net supports the identification, design, and implementation of multicenter clinical research while incorporating standardization of multiple study procedures, utilization of novel technology, extensive integration of information technology, and the ability to leverage its resources to bring promising new therapies to evaluation that might otherwise not exist. Principal emphasis is placed on clinical trials, including comparative effectiveness trials, but epidemiology, outcomes, and other research approaches may be supported as well. Diabetic retinopathy is a complication associated with both type 1 and type 2 diabetes; DRCR.net, which is funded in part by the *Special Diabetes Program*, enrolls both type 1 and type 2 diabetes patients. In soliciting site participants, involvement of community-based, as well as academic-oriented partners, has been encouraged.

HIGHLIGHTS OF PROGRESS

- Establishment of a nationwide network that currently includes 112 clinical sites, 1,165 personnel, and spans 36 states. Community-based clinical sites comprise 81 percent of the network, representing about one-third of the U.S. retina specialists; most major research institution-based programs are also involved.

- Rapid implementation of 15 protocols (both large and small) since inception, in response to basic research and applied technological developments in the field of diabetic retinopathy. Four protocols are currently recruiting and four additional protocols are in development.

- Landmark comparative effectiveness trial demonstrating that a new combination therapy of ocular injections of a U.S. Food and Drug Administration (FDA)-approved drug, ranibizumab (Lucentis®), and laser treatment was definitively superior to the standard practice of laser treatment alone. With the potential to slow progression, and in many cases, reverse vision impairment from diabetic retinopathy, this is the biggest advance in diabetic retinopathy in 25 years, since a previous NIH study established the standard laser therapy. Nearly 50 percent of patients who received the combination treatment experienced substantial visual improvement after 1 year, compared to 28 percent who received the standard laser treatment, while fewer than 5 percent experienced substantial visual loss with the combination treatment compared with almost 15 percent who received the standard laser treatment.

- Determined that focal/grid laser photocoagulation for diabetic macular edema can lead to substantial improvement of visual acuity far more often than was previously thought.

- Demonstrated that steroid injections into the eye, although effective in reducing diabetic macular edema, were not superior to focal/grid laser alone, and had considerable side effects.

- Compared the safety of a single panretinal laser treatment, versus multiple treatments, the standard course employed for over 30 years. If preliminary results indicating similar safety profiles are confirmed in a larger trial, they would have far-reaching implications for the cost and convenience of one of the most common treatments for diabetic retinopathy.

- Completed study measuring variability in retinal thickening throughout the day in patients with diabetic macular edema.

- Distributed electronic visual acuity testing devices to all sites. This FDA-approved test is faster to administer than the standard version, and results are easily incorporated into a database.

- Collaborated with industry on an innovative protocol to create a drug that would not otherwise be commercially pursued (preservative-free intraocular steroid).

- Compared new therapies across multiple industries. This effort included negotiations for clinical site funding costs with these industries, utilizing the Network's industry collaboration guidelines.

- Developed an online system for collecting, reviewing, maintaining, and publicly reporting financial relationships of investigators with industry.

- Publication of 24 manuscripts by various journals, with an additional six manuscripts accepted for publication, three currently under review, and 11 currently in development. DRCR.net investigators also gave 16 poster or platform presentations on behalf of the Network at national and international conferences in 2009 alone. The Network Web site provides free public access to these publications (http://drcrnet.jaeb.org/Publications.aspx).

Anticipated Outcomes

Diabetes (type 1 and type 2) is the leading cause of new blindness in people 20-74 years old, and diabetic retinopathy causes 12,000 to 24,000 new cases of blindness each year.[38] Laser photocoagulation is an effective technique that uses the heat of a laser beam to seal abnormal leaky blood vessels in the retina. While laser photocoagulation can prevent blindness, the technique itself can lead to impaired vision. Therefore, improved technologies are being developed and tested by DRCR.net. The network provides infrastructure for conducting multiple concurrent and consecutive studies, with the ability to rapidly develop and initiate new protocols. Already, DRCR.net has made several significant contributions to the treatment of diabetic retinopathy, including results of a landmark combination therapy trial (described above), which are already being implemented in clinical practice to slow progression and in some cases reverse the vision impairment from diabetic retinopathy.

One of the most important DRCR.net priorities is to have a portfolio of ongoing clinical trials that not only encompasses a broad diversity of promising new therapeutic approaches, but also addresses the full spectrum of patients with diabetic eye disease. The Network is actively pursuing identification and design of important clinical trials that complement each other in

---

[38] Centers for Disease Control and Prevention. National diabetes fact sheet: general information and national estimates on diabetes in the United States, 2007. Atlanta, GA: U.S. Department of Health and Human Services, Centers for Disease Control and Prevention, 2008. Accessed from www.cdc.gov/diabetes/pubs/factsheet07.htm

terms of patient eligibility and therapeutic approach. This approach prevents competition between studies for similar patients and expands the opportunities for patients to participate in these investigations. Ultimately, the goal is for any person with diabetes to be potentially eligible for a DRCR.net study protocol. As a large-scale multicenter network, DRCR.net has been successful at leveraging its resources to work with industry in developing therapies that might not have been otherwise pursued. Appreciation of the Network's benefits have prompted numerous inquiries from commercial entities regarding evaluation of new therapies by DRCR.net. These opportunities are being carefully considered to ensure that any such study would assess a need judged timely and critical by DRCR.net and would maintain rigorous scientific and ethical guidelines.

DRCR.net contributes to the training and knowledge of the ophthalmologic community with regard to rigorous clinical trials. This is one of the reasons for including a large number of community-based sites, offering them an opportunity to participate and become experienced in these efforts. Such expansion of quality clinical centers helps not only the Network, but patients throughout the country and the overall education of the ophthalmologic community.

Ongoing Evaluation

The DRCR.net Data and Safety Monitoring Committee (DSMC) has a dual role of external monitoring of the Network's protocols and providing input to NEI on the merits of the protocols proposed by the Network as well as the Network's progress. The Committee meets in person at least twice a year and by conference call as needed throughout the year. Furthermore, new protocols for large randomized trials are presented to an External Protocol Review Committee, which provides input to NEI on the merits of the concept behind the protocol.

The DRCR.net Executive Committee is involved in policy decisions and oversees the scientific direction of the Network. Executive Committee membership includes broad leadership across the Network including the current and past Network Chairs, the Director and Executive Director of the Coordinating Center, the current and past Principal Investigators of the Reading Center, three rotating clinical site investigators and one clinical site coordinator, as well as representation from the NEI. The Executive Committee has monthly conference calls and meetings in person at least twice per year.

The DRCR.net Operations Group is responsible for the day to day management and monitoring of the Network. The Group consists of the current and past Network Chairs, three Network Vice-Chairs, an NEI representative, and the Coordinating Center Principal Investigator and Executive Director. The Operations Group reviews preliminary protocol ideas and monitors clinical site performance including quality of enrollment, follow-up, adherence to protocol, and timeliness of response to data queries.

Additional committees have developed organizational structure policies: editorial policies, publicity and presentation policies, industry collaboration guidelines, financial disclosure and conflict of interest policies, competing studies policies, ancillary study policies, confidentiality policies, policies on maintenance of activity for a site or investigator, and DSMC standard operating procedures. Each committee enjoys broad representation from Network investigators.

In addition, DRCR.net has been evaluated by external panels of scientific and lay experts at *ad hoc* evaluation meetings convened by NIDDK in January 2005 and April 2008. These meetings were an opportunity for external experts to evaluate progress and provide input on future research directions (for more information, see the Executive Summary and Appendix B). Through *ad hoc* evaluation meetings and other meetings described above, NEI continually seeks external input to inform current and future directions for the DRCR.net.

Program Enhancements

Because of the evolving nature of science, consortia supported by the *Special Diabetes Program* have evolved over time and have undergone enhancements to take advantage of new technologies and research findings, and to accelerate progress. Some enhancements have been made in response to external input and others have been initiated by the consortium members. Examples of program enhancements for DRCR.net include:

- Major randomized clinical trial proposals are reviewed for scientific merit by the External Protocol Review Committee and the Network's DSMC. To expedite the review process, mechanisms have been implemented to provide for a 2-week turnaround time by the External Protocol Review Committee.

- Patient retention beyond 1 year had been a challenge for DRCR.net in the past. To address this issue, the Network emphasizes to investigators and coordinators how enrollment and retention are equally important to the success of the Network. Although, most protocols now have at least a 90 percent 1-year retention rate, the Network strives for higher rates.

Coordination with Other Research Efforts

The Network also provides funding for small projects judged critical to the development or implementation of its trials. For example, a phase 2 study on bevacizumab was conducted to provide preliminary evidence of anti-vascular endothelial growth factor (VEGF) effect in macular edema, prior to embarking on a large phase III study.

DRCR.net Administrative History	
Date Initiative Started	2002
Date *Special Diabetes Program* Funding Started	2002
Participating Sites (Offices)	134
Participating Physicians	469
Participating Components	NEI, JDRF, NIDDK
Web site	www.drcr.net

DRCR.net consists of two cooperative agreements including the Coordinating Center and the Operations Center; clinical site participation is open to all qualified investigators/clinicians whose sites have the requisite equipment to conduct a study protocol.

APPENDIX D

TYPE 1 DIABETES
CONSORTIA COORDINATION

This Appendix provides an overview of the numerous collaborative efforts among the type 1 diabetes research consortia and networks.

PROMOTING COORDINATION AMONG TYPE 1 DIABETES RESEARCH CONSORTIA AND NETWORKS

The research efforts supported by the *Special Statutory Funding Program for Type 1 Diabetes Research* span a wide range of scientific areas. However, many of the large-scale research efforts have elements in common. For example, several research consortia are studying the genetics of type 1 diabetes or of specific complications; multiple consortia are enrolling newborns in studies and following them to examine different environmental triggers; and clinical trials networks are testing different strategies to slow disease progression in newly diagnosed patients. Coordination helps to prevent duplicative work by promoting the sharing of resources and methodology as well as by facilitating cross-disciplinary research approaches. Furthermore, collaboration between researchers with distinct interests facilitates the pursuit of novel research directions.

Panels of external scientific and lay experts convened by NIH to provide input on progress and future directions have strongly encouraged NIH to capitalize on existing research efforts by maximizing connections among research groups with both related and distinct interests. The panels encouraged NIH to enhance strong existing coordination across consortia to synergize research efforts. Based on this input and in order to maximize research progress, NIH has facilitated and enhanced coordination among research consortia with both overlapping and distinct interests. The NIH has organized meetings to facilitate broad coordination efforts as well as focused meetings of consortia that share common interests. For example, research consortia studying newborns (TEDDY, TRIGR, TrialNet) have met to discuss opportunities for collaboration, and have also coordinated patient recruitment to ensure that they are not adversely competing for patient participants in their studies. This helps all studies achieve their goals in the most streamlined and cost-efficient manner. In another example, a research consortium studying continuous glucose monitoring in children (DirecNet) and a clinical trials network testing strategies for treating newly diagnosed patients (TrialNet) are collaborating on a clinical trial testing early intensive blood glucose control using a closed-loop system in new-onset patients. Thus, the strengths and expertise of both networks are being utilized to conduct this joint trial.

ENHANCING INFORMATION SHARING

To enhance information sharing, NIDDK, with input from external experts, spearheaded the development of Web sites for people with or at risk for type 1 diabetes and their family members (www.T1Diabetes.nih.gov/patient) and researchers (www.T1Diabetes.nih.gov/investigator). The Web site for patients describes clinical research studies recruiting patients and has contact information for the studies if patients are interested in enrolling. The Web site for investigators includes information on research consortia and clinical trial networks; research resources available to the broad scientific community; and information on research funding opportunities. These Web sites not only enhance patient recruitment efforts, but also provide researchers with access to information, data, and protocols generated by the type 1 diabetes research consortia, thereby facilitating resource sharing and coordination.

The NIDDK is also spearheading a new Web site to advertise the availability of biosamples and data from type 1 diabetes research consortia. Through consortia Web sites, the NIH Guide for Grants and Contracts, and other methods, NIH has already advertised the availability of samples and data. However, the new Web site will serve as a "one stop shop" for information on research resources that are currently available, as well as resources that are expected to be available in the future.

HIGHLIGHTS OF TYPE 1 DIABETES CONSORTIA COLLABORATION AND COORDINATION

A summary of interactions between research consortia is presented in Table D1. The "at a glance" matrix shows consortia that have ongoing or past collaborative activities. For a description of the collaborative activities, please see sections in each consortium's evaluation called "Coordination with Other Research Efforts" in Appendix C.

Table D1: "At a Glance" Matrix of Past and Ongoing Type 1 Diabetes Consortia Coordination Activities

Blue-shaded squares indicate collaboration between the consortia

	AMDCC	Prevention Centers	BCBC	CIT	CITR	DirecNet	EDIC	FIND	GoKinD	ITN	ICRs/IIDP	T1D Mouse Resource	NHPCSG	SEARCH	Standardization Programs	TEDDY	TRIGR	T1DGC	T1D-RAID	TrialNet
Animal Models of Diabetic Complications Consortium (AMDCC)	■						■	■	■										■	
Autoimmune Disease Prevention Centers		■									■									
Beta Cell Biology Consortium (BCBC)			■								■	■								
Clinical Islet Transplantation (CIT) Consortium				■	■					■	■		■		■			■	■	■
Collaborative Islet Transplant Registry (CITR)				■	■															
Diabetes Research in Children Network (DirecNet)						■														■
Epidemiology of Diabetes Interventions and Complications (EDIC)	■						■	■	■						■			■		
Family Investigations of Nephropathy and Diabetes (FIND)	■						■	■	■				■							
Genetics of Kidneys in Diabetes Study (GoKinD)	■						■	■	■											
Immune Tolerance Network (ITN)				■	■					■								■	■	■
Islet Cell Resource Centers (ICRs)/ Integrated Islet Distribution Program (IIDP)		■	■	■							■		■						■	
Type 1 Diabetes Mouse Resource	■		■									■								
NHP Transplantation Tolerance Cooperative Study Group (NHPCSG)				■				■			■		■	■					■	
SEARCH for Diabetes in Youth													■	■	■	■	■	■		
Standardization Programs (C-peptide, HbA1c, DASP)				■			■							■	■	■	■	■	■	■
The Environmental Determinants of Diabetes in the Young (TEDDY)				■										■	■	■	■			
Trial to Reduce IDDM in the Genetically At Risk (TRIGR)														■	■	■	■	■		
Type 1 Diabetes Genetics Consortium (T1DGC)				■	■		■			■				■	■		■	■		■
Type 1 Diabetes-Rapid Access to Intervention Development (T1D-RAID)	■			■						■	■				■				■	■
Type 1 Diabetes TrialNet				■		■				■					■	■	■	■	■	■

APPENDIX E

SUPPLEMENTAL MATERIAL
ON SCIENTIFIC CONFERENCES,
WORKSHOPS, AND MEETINGS
RELEVANT TO TYPE 1 DIABETES
AND ITS COMPLICATIONS

In addition to input that NIH and CDC receive at meetings specifically focused on research supported by the *Special Statutory Funding Program for Type 1 Diabetes Research* (*Special Diabetes Program* or *Program*) the agencies also obtain input at scientific conferences, workshops, and meetings that are relevant to type 1 diabetes and its complications. This input informs the planning process for use the *Special Diabetes Program*.

RESEARCH CONFERENCES AND WORKSHOPS

This listing provides information on scientific conferences and workshops with relevance to type 1 diabetes and its complications that have occurred since the development of the 2007 *"Evaluation Report"* on the *Special Statutory Funding Program for Type 1 Diabetes Research* (www.T1Diabetes.nih.gov/evaluation) through March 1, 2010. Please see Appendix 4 of the 2007 report for a list of previously held conferences and workshops.

Advances Toward Measuring Diabetic Retinopathy and Neuropathy: From the Bench to the Clinic and Back Again
April 4-5, 2007, sponsored by NIDDK
This conference focused on promoting advances in phenotyping diabetic retinopathy and neuropathy in animal models. Sessions included presentations describing clinical and animal studies in diabetic retinopathy and neuropathy; current methods for identifying, quantifying, and measuring these complications; and new advances in other scientific areas that may lead to improvements in phenotyping these conditions. A series of plenary talks and discussion sessions involving international leaders in their respective fields provided a forum for evaluating the current state of the art, and for identifying needs and research

opportunities, which helped to inform a pilot and feasibility program sponsored by the Mouse Metabolic Phenotyping Centers.

Clinical Proteomics in Diabetes and its Complications
July 20, 2007, sponsored by NIDDK
The main focus of this workshop was the application of proteomic technologies to clinical research relevant to diabetes and its complications. Particular emphasis was placed on research aimed at the identification of novel protein markers of diabetes and pre-diabetes, but more generally the application of proteomics to clinical studies. This workshop also provided a venue to bring together researchers with expertise in proteomics with clinical researchers interested in applying this technology to problems related to diabetes and its complications, in order to foster new collaborations.

miRNA and Epigenetic Regulations of the Immune Response
December 11-12, 2008, sponsored by NIDDK, NIAID, NIAMS, JDRF
Epigenetics is the study of stable genetic modifications that result in changes in gene expression and function without a corresponding alteration in DNA sequence. microRNAs (miRNAs) are naturally occurring molecules that can specifically silence the expression of a gene or a family of genes by blocking translation of the proteins they encode; they are involved in the regulation of a wide variety of cellular functions. Research has shown that epigenetic mechanisms and miRNAs are critically involved in immune responses. The purpose of the workshop was to bring together researchers interested in studying epigenetic and miRNA-mediated regulation of T cell development and function and their role in the immune and autoimmune responses in diseases such as type 1 diabetes.

Non-adherence in Adolescents with Chronic Illness

September 22-23, 2008, sponsored by NIDDK

Adherence to a prescribed treatment regimen can be a matter of life and death for people with chronic diseases, including people with type 1 diabetes who must check blood glucose levels several times each day and administer insulin. When seemingly rigid requirements are ignored by the adolescent going through the sometimes difficult transition to adulthood, the results can be tragic. The purpose of this workshop was to explore the risk factors for non-adherence in adolescents with kidney disease, diabetes, or gastrointestinal disease and determine ways to promote better adherence.

Towards an Artificial Pancreas: An FDA-NIH-JDRF Workshop

July 21-22, 2008, sponsored by FDA, NIH, JDRF

This workshop provided a public forum for discussing the progress and remaining challenges in the development of closed-loop systems designed to regulate blood glucose control in people with diabetes. The workshop also provided stakeholders with information to accelerate the development of an artificial pancreas. Session topics included: state-of-the-art design of closed-loop glycemic control systems; results of recently conducted clinical trials; design of clinical trials, including how to define success and failures of a closed-loop system; algorithms and *in silico* models; engineering challenges; patient considerations; metabolic monitoring; and paths for developing a marketable closed-loop system. In December 2008, with support of the *Special Diabetes Program*, NIDDK issued solicitations to support research conducted by small businesses toward the development of new technologies for an artificial pancreas.

Imaging the Pancreatic Beta Cell, 4th Workshop

April 6-7, 2009, sponsored by NIDDK

The purpose of the workshop was to explore the considerable progress and foster collaborative research in the field of imaging the pancreatic islet cell mass, function, or inflammation in health and disease. The overall intended goal of the field is to develop clinically useful imaging approaches for monitoring the mass, function, and inflammation of endogenous and transplanted islets and beta cells in people with type 1 or type 2 diabetes and those at risk for these diseases, in order to understand the natural history of disease and to monitor therapy.

Inflammation, Immunity, and Metabolism at the Interface of Type 1 and Type 2 Diabetes

May 5-6, 2009, sponsored by NIDDK

Diabetes is a heterogeneous disease that is affected by a wide spectrum of inflammatory reactions. Whereas chronic and destructive inflammation of the pancreatic islets (insulitis) is a defining causal feature of type 1 diabetes, low-grade systemic inflammation and activation of innate immunity contribute to the pathogenesis of type 2 diabetes. Recent research suggests, however, that systemic inflammation and insulin resistance also may contribute to type 1 diabetes, and the reduced beta cell mass observed in people with type 2 diabetes may in part be due to insulitis and enhanced programmed cell death. The composition and texture of these innate and adaptive immune responses and the interface with metabolic disturbances determine the inflammatory phenotype observed in the diabetes syndromes. The purpose of the workshop was to discuss: (1) the reciprocal regulation of innate and adaptive immunity, highlighting a possibly significant role in the pathogenesis of diabetes; (2) insulin resistance and chronic activation of the innate immune system in both major forms of diabetes, and the contribution to the metabolic derangement that is common to both diseases; (3) convergence of the inflammatory and autoimmune processes on the function and survival of the beta cell, and the differences and commonalities between type 1 and type 2 diabetes; and (4) lessons learned from the investigation of other chronic autoimmune/inflammatory disorders, with an emphasis on how this information might help investigators understand diabetes pathogenesis and potential treatments.

Typology of Diabetes in Children and Young Adults
September 16-17, 2009, sponsored by NIDDK, CDC
The purpose of the meeting was to review knowledge related to the typology of diabetes in childhood, with a particular focus on the potential overlap between type 1 and type 2 diabetes. The aims of the workshop were to: review the basis of current classification methods; identify areas of uncertainty in diabetes classification; explore new data related to the typology of diabetes in childhood; and identify new areas for research, with the goal of establishing improved paradigms for the classification of pediatric diabetes.

Next Generation Beta Cell Transplantation
November 9, 2009, sponsored by NIDDK, FDA, JDRF
The success of clinical islet transplantation as a curative therapy for type 1 diabetes has been hampered by concerns regarding durability of the transplanted islets, shortages of cadaver donor pancreata, the toxic effects of chronic immunosuppression, and recurrent autoimmunity. To hasten progress and circumvent these limitations, adult human beta cell replacement alternatives are being developed for clinical investigation using both porcine islets and differentiated human stem cells. In addition, encapsulation materials designed to shield transplanted cells from destructive immunity are being evaluated. At this workshop, regulatory authorities, academia, industry, and funding bodies convened to discuss the translational landscape and technology platforms required for the next generation of beta cell transplantation. It provided an interactive venue for identifying the hurdles that need to be overcome to achieve clinical success.

Diabetes Mellitus Interagency Coordinating Committee (DMICC) Meetings Relevant to Research on Type 1 Diabetes and Its Complications

This listing provides highlights of recent DMICC meetings relevant to type 1 diabetes that have occurred since the development of the 2007 *"Evaluation Report"* on the *Special Statutory Funding Program for Type 1 Diabetes Research* (www.T1Diabetes.nih.gov/evaluation) through March 1, 2010. For descriptions of previous DMICC meetings focused on the *Special Diabetes Program* or with relevance to type 1 diabetes, please see Appendices 3 and 4 of the 2007 report.

Opportunities for Diabetes Clinical Research
January 18-19, 2007

The purpose of this meeting was to solicit input from DMICC members and external experts on opportunities for clinical research on type 1 and type 2 diabetes. Many past and present NIH-supported diabetes clinical trials have been collaborative efforts involving more than one component of NIH, CDC, and FDA, for example. Thus, the DMICC provided an ideal venue to conduct a trans-NIH and trans-HHS discussion about opportunities for agencies to work together to conduct future clinical trials. The meeting also provided an opportunity for the Committee to obtain input from external experts in diabetes and diabetes clinical trials about key areas in which a well-designed trial could make a difference in the lives of people with diabetes.

The meeting began with a series of presentations to the Committee made by external experts on the current state-of-the science, as well as on unanswered questions related to the treatment and prevention of type 2 diabetes, the treatment of type 1 diabetes, and the treatment of older people with diabetes. After the presentations, the participants formed two break-out groups focused on the areas of diabetes management and diabetes prevention to discuss a list of possible trials in each area that had been distributed prior to the meeting. The list was developed based on external input obtained before the meeting. Related to treatment of type 1 diabetes, the participants discussed opportunities to develop a closed-loop insulin pump.

The second day of the meeting included presentations by a representative from each break-out group who summarized the group discussions for all meeting participants. Participants further discussed the trials and provided additional input on all of the possible trials. External input, such as input obtained at this meeting, is critically important to inform decisions made by NIDDK and other DMICC member organizations about future diabetes clinical trials supported by regular appropriations and the *Special Diabetes Program*.

DMICC Member Overview of Diabetes-Related Activities
September 20, 2007

This meeting provided an opportunity for DMICC member agencies, with emphasis on NIH Institutes and Centers, to share their plans for new and ongoing initiatives in diabetes research. In particular, members were encouraged to present research or programs that related to the Diabetes National Plan for Action (DNPA), developed under the auspices of the U.S. Department of Health and Human Services. DNPA, which was published in December 2004, focused on both type 1 diabetes and type 2 diabetes. It can be found at: http://aspe.hhs.gov/health/NDAP/NDAP04.pdf. The goals of DNPA are to increase national awareness of diabetes and its impact and what can be done to prevent and manage the disease; reduce the prevalence of diabetes and its risk factors; promote improved detection, monitoring, and treatment; and coordinate public and private efforts and leverage existing resources. Topics in the DNPA include strategies for addressing type 1 and type 2 diabetes for individuals and families, schools, health care providers, employers, communities, health insurance providers, media, researchers and educators, and governments. The DMICC is integral to the federal response to the DNPA.

In addition to presentations on type 2 diabetes research from NIDDK, cardiovascular clinical trials from NHLBI, and diabetes surveillance and prevention and control programs from CDC, the Centers for Medicare & Medicaid Services presented information on physician-focused care improvement initiatives to improve quality and efficiency within the Medicare system. The Agency for Healthcare Research and Quality, Health Resources and Services Administration, and Indian Health Service (IHS) also provided updates of diabetes-related initiatives. With regard to type 1 diabetes, NICHD discussed TRIGR and DirecNet. The NIDDK also provided an update on the *Special Diabetes Program* and reminded DMICC members that both *"Advances and Emerging Opportunities in Type 1 Diabetes Research: A Strategic Plan"* and the *"Evaluation Report"* on the *Special Statutory Funding Program for Type 1 Diabetes Research* can be found on NIDDK's Web site. Additionally, future plans for an external evaluation meeting to evaluate major clinical projects were discussed.

Expanding Collaborations To Translate Research into Practice
April 1, 2008
The DMICC provides a venue for discussion of current and future projects conducted by member agencies. Presentation of projects helps members to identify opportunities for collaboration and allows them to make use of each other's expertise and resources. This meeting focused on fostering new collaborations among DMICC member agencies; speakers highlighted potential opportunities at their agency or institute which could involve the participation of other DMICC member agencies. For example, it was suggested that research agencies, such as NIH and CDC, could collaborate with service provider agencies, like IHS, on the design of research studies. Early input from service provider agencies could assist in the translation of research results and dissemination of information into practice.

The NIDDK provided an update on the *Special Statutory Funding Program for Type 1 Diabetes Research* including announcement of the extension of the *Program* and the *Special Diabetes Program for Indians* through FY 2009. In response to challenges to most effectively using funds in a single year with the typical NIH funding mechanisms, NIDDK, which oversees the *Special Diabetes Program*, received NIH approval for a new multiyear funding mechanism called the DP3. In FY 2009, this funding mechanism was used to solicit applications for research on the newly discovered type 1 diabetes genes and the mechanisms by which they cause susceptibility to disease. Finally, NIDDK has organized an evaluation meeting for April 2008 for an external panel of scientific experts to review the clinical research efforts supported by the *Special Diabetes Program* and to guide future efforts of these ongoing programs.

Strategic Planning To Enhance Federal Diabetes Programs

August 11, 2008

This meeting included several different topics, including an update on the *Special Statutory Funding Program for Type 1 Diabetes Research* from NIDDK and an update on the *Special Diabetes Program for Indians* by IHS. Regarding the type 1 diabetes *Program*, NIDDK asked for input on plans for supporting type 1 diabetes research with the funds, which had recently been extended through FY 2011. To inform decisions, NIDDK will continue to be guided by the 2006 strategic plan for Type 1 Diabetes Research, by a new diabetes strategic planning effort (described below), and by input obtained from an external evaluation panel convened in April 2008 to assess the large clinical projects that were previously funded through the *Program*. A similar meeting is planned for 2009 to discuss pre-clinical projects; the input obtained at that meeting will also guide the use of the funds. The NIDDK also reported on recent initiatives made possible by the *Special Diabetes Program*, such as the Type 1 Diabetes Pathfinder Award to attract new talent to type 1 diabetes research.

The parallel *Special Diabetes Program for Indians* had also been recently extended through FY 2011. The IHS provided an update on plans, which included a tribal consultation concerning how best to utilize the funding to the benefit of American Indians with or at risk for diabetes. In general, communities are free to determine how to direct the funds to accomplish

program goals and to expand the diabetes-fighting infrastructure they already have. Already, dramatic success has been achieved in reducing the diabetes burden in the American Indian community, as evidenced by the lowering of average hemoglobin A1c (HbA1c) levels. In the future, IHS will be working to identify the approaches that are most effective in realizing these health improvements so that successes can be replicated at other sites.

Another topic of discussion was an NIDDK proposal to begin a new diabetes strategic planning process under the auspices of the DMICC to help guide the federal investment in diabetes research. In 1999, the Congressionally-mandated Diabetes Research Working Group developed and published "*Conquering Diabetes: A Strategic Plan for the 21st Century*," a comprehensive diabetes research plan that has served as a blueprint for discovery. Since that time, major changes have taken place in the understanding of diabetes. At the same time, significant data have emerged on the national burden of pre-diabetes and on the alarming increase of diabetes in children. Thus, the Committee decided that the time was right to identify high-priority opportunities for diabetes research that can be accomplished in the next 5 to 10 years. The NIDDK, as chair of the DMICC, would spearhead the new strategic planning effort with broad external input. The plan is envisioned to guide NIH, other federal agencies, and the investigative and lay communities in their pursuit of the goal of conquering diabetes. Additionally, the new plan would help to guide type 1 diabetes research supported by the *Special Statutory Funding Program for Type 1 Diabetes Research*.

Federally Supported Diabetes-related National Education Programs

May 6, 2009

Presentations at this meeting were centered on diabetes-related national education programs. The NEI's National Eye Health Education Program ensures that vision is a public health priority through the translation of eye and vision research into public and professional education programs and includes diabetic eye disease as one of its main program areas. The NIDDK and CDC's National Diabetes Education Program disseminates research results through its two campaigns, "*Control Your Diabetes. For Life*," based on the findings of the Diabetes Control and Complications Trial, and "*Small Steps. Big Rewards. Prevent type 2 Diabetes*," which translates the results of the Diabetes Prevention Program clinical trial into materials for health care providers and patients. The NIDDK's National Kidney Disease Education Program aims to reduce the morbidity and mortality caused by kidney disease and its complications through its campaigns. The NLM's Medline Plus is a resource for health information, including diabetes-related information, for patients, family, friends, and professionals. The meetings also included discussions of education activities from providers such as Veterans Health Administration and IHS.

APPENDIX F

ADVANCES AND EMERGING

OPPORTUNITIES IN DIABETES RESEARCH:

A STRATEGIC PLANNING REPORT OF

THE DIABETES MELLITUS INTERAGENCY

COORDINATING COMMITTEE

The statutory Diabetes Mellitus Interagency Coordinating Committee (DMICC), with leadership from NIDDK, developed a Diabetes Research Strategic Plan to serve as a scientific guidepost to NIH, other federal agencies, and to the investigative and lay community by identifying compelling research opportunities. These scientific opportunities will inform the priority-setting process for the diabetes research field and propel research progress on the understanding, prevention, treatment, and cure of diabetes and its complications. It will also serve as an important guide for research supported by the *Special Statutory Funding Program for Type 1 Diabetes Research*. The Plan addresses extraordinary opportunities in 10 major diabetes research areas listed below.

- Genetic Basis of Type 1 Diabetes, Type 2 Diabetes, Obesity, and Their Complications

- Type 1 Diabetes and Autoimmunity

- The Beta Cell

- Type 2 Diabetes as a Multi-Dimensional Disease

- Obesity

- Bioengineering Approaches for the Development of an Artificial Pancreas To Improve Management of Glycemia

- Clinical Research and Clinical Trials

- Special Needs for Special Populations

- Diabetes Complications

- Clinical Research to Practice: Translational Research

The Strategic Plan also includes a chapter that outlines resource and infrastructure development needs to support the implementation of the future directions for diabetes research identified in the Plan.

This Appendix includes specific research questions and future research directions that have been excerpted from the Strategic Plan. Included are chapters with relevance to type 1 diabetes and its complications. Therefore, chapters on "Type 2 Diabetes as a Multi-Dimensional Disease" and "Obesity" are excluded; some sections from other chapters are also excluded if they are not relevant to type 1 diabetes. Some sections cover both type 1 and type 2 diabetes and were included in their entirety. The key questions and future directions, listed under the chapter subheadings, were identified in the strategic planning process as being critically important for overcoming current barriers and achieving progress in diabetes research relative to the chapter's area of focus over the next 10 years. For the complete Plan, please see: http://diabetesplan.niddk.nih.gov.

GENETIC BASIS OF TYPE 1 DIABETES, TYPE 2 DIABETES, OBESITY, AND THEIR COMPLICATIONS

Genes and Pathways
Key Questions:

- What are the causal genes and variants influencing or residing within each candidate susceptibility locus?

- Are the candidate genes/regions identified in European-origin populations (where most of the studies have been performed) also operative in other, ethnically diverse populations?

- Do candidate genes/risk variants interact to modify risk, and how is the penetrance of disease alleles affected by environmental factors?

- Are there subsets of genes that, taken together, represent a causal pathway that could define a therapeutic target?

- What are the effects of identified genetic variants on integration of genomic, expression, and proteomic profiling on disease risk?

- Can genetic variation be coupled with gene expression profiles at the RNA and protein levels to catalog target tissues at the population, individual, and cellular levels for both humans and animal models?

- Can model organisms be utilized to advance research from human genetic studies, and can results from model organisms direct targeted human studies?

Future Directions:
➢ Develop standardized and emergent protocols for assessing phenotypic characteristics of populations, both clinical and epidemiologic, for use in genetic studies.

➢ Understand how candidate genes contribute to disease risk.

➢ Elucidate the interactions among genes at the cellular level and discover common pathways of risk.

Detection of Rare Variants
Key Questions:
- How can sequence variation that is rare in populations, yet accounts for familial risk of disease, be identified?

- Can genomic sequence data from many individuals with known phenotypes provide insight into the effect that natural variation in genome structure has on susceptibility to diabetes and obesity?

- What is "normal" sequence variation compared to "risk" variation in the context of environmental triggers that lead to diabetes and obesity?

- Can population-specific DNA sequences be identified that are associated with disease risk and that are predictive of response to therapies?

Future Directions:
➢ Perform DNA sequencing in tens of thousands of participants with type 1 diabetes, type 2 diabetes, and obesity to detect all sequence variants that may be associated with risk of these conditions.

➢ Correlate sequence variants with the level of risk for development of diabetes, obesity, and their complications.

Gene-Environment Interactions
Key Questions:
- What kinds of sample and data resources are needed for analyzing genetic variation in groups of participants with diabetes and obesity or in healthy populations before they develop complications, so that environmental triggers can be identified in those at high genetic risk?

- How and to what extent will information be collected on environmental triggers, especially unknown/ potential triggers for diabetes, obesity, and their complications?

- Can research tools used in mouse models of disease be used to identify potential modifier effects in human genetic data?

- How can genetically determined epidemiologic risk factors be identified and monitored as biomarkers of exposures that interact with genetic risk variants?

- What recent changes in human exposures, diets, or social and behavioral activities contribute to onset of disease in genetically predisposed individuals? Can any of these factors be modified to lower risk?

Future Directions:

➢ Determine how candidate genes or sequence variants interact with environmental risk factors that can lead to disease outcome.

➢ Develop resources and technologies to study gene-environment interactions.

Epigenetic Contributions to Risk

Key Questions:

• Do DNA methylation and other aspects of epigenetic modification contribute to inter-individual variation in the risk of diabetes, obesity, and diabetes complications?

• Do epigenetic mechanisms correlate with risk and serve as therapeutic targets?

• What is the potential interaction between epigenetic modification and a pro-inflammatory environment and oxidative stress, and how does this interaction affect the risk of diabetes and obesity?

Future Directions:

➢ Identify epigenetic markers that influence susceptibility to diabetes, obesity, and/or diabetes complications.

Translation of Genetic Research from Bench to Bedside

Key Questions:

• How can the development of diabetes and obesity investigators who are well-trained, multidisciplinary and interdisciplinary, and able to form research teams be fostered?

• Can an incubator be created for innovative research tools and information technologies focused on translational and behavioral research in diabetes and obesity?

• Will current guidelines on human participants research permit synergism of multidisciplinary and interdisciplinary clinical and translational research to facilitate the application of new knowledge and techniques in clinical practice?

• Can opportunities be developed to bring physiologists (both animal and human) into a productive collaboration with geneticists to bridge research gaps?

• What methods can be developed to translate novel techniques of prediction, prevention, and treatment into the general community?

Future Directions:

➢ Optimize the use of genetic and environmental risk factor data in the design of translational and clinical research programs for diabetes and obesity.

TYPE 1 DIABETES AND AUTOIMMUNITY

Human Type 1 Diabetes Trials (Prevention/Reversal/Transplantation)

Key Questions:

• Will additional information about genetic underpinnings of type 1 diabetes allow therapies to be targeted to homogeneous populations, thus increasing their effectiveness?

• Will antigen-specific versus non-specific tolerance induction protocols be safe and effective in preventing progression to overt type 1 diabetes in individuals deemed to be at high future disease risk?

• How can combination therapies using short-course immunosuppressants, cellular mobilization agents, insulin sensitizers, anti-inflammatories, islet antigens, and/or molecules capable of inducing beta cell replication *in vivo* be tested?

- How can multi-center, international collaborative trials that support biomarker and discovery studies best be accomplished?

- How can very long-term follow-up (*i.e.*, beyond the 1 to 2 year standard for current studies), including metabolic and mechanistic studies, as well as monitoring of adverse events of patients in trials for the prevention of beta cell loss, be accomplished?

- Can biomarkers be developed to stratify patients for trials and to obtain an early indication of therapeutic effectiveness?

- Will drugs designed for the treatment of other disorders, especially autoimmune disorders, and possessing a highly favorable safety profile, prove efficacious as treatment(s) for type 1 diabetes?

- Is it possible that intervention may provide a clinical benefit in patients months or even years after diagnosis?

- Could the principles of "disease staging," often used in oncology, be applied to settings of type 1 diabetes both prior to and well beyond the diagnosis of this disease?

Future Directions:

➢ Conduct coordinated clinical trials to test therapies to prevent or reverse type 1 diabetes.

Natural History and Pathogenesis of Human Type 1 Diabetes

Key Questions:

- What is the natural history of type 1 diabetes, including the precise sequence of events leading to the initiation of insulitis, and continuing on to clinical diabetes?

- Why is type 1 diabetes increasing in incidence and occurring more often at younger ages?

- What is the basis of the observed heterogeneity in type 1 diabetes and is there additional heterogeneity yet to be discovered?

- Is noninvasive imaging of beta cell mass and associated insulitis achievable?

- Can autoimmune pathogenesis at the islet, whether in people in pre-clinical stages of pathology or in autoimmune recurrence in transplant recipients, be measured indirectly in the blood, for example by a measurement of T cell responses to diabetes-relevant antigens? Can such biomarker assays be developed to enhance prediction of type 1 diabetes, facilitate studies of natural history, and serve as surrogate markers in therapeutic trials?

- What is the role of the gut microbiome in disease etiology?

Future Directions:

➢ Discover triggering factors for islet autoimmunity and environmental factors responsible for the recent increase in incidence of type 1 diabetes.

➢ Better define the heterogeneity and diagnosis of type 1 diabetes and foster the development of therapies specific to different forms of the disease.

➢ Delineate the natural history, or histories, of type 1 diabetes.

➢ Elucidate the impact of environmental or other non-genetic factors on development of type 1 diabetes.

➢ Study role of innate immunity in diabetes.

Animal Models/Translational Efforts from Pathogenesis to Therapy

Key Questions:

- Can higher fidelity mouse models of human disease be developed that will improve the ability to predict the efficacy of new therapies in patients?

- Can non-obese diabetic (NOD) mice (and/or higher fidelity mouse models of human disease) be used to:

  - Perform systematic screening of small molecules or other potential therapies for prevention or reversal of type 1 diabetes?

  - Identify environmental agents that precipitate or prevent type 1 diabetes?

  - Identify biomarkers in the blood that can monitor islet cell mass or autoimmunity?

- Can the function of human diabetes susceptibility or protective genes be effectively studied in mouse models?

- Can common pathogenic mechanisms be identified among different autoimmune diseases and in different disease models that may inform the search for new therapeutic targets and strategies?

Future Directions:

➤ Rapidly translate new findings on disease pathogenesis in animal models into potential therapies.

➤ Use animal models to identify and validate biomarkers of type 1 diabetes.

➤ Develop a higher fidelity mouse model of human disease that develops type 1 diabetes.

➤ Develop *in silico* models for type 1 diabetes.

Beta Cell Function in Type 1 Diabetes: Autoimmune Attack and Prospects for Recovery

Key Questions:

- What is the beta cell mass/function at onset of type 1 diabetes?

- How much residual beta cell mass/function is required for reversal after immunotherapy? Does it differ with different treatments?

- Can mechanisms that protect mouse cells from autoimmune destruction also protect human islets from autoimmune attack?

- Why is pancreas volume greatly reduced in people with type 1 diabetes? Does this reduction have an influence on disease parameters? Can it be used as a biomarker of disease development or potential for success in therapeutic intervention?

- Are there diabetes-susceptibility genetic variants that determine the ability of beta cells to resist autoimmune attack, or to regenerate or recover function once autoimmunity is controlled?

Future Directions:

➤ Develop metabolic tests to detect early signs of beta cell dysfunction.

➤ Examine the effect of insulin resistance on the development of type 1 diabetes.

➤ Identify genes and mechanisms that protect beta cells from autoimmune dysfunction and/or destruction, in animal models or in humans when possible.

> Define specific and sensitive surrogate markers of physical and/or functional beta cell recovery in response to immunotherapy and determine if beta cell mass can regenerate without reactivating autoimmunity.

Immune Mechanisms of Pancreatic Pathology

Key Questions:

- How diverse are the T and B cell responses to individual diabetogenic antigens, and how can the dominant effect of major histocompatibility complex (MHC) sequence on diabetes susceptibility be explained?

- What are the respective roles of CD4+ and CD8+ T cells, as well as other immune cell subsets (*e.g.*, B cells, NK cells, dendritic cells, and mast cells), in pathogenesis?

- What is the role of regulatory cell populations in diabetes pathogenesis or protection?

- What is the relationship between autoimmunity and inflammation in type 1 diabetes, and what are the roles of other organs such as gut, liver, fat, or others?

- What underlies the variability of attack on different islets within the same pancreas, and can that understanding be used to interdict the disease process?

Future Directions:

> Identify the range of tolerance mechanisms defective in type 1 diabetes models and patients (*e.g.*, genetic polymorphisms in immune system genes) and delineate precisely where the cellular and molecular defects lie.

> Define how auto-inflammatory infiltrates and beta cells communicate with each other in controlling type 1 diabetes progression.

> Understand the repertoires of responding lymphocytes, including T cells and B cells.

> Identify the range of regulatory cell populations potentially defective in type 1 diabetes and learn which regulatory populations—defective or not—provide good therapeutic opportunities.

> Define which pathways are shared by different autoimmune diseases and which are disease-specific.

> Extend and preserve existing pancreas repositories and data banks, which are critical for direct examination of pancreatic pathology.

THE BETA CELL

Integrated Islet Physiology

Key Questions:

- What is the full communication network that exists between the five endocrine cell types regulated in the islet? What is its role in disease progression?

- Are novel receptors and paracrine factors present in the endocrine pancreas?

- What are the functional interactions among the exocrine, ductal, and endocrine cell types?

- How does islet vasculature affect islet function and engraftment after transplant?

- How is islet innervation established? Does it change over time and/or in response to physiological cues and disease states? How does it affect islet function?

- What is the integrated physiology of the human islet? How does this differ from regulation in rodent islets?

Future Directions:

➢ Investigate integrated islet paracrine regulation.

➢ Develop drug therapies targeting islet signaling pathways.

➢ Develop scaffolds and other support systems for beta cells.

➢ Increase understanding of human (versus rodent) islet physiology.

➢ Determine the influence of the intrauterine environment on islet development and function.

Beta Cell Dysfunction and Failure

Key Questions:

• What are critical steps of unfolded protein response (UPR) that could be manipulated to improve beta cell function and survival?

• Which of the nutrient sensing pathways contribute to beta cell loss?

• Which of the intracellular signaling pathways can be manipulated to preserve beta cell function and mass?

• What are the initiating events, participating cells, and destructive processes underlying the intra-islet inflammatory response?

• What are common features of immune-mediated damage in type 1 and type 2 diabetes, and how might this potential mechanistic overlap inform the development of new therapeutic approaches for both diseases?

Future Directions:

➢ Discover ways of modulating intra-islet inflammatory mediators in order to prevent insulitis in type 2 diabetes.

➢ Develop pharmacological agents to modify key signaling molecules to preserve and protect beta cell function.

Cellular Replacement Therapies for Diabetes

Key Questions:

• Are there ways to promote successful islet engraftment and survival so that people require fewer islets and/or transplants to produce sufficient amounts of insulin?

• Can researchers harness the information from a fundamental understanding of the developmental biology of the endocrine pancreas to generate fully functional beta cells from stem cells *in vitro*?

• Can induced pluripotent stem (iPS) cells be generated safely for patient-specific cell replacement therapy, eliminating the concern of genome integration by the associated viral vectors?

• What are the underlying principles of cellular reprogramming, and under what physiological or pathophysiological conditions will transdifferentiation, transdetermination, and reprogramming occur?

• What are developmental and/or epigenetic factors that affect pancreatic endocrine fate?

• Given the number of ways to increase beta cell mass in rodent models, can these findings be translated into increasing beta cell mass in humans?

• What are common features in beta cell replication between rodents and humans at the physiological periods when replication is known to take place (neonate, puberty, and pregnancy)?

Future Directions:

➤ Improve islet transplant procedures by determining the optimal sites for islet transplantation and developing novel islet survival strategies.

➤ Define a molecular signature for endogenous human beta cells, as well as for human stem cell-derived beta cells, and their progenitors.

➤ Discover late developmental pro-beta cell signals and use these signals to produce large numbers of functional human beta cells from stem/progenitor cells.

➤ Generate large quantities of fully functional beta cells through the transdifferentiation or direct reprogramming of other adult or progenitor cell types *in vitro* and/or *in vivo*.

➤ Develop animal models to test the engraftment, survival, and metabolic impact of human beta cells or islets derived in culture from stem/progenitor cells.

➤ Create new animal models of human diabetes.

➤ Understand the cell types, signaling pathways, and genes that control islet cell mass and beta cell replication and are relevant to the regenerative capacity of the human islet.

Imaging the Pancreatic Islet

Key questions:

• What are the best technologies, reagents, and targets for noninvasive imaging of pancreatic beta cell mass and function? For islet inflammation?

• How best can transplanted islets be monitored *in vivo*? Can angiogenesis and neurogenesis in these islets be visualized directly, and can imaging be used to monitor the life cycle and common causes of loss of the transplanted tissues?

• How does beta cell mass change throughout the normal human lifespan? What are the effectors and natural history of cell loss in diabetes? What is the relationship between mass and function in health, pregnancy, obesity, insulin resistance, etc.?

Future Directions:

➤ Assemble interdisciplinary environments and teams to work on imaging the beta cell, and invite cross-pollination from related fields such as cancer and neuroimaging.

➤ Identify cell-specific beta cell surface proteins as molecular imaging targets and use high-throughput methods to find or produce highly specific, tight-binding, small molecule or peptide imaging agents.

➤ Recruit chemists to design imaging agents for beta cell targets, or to improve the kinetic and imaging properties of existing promising agents.

➤ Develop novel, noninvasive technologies to monitor islet cell function, islet angiogenesis, nerve function and growth, and inflammation.

➤ Define the biology of promising imaging agents and their cell targets, such as the expression in development and islet life cycle, cellular location during function, and other fundamental properties.

BIOENGINEERING APPROACHES FOR THE DEVELOPMENT OF AN ARTIFICIAL PANCREAS TO IMPROVE MANAGEMENT OF GLYCEMIA

Glucose Sensors

Key Questions:

• Can accuracy and reliability of glucose sensors be improved?

- Can new glucose-sensing technologies be developed?

- Will the incorporation of nanotechnology strategies and the use of smart biomaterials be able to improve reliability and durability of sensors?

- Will it be possible to develop a reliable and durable implantable sensor?

- Will it be possible to develop new technologies/ strategies for a noninvasive, reliable, low cost, continuous glucose sensor?

- Will universal design strategies for sensor development be applied to facilitate use by people with diabetes?

Future Directions:

➢ Develop improved glucose sensors.

➢ Validate glucose-sensing technologies.

➢ Translation.

Algorithm Development—*In Silico*/ Simulation Models

Key Questions:

- What outcome measures are suitable for judging the effectiveness of closed-loop control in relatively short-duration clinical trials? What would be the "standard" performance criteria? What degree of control error is acceptable?

- What are the requirements for designing control modules?

- Can *in silico* models of human metabolism be improved by making them more powerful in terms of generating "virtual participants" for *in silico* trials? Can a rich tracer database on type 1 diabetes (adult and children) be developed? Can counter-regulation

and exercise be incorporated? Can a type 2 diabetes simulator be developed?

- What safety features can be incorporated into controllers?

Future Directions:

➢ Using system biology approaches, develop a comprehensive computer simulation environment allowing for efficient and cost effective *in silico* experiments with diabetes treatments.

➢ Develop effective closed-loop algorithms for clinical and outpatient use.

Insulin—Improving Delivery and Formulation

Key Questions:

- Which insulin delivery approaches result in clinically relevant improvements and are acceptable to the user?

- How do market-specific cost constraints influence the optimization of novel delivery methods, devices, and insulins?

- What changes in insulin chemistry and/or physical properties would most likely improve its use in alternative delivery routes, devices, and/or materials?

- How can the potential risk of alternative delivery sites and insulin chemistries to produce unwanted metabolic, toxic, or immunogenic effects be quantified and reduced?

- How may the automated delivery of insulin counter-regulatory hormones such as glucagon be integrated into current or future closed-loop systems? What changes in glucagon chemistry and/or physical properties are needed to have more effective and stable glucagon formulations for delivery by pumps?

Future Directions:

➢ Establish standardized pre-clinical models for safety and efficacy testing of alternative insulin delivery methods, materials, and devices that dependably predict their potential clinical utility.

➢ Develop integrated insulin delivery systems that improve the quality of life.

➢ Develop failsafe devices or biomaterials that respond based on low glucose levels to release glucagon or other insulin-counteractive therapeutics to prevent hypoglycemia.

➢ Reduce immune responses to facilitate alternative site and/or long-acting polymeric insulin delivery systems.

➢ Develop new insulins with increased stability at high concentrations and minimal, reproducible subcutaneous absorption delay time.

➢ Develop a family of non-toxic, non-antigenic, low molecular weight molecules that effectively and specifically bind glucose in the presence of serum components and across the physiological range of glucose concentrations, from hypoglycemic to hyperglycemic levels.

Telemedicine

Key Questions:

• What are the best technological solutions (both hardware and decision-support software) to best enable telemedicine to be easily and effectively applied in clinical practice?

• What types of behavioral modification tools or incentives can be developed to facilitate communication and adherence to telemedicine-generated instructions?

• Can high blood glucose or low blood glucose alerts be sent automatically from a glucose meter to a health care provider by way of a Web server to elicit an immediate assistance response that could reduce emergency room visits?

• Can personal digital assistant (PDA) applications ("apps") for diabetes management, which track blood glucose, food intake, insulin, and exercise, improve outcomes?

• How can telemedicine platforms be integrated into an automated closed-loop system?

Future Directions:

➢ Develop telemedicine approaches that can be incorporated as components and/or adjuvants of an artificial pancreas.

➢ Determine whether online peer-to-peer management can improve diabetes outcomes.

Tissue Engineering for Replacement of Pancreatic Islets

Key Questions:

• Will the development of novel biomaterials contribute to more effective immunobarrier/encapsulation methods to establish and maintain a functional bioartificial pancreas using transplanted islets from different sources?

• What methods can be developed for effective vascularization of islets after implantation?

Future Directions:

➢ Improve perfusion of islet cells within a graft site.

➢ Develop new biomaterials and immunobarrier protection for transplanted islets.

Impact of Closed-Loop Control on the Pathophysiology of Diabetes

Key Questions:

- Can an artificial mechanical pancreas or islet replacement restore glucose counter-regulation and hypoglycemia awareness and preserve brain function in people with type 1 diabetes, especially young children?

- Can early intensive insulin therapy increase beta cell survival and prevent the loss of the glucagon response to hypoglycemia in people with new-onset of type 1 diabetes?

- What are the short- and long-term consequences of the route of delivery of insulin on glycemic outcome, vascular complications, and body weight?

- Is glucose the only target that should be used in developing closed-loop systems? Should additional compounds be measured online, *e.g.* insulin, glucagon, other metabolites?

- Are the differences between systemic and portal administration significant enough to favor technologies (mechanical or cellular) that deliver insulin to the liver—its primary site of action?

- Can incorporation of automated glucagon delivery increase defenses against hypoglycemia without excessively raising blood glucose?

Future Directions:

- Determine the impact of an artificial mechanical pancreas on brain function, fuel metabolism, and structure, especially in children.

- Pursue approaches to scale up and commercialize production.

- Determine if a closed-loop system artificial mechanical pancreas is sufficient to restore normal glucose counter-regulation and reverse hypoglycemia unawareness.

- Determine whether an artificial mechanical pancreas (or implanted engineered islets) can preserve beta cells and maintain alpha cell responses to hypoglycemia in type 1 diabetes if given early, when some insulin secretion is still present.

- Determine whether insulin delivery via the portal vein will be more effective in achieving normoglycemia by reducing insulin resistance and enhancing portal sensing of glucose and gut peptides.

- Develop methods to measure insulin levels in real time, to provide input to closed-loop feedback algorithms.

Behavioral Aspects

Key Questions

- What are the challenges and benefits of new diabetes technologies for individuals with the disease, including physical (*e.g.*, complexity of use, ease of availability), behavioral (*e.g.*, cognitive load, adherence, time requirements), psychological (*e.g.*, quality of life, fear of hypoglycemia), and social (vocational and family functioning) impacts?

- What factors contraindicate the use of specific diabetes technologies for individuals with diabetes (*e.g.*, age, knowledge, psychological status, cognitive development, functional status, treatment regimen, type and stage of diabetes, and home environment and disease management support)? How can accessibility and usability be increased across populations?

- How can these technologies be more accessible to people from different backgrounds and those with educational, sensory, motor, and cognitive limitations? Has the human/technology interface been designed to be easy to use for people with limited literacy and numeracy skills?

- What are the most effective ways for health care providers to incorporate new technologies and the data they produce into practice?

Future Directions:

➢ Quantify the broad-ranging impact of new diabetes technologies on people with diabetes.

➢ Increase accessibility and usability of technologies by people with diabetes-related (and non-diabetes-related) functional impairments and disabilities.

➢ Increase adoption and effective use of technologies across the lifespan.

➢ Increase employment of generic new technologies to promote positive health behavior change in people with diabetes.

➢ Develop more effective information and educational and training methods for health care providers in use of diabetes technological advancements.

Design of Clinical Trials and Clinical Outcomes
Key Questions:

- What are appropriate outcome measures (*e.g.*, HbA1c, reduction in hypoglycemia, reduction in glycemic variability) for clinical trials of artificial mechanical pancreas technologies in people with type 1 or type 2 diabetes?

- Can continuous glucose monitors (CGM) or an artificial mechanical pancreas be used successfully in insulin-requiring patients with type 2 diabetes to maintain HbA1c targets with less hypoglycemia?

- Can reduction of glycemic variability in people with type 2 diabetes who are insulin-dependent lead to improved outcomes, such as reduced diabetic nephropathy, reduction in cardiac arrhythmias in people at high risk for cardiac mortality, and/or reduction of systemic inflammation and oxidative stress?

- What is the value of CGM and/or closed-loop insulin delivery devices in the intensive care unit?

- Can an artificial mechanical pancreas prevent hypoglycemia and/or diabetic micro- and macrovascular complications?

- Should the measurement of vital signs such as heart rate, temperature, and breathing rate be monitored together with glucose monitoring in clinical studies to prevent hypoglycemia and excessive glycemic postprandial excursions?

Future Directions:

➢ Study the impact of closed-loop glucose control on exercise and nocturnal hypoglycemia.

➢ Determine the efficacy of CGMs and eventually of closed-loop glucose control to improve disordered fuel metabolism and reduce hypoglycemia and diabetic complications in people with type 2 diabetes who require insulin treatment.

➢ Determine whether closed-loop glucose control can preserve beta cell function in people with new-onset type 1 diabetes or with type 2 diabetes.

- Conduct long-term studies of closed-loop glucose control in children and adolescents.

- Study use of continuous glucose monitoring and closed-loop insulin delivery systems in people with gastroparesis.

- Study use of closed-loop technologies in the intensive care unit (ICU).

CLINICAL RESEARCH AND CLINICAL TRIALS

Treatment

Key Questions:

- Are there approaches to the initial treatment of type 2 diabetes that will reverse or slow the decline in beta cell function that has been shown to occur over time?

- What is the optimal timing for diabetes interventions? Do specific treatments have maximum benefit at different stages of the disease?

- What genetic factors or other patient characteristics influence the choice of initial therapy for individuals?

- How can adherence to diabetes treatments be improved?

Future Directions:

- Conduct studies to preserve endogenous insulin secretion or induce "remissions" of diabetes.

- Determine whether preventing or delaying diabetes can also delay or prevent the chronic complications of the disease.

- Evaluate the effect of bariatric surgery procedures on obesity, diabetes, and underlying pathophysiology.

- Evaluate early effects and duration of action of commonly used anti-diabetic drugs for the initial treatment of early type 2 diabetes.

- Identify biomarkers.

- Design well-powered, comprehensive clinical trials aimed at individualizing therapy of type 2 diabetes.

- Examine the causes of and means of improving poor adherence to diabetes treatment regimens.

- Describe the epidemiology of hypoglycemia.

- Determine whether hypoglycemia unawareness can be prevented or reversed.

Etiology of Diabetes and Its Complications

Key Questions:

- Can genetic information improve disease prediction over currently available clinical markers?

- Can genetic information predict response to lifestyle or pharmacological interventions in disease prevention or treatment?

- Can genetic information predict the development of diabetic complications? For instance, do genetic predictors of hyperglycemia also influence risk of coronary heart disease?

- What are the etiologic factors that explain clinical heterogeneity and provide a rational molecular basis for disease taxonomy, particularly in type 2 diabetes?

- What are the mechanisms underlying the impact of intrauterine exposures or diet and exercise on the risk of developing type 2 diabetes?

- What is the impact of environmental exposures on the risk of developing type 1 diabetes?

- What is the role of sleep disturbances in increasing the risk of type 2 diabetes? What is the effect of treating obstructive sleep apnea in the prevention and therapy of type 2 diabetes?

Future Directions:

➤ Continue to expand knowledge of the genetic basis for type 1 and type 2 diabetes.

➤ Continue to incorporate newly discovered variants into genetic prediction models using existing prospective population cohorts.

➤ Conduct studies to assess how environmental and genetic factors interact to produce type 2 diabetes and affect responses to interventions.

➤ Identify factors that influence the evolution of type 1 diabetes.

➤ Harness genetic information to characterize individual susceptibility to diabetic complications.

➤ Conduct studies to improve understanding of both the relative importance and the mechanism(s) by which sleep disturbances increase the risk of type 2 diabetes.

➤ Evaluate whether treating obstructive sleep apnea has an effect on the prevention and treatment of type 2 diabetes.

Complications

Key Questions:

• How does the pathophysiology of atherosclerosis differ in people with type 1 diabetes, in people with type 2 diabetes, and in non-diabetic populations?

• How important is insulin resistance in the development of macrovascular complications in people with type 1 diabetes?

• What are the principal mediators of atherosclerosis in people with type 2 diabetes and can specific targeted interventions be developed?

• How important is aggressive and sustained blood pressure and lipid lowering in reducing the risks of micro- and macrovascular complications in people with type 1 diabetes, and when should they be implemented in the course of the disease?

• What is the mechanism of the adverse impact of renal disease on cardiovascular disease (CVD) in individuals with type 1 and type 2 diabetes?

• Can reliable biomarkers of disease, including the long-term microvascular and cardiovascular complications, be identified to make clinical trials more efficient and guide therapy?

Future Directions:

➤ Define optimal treatment to reduce CVD risk in people with type 1 diabetes.

➤ Assess the rate of development of atherosclerosis in people with type 1 diabetes and investigate which interventions will have the most salutary effects and when they should be applied.

➤ Examine the role of coagulation abnormalities as risk factors for CVD in type 1 and type 2 diabetes patients.

➤ Assess how neuropathy contributes to unique CVD risk in people with diabetes.

➤ Examine the role of nephropathy in contributing to CVD in people with diabetes.

➤ Develop surrogate end points and biomarkers that can be used in studying interventions to decrease vascular complications in diabetes.

➤ Study the effect of glycemia and insulin resistance on cognitive function.

SPECIAL NEEDS FOR SPECIAL POPULATIONS

Pregnancy and the Intrauterine Environment
Key Questions:

- What are the immediate- and long-term health outcomes for offspring of women treated for diabetes or placed on weight maintenance or weight loss regimens during pregnancy?

- What noninvasive fetal measurements can be used to quantify diabetic "fetopathy" *in utero*? How can such measurement(s) be applied clinically to identify pregnancies in need of intensified maternal glucose control?

- Which anti-diabetic treatments work to mitigate perinatal and/or long-term complications in such pregnancies?

- By what mechanisms does the intrauterine environment increase the risk of the offspring developing obesity and diabetes?

- What biomarkers can be used to monitor women who have had gestational diabetes to determine if their glucose homeostasis is deteriorating, even before glucose levels become impaired? What interventions can actually stop progression to diabetes?

Future Directions:

- Identify the safest and most effective approaches to achieve optimal glycemic control during pregnancy.

- Determine the effects that different interventions for diabetes and/or obesity in mothers have on the long-term health outcomes for offspring.

- Develop new approaches to antepartum monitoring and management of gestational diabetes.

- Develop effective clinical approaches to prevent birth defects in diabetic pregnancies.

- Investigate the progression to type 2 diabetes and its mitigation in women with prior gestational diabetes.

Diabetes in Children and Youth
Key Questions:

- What is the role of overweight and obesity in the development of diabetes—including hybrid diabetes—in children and youth? Are there racial and ethnic differences?

- How does the development of overweight/obesity in children or youth affect diabetes management and outcomes, and contribute to patterns of disordered eating?

- Do children with hybrid diabetes have the same genetic, environmental, and cultural risk factors as those with type 1 diabetes?

- How can children and youth be more successfully transitioned to adult management of diabetes? What are the most effective and affordable ways for parents, caregivers, and individuals with diabetes to become motivated and competent to manage diabetes?

- How can children and youth with diabetes obtain optimal support for their diabetes care from environments outside the home (*e.g.*, day care, schools, colleges, community organizations)?

- What complications and risk factors for complications are present in youth with diabetes?

- Can diabetic ketoacidosis (DKA) rates be significantly reduced in the United States, at presentation and over the course of childhood diabetes?

- How can the interactions between the four main modifiable parameters influencing glucose control (insulin administration, diet, physical activity, and stress) be better understood? What types of interventions would be successful and cost effective at achieving optimal glycemic control and improving quality of life?

- Can pre-diabetes be identified (by a cost effective strategy) and the development of type 2 diabetes in children and adolescents be delayed or prevented?

Future Directions:

➤ Determine whether the increase in type 1 diabetes in younger children is due to increases in obesity/overweight.

➤ Characterize the role of obesity in contributing to inflammation and insulin resistance in all forms of childhood diabetes.

➤ Develop effective weight loss strategies, in the context of the growing and developing child, for children with all forms of diabetes who are overweight.

➤ Develop cost effective methods for assessing and tracking diabetes complications and risk factors for complications in children and youth with diabetes.

➤ Study behavioral methods to improve treatment adherence in the context of a chronic disease, including a better understanding of the way treatment approaches need to evolve with the maturation of the child.

➤ Determine risk factors for the development of DKA and establish approaches to reduce rates of DKA in the United States.

Diabetes in Older Adults

Key Questions:

- What are the optimal strategies for motivating older people to improve and sustain lifestyle changes that can help prevent or control diabetes?

- What are the appropriate (optimal) glycemic, blood pressure, and cholesterol targets across the spectrum of health for older adults to help prevent diabetes complications (and maintain quality of life)?

- If it is not feasible to reach targets for all three risk factors (glycemia, blood pressure, and cholesterol) due to therapeutic complexity, polypharmacy, costs, and/or competing medical conditions, how should risk factor control be prioritized to limit morbidity and mortality in older adults?

- How does diabetes and its treatment affect other health issues faced during aging, such as falling, osteoporosis, incontinence, polypharmacy, and declines in functional status?

- For the frail, older adult with diabetes and limited life expectancy, what are the most important treatment priorities if the goal is to maintain quality of life and decrease the risk of the geriatric syndromes?

Future Directions:

➤ Determine how to activate older adults with or at risk for diabetes to improve and sustain lifestyle modification.

➤ Determine the optimal strategy to manage hyperglycemia and minimize cardiovascular risk in older adults with diabetes.

➤ Study differential drug clearance in older adults, as well as across the lifespan and across different races and ethnicities.

DIABETES COMPLICATIONS

Metabolic, Biochemical, and Signaling Pathways

Key Questions:

- How do the identified molecular pathways associated with diabetes interact within the cell and does this vary for different cell types?

- Are there undiscovered molecular pathways that contribute to diabetes complications?

- What protective pathways are present and how do they interact with other pathways? Do complications arise from an imbalance of maladaptive to adaptive responses?

- What are the relative contributions of hyperglycemia versus impaired insulin and other growth factor signaling in the development of diabetes complications?

- What is the effect of large dynamic changes in the levels of glucose and other metabolites in comparison to sustained elevations?

- Why do cells exposed to the same systemic factors have different pathologies? Why does the apparently global pathogenic mechanism of increased mitochondrial activity have variable consequences in different cell types?

- What is the clinical significance of the identified biochemical changes in the cell induced by diabetes?

Future Directions:

- ➤ Develop better tools to assess mitochondrial function, transport, number, fission/fusion states, transcription factors, and DNA.

- ➤ Improve mitochondrial function in tissues in which mitochondrial dysfunction contributes to complications.

- ➤ Develop a better understanding of the immunologic pathways common to type 1 and type 2 diabetes and diabetes complications.

- ➤ Develop better tools to study glycation and lipoxidation of proteins.

- ➤ Determine if modulators of autophagy affect diabetes complications.

- ➤ Develop tools and approaches that produce a more global understanding of the cellular effects of diabetes and a more specific understanding of the effects of diabetes on individuals.

Genetics and Epigenetics

Key Questions:

- What are the genes that predispose or protect people from developing end-stage renal disease, diabetic retinopathy, neuropathy, and other diabetes-associated complications?

- How do candidate genes identified by genome-wide studies contribute to the pathogenesis of diabetic complications?

- How do epigenetic mechanisms fit within the context of other known cellular mechanisms for diabetes complications?

- Are epigenetic changes in chromatin responsible for metabolic memory? How do they interact with other persistent effects of glucose control, such as glycation and oxidation of long-lived macromolecules?

- Is epigenetics the mechanism by which birth weight determines adult susceptibility to diabetes and coronary heart disease?

- What is the role of small regulatory RNA, in particular the microRNA, in the development of diabetes complications?

Future Directions:

➤ Identify the key genetic factors predisposing to or protecting from diabetic complications and define the population genetic architecture underlying this risk.

➤ Test the role of genes identified from genome-wide association studies (GWAS).

➤ Incorporate new genomic and epigenomic technologies to evaluate diabetic complications.

➤ Characterize epigenetic changes or patterns of changes that can be used in population studies to probe the questions of metabolic memory.

➤ Investigate the changes in microRNA profiles associated with diabetes complications and the downstream effects of identified microRNA.

Tissue and Organ System Injury

Key Questions:

• How does systemic inflammation from dysregulation of the innate and adaptive immune systems affect specific tissues, such as the periodontium, bone and endothelium?

• What are the mechanisms of injury in specialized cells, such as podocytes, pericytes, Müller cells and interstitial cells of Cajal?

• What distinguishes cardiovascular, kidney, and urologic disease associated with diabetes from non-diabetes related forms of these diseases? Does diabetes accelerate the same pathologic processes or have unique components?

• What mechanisms are responsible for the increased mortality in people with diabetes and end-stage renal failure?

• Is there a point in the progression of diabetes complications when the pathologic process becomes relatively independent of the diabetes-related factors that initiate it? Is there a point when the progression becomes irreversible?

• What are the pathological and molecular correlates of autonomic neuropathy? What are the biologic mechanisms involved in the bi-directional associations of depression and diabetes and Alzheimer's disease and diabetes?

• To what extent does the pain associated with diabetes reflect peripheral tissue injury versus altered central nervous system (CNS) processing and perception of pain?

Future Directions:

➤ Develop *in vitro* models to study vascular complications.

➤ Establish bio-repositories of human cells and tissues.

➤ Determine the mediators of dyslipidemia-induced renal and neuronal injury.

➤ Pursue cross-disciplinary research to understand the basic science for neurovascular disease related to diabetes.

➤ Understand the mechanisms by which diabetes affects the enteric nervous system and related elements in the gastrointestinal system.

➤ Explore the "temporal theory" of urinary incontinence and diabetic uropathy.

➤ Incorporate measures of depression, cognitive impairment, brain vascular lesions, and Alzheimer's disease in longitudinal studies of diabetes complications.

Tissue Repair and Regeneration

Key Questions:

- Can the complications of diabetes be reversed by stimulating formation of normal new vessels and re-growth of nerves? Is this possible despite continued hyperglycemia?

- How do the various pathways leading to abnormal vascular proliferation, loss, and permeability contribute to complications in different tissues?

- Can restoration of the regulation and oxygen sensing of hypoxia inducible factor (HIF)-1 alpha rescue the diabetic impairments in neovasacularization?

- How do dysfunctional repair mechanisms contribute to poor recovery from maternal injuries of childbirth and the resultant increased risk of stress incontinence and female pelvic floor disorders?

- How are specific populations of stem/progenitor cells affected by diabetes? Are these abnormalities reversible through optimal diabetes treatment or therapies targeted to stem/progenitor cells?

- Will new cell reprogramming techniques, such as induced pluripotent stem (iPS) cells, lead to individualized cell therapy?

Future Directions:

- ➤ Elucidate the mechanisms underlying the poor revascularization response to ischemia in diabetes.

- ➤ Characterize the impairments in stem and progenitor cell populations.

- ➤ Develop cell-based therapies.

Biomarkers, Imaging, and Bioinformatics

Key Questions:

- Can early diabetes-induced changes in tissues and organs be detected by noninvasive imaging?

- Will computational models that incorporate several biomarkers and imaging results create a composite analysis that is a better measure of disease progression than the individual components?

- What are the indicators that predict an irreversible step in the progression of diabetes complications such as the identification of a vulnerable atherosclerotic plaque that is likely to rupture?

- Why do agents that prevent the onset of diabetes complications in rodent models not prevent complications progression in humans? Are intermediate models such as swine or nonhuman primates key steps in paths to translation?

- How can the large amount of data generated by genomic, epigenomic, and high-throughput screening experiments be synthesized into new, testable hypotheses on diabetes complications?

Future Directions:

- ➤ Develop biomarkers for diabetes complications.

- ➤ Leverage technological advances in noninvasive imaging.

- ➤ Improve animal and cell models.

- ➤ Transform high-throughput screening to elucidate the complexity of diabetes complications.

- ➤ Apply systems biology and bioinformatics tools to the analysis of data generated on human samples and experimental models.

Therapeutic and Preventive Strategies

Key Questions:

- Do treatments that prevent the development of complications also prevent the progression of complications?

- What is the impact of diabetes duration and pre-existing tissue damage on the ability to respond to therapies?

- What behavioral interventions improve diabetes self-management and prevent complications?

- Will combination therapies be more effective than single therapies? Can mechanisms for testing combination therapies be developed?

- What are approaches that will lead to individualizing therapies? For example, which diabetic individuals will benefit from a therapy that uncouples oxidant and carbonyl stress from hyperglycemia?

- How can therapies be targeted to specific tissues?

Future Directions:

- ➤ Personalize drug development and treatment.

- ➤ Improve behavioral approaches to treating co-morbid depression and diabetes.

- ➤ Identify novel therapeutic targets and develop more effective approaches for the prevention and treatment of diabetic complications.

- ➤ Target therapies to specific compartments.

- ➤ Establish a mechanism for early evaluation of therapeutic agents parallel to the pharmaceutical industry.

CLINICAL RESEARCH TO PRACTICE: TRANSLATIONAL RESEARCH

Diabetes Clinical Care

Key Questions:

- What are the best approaches to optimize cardiometabolic risk reduction in diverse populations with pre-diabetes or type 2 diabetes?

- How can diabetes management and outcomes be improved in older persons with diabetes who often have serious comorbidities?

- How can diabetes management processes be improved to alleviate the burden of disease in younger people with diabetes?

- What is the most appropriate sequence, rate of intensification, and tailoring of therapeutic goals to individual patient characteristics to optimize health outcomes and safety?

Future Directions:

- ➤ Develop individualized care approaches to optimize outcomes.

- ➤ Identify methods to improve the quality of life and outcomes of older persons with diabetes.

- ➤ Identify strategies for attaining optimal health outcomes in youth with type 1 diabetes.

- ➤ Determine systems of care that optimize processes and improve outcomes for people with diabetes.

- ➤ Find ways to make clinical trials more generalizable to diverse populations in different settings.

Patient-Centered Care

Key Questions:

- What self-management approaches support clinical care and ensure better outcomes for those whose diabetes is accompanied by multiple comorbidities?

- Which factors unique to the individual with diabetes, intervention, health care system, and context outside of the health care setting contribute to the success of self-management approaches?

- How can people with diabetes become more effectively engaged in the self-management of their disease in concert with their health care provider's efforts?

- How can evidence-based self-management interventions, using cognitive behavioral approaches, be incorporated into clinical and community-based care?

Future Directions:

- ➢ Identify a concise, practical set of behavioral and psychosocial factors, including both process and outcome measures, that can be collected and used on a routine basis to inform patient-centered care.

- ➢ Understand the long-term effects of diabetes interventions with regard to sustained behavioral change (patient and/or provider) and diabetes health outcomes.

- ➢ Understand how to increase diabetes self-management.

Systems of Care

Key Questions:

- How can multi-level interventions, combining policy/marketing, community, organization, delivery system, provider, and patient/family components, be implemented and sustained to improve diabetes care and outcomes?

- What are the key principles for adapting evidence-based interventions to real world settings in ways that make them locally relevant, preserve their effectiveness, and expand their reach to a higher proportion of people with diabetes?

- How do novel mechanisms for payment of health care services impact the process and outcomes of diabetes care?

- How can interventions to control diabetes be cost effective for society and financially feasible from the perspective of individual payers and health care organizations?

- What practical measures of the quality/processes of diabetes care bear the strongest relationship with better downstream outcomes? Can reporting of such measures and novel methods of payment improve these outcomes?

- Can decision support tools or other health information technologies be used to facilitate breakthroughs in clinical performance related to diabetes care and quality improvement?

Future Directions:

- ➢ Understand how changes in the structure of health care delivery systems can lead to improvements in diabetes care and prevention.

- Develop strategies to implement and sustain organizational efforts to improve diabetes care and outcomes.

- Integrate multi-level interventions (combined policy/marketing, organization, provider, patient/family, community) synergistically to enhance the likelihood of success and sustainability.

- Identify optimal settings for delivery of diabetes interventions.

- Evaluate "natural experiments" that occur when policy or care changes are instituted in health care settings that impact large numbers of people with diabetes.

- Develop new approaches to study the impact of system- and policy-level interventions on diabetes control and prevention.

- Identify promising strategies, such as pay-for-performance and public reporting of performance measures, to bridge the persistent gap in quality of diabetes care and outcomes.

- Identify new uses of health information technology to improve diabetes care.

RESOURCE AND INFRASTRUCTURE NEEDS FOR DIABETES RESEARCH

Research Training and Human Resource Development

Key Questions:

- How can training and career development in all aspects of diabetes research be enhanced?

- What programs can be developed to train multidisciplinary researchers capable of examining interactions among biological, psychological, behavioral, social, and environmental factors that impact diabetes and obesity?

- How can biomedical engineers, computational biologists, mathematicians, and experts in disciplines not traditionally applied to the problems of diabetes, obesity, and complications be encouraged to pursue research on these diseases?

- How can training of physician-scientists be supported in critical areas such as genetics/genomics and biostatistics, population-based methods, and interventional research?

- How can investigators from underrepresented minority groups be more effectively encouraged to pursue research careers that are focused on diabetes and obesity?

- What educational opportunities can be developed for clinical practitioners and for the general public to encourage participation in clinical research?

Future Directions:

- Incorporate transdisciplinary research opportunities into training programs related to diabetes and obesity.

- Create training programs that encourage the application of new fields of study to key problems in diabetes.

- Enhance training opportunities for basic and clinical investigators and establish opportunities for translational research in all aspects of diabetes and obesity research.

- Develop programs to educate the medical community and the general public on clinical research.

Diabetes Research Resources

Key Questions:

- How can access to high-quality human islets and pancreatic tissue for research be improved?

- What data registries or biobanks of human tissues and cell lines from people with and without diabetes would best support diabetes research?

- How can long-term studies of diabetes and its complications be optimized to provide research data and resources to the diabetes research community?

- How can transdisciplinary research and collaboration be encouraged, publicized, and supported across departments, institutions, and methodological fields?

Future Directions:

➤ Establish biobanks of annotated human tissue samples related to diabetes and obesity etiology and diabetic complications.

➤ Follow cohorts of individuals with type 1 diabetes and youth with type 2 diabetes longitudinally.

➤ Develop mechanisms to foster communication and collaboration among researchers and clinicians with an interest in diabetes and obesity.

➤ Promote interactions between NIH-supported Centers for diabetes and obesity research and other research institutions to maximize access to state-of-the-art resources and training.

New Technologies, Methodologies, and Measurements for Research

Key Questions:

- What DNA/RNA/protein sequencing and other technologies are needed to identify and study diabetes candidate genes and to better correlate genotypes with phenotypes in humans?

- How can mouse or cellular models be developed that are informative about the functional consequences of genetic differences associated with diabetes or obesity?

- How should evolving proteomic and metabolomic approaches be harnessed for diabetes research?

- What imaging technologies and resources are needed to advance research on diabetes, obesity, and related complications in humans?

- What bioinformatics resources and statistical approaches need to be developed or made more accessible to facilitate diabetes research?

- What tools are needed to measure energy balance in free-living humans?

- What new analytic methods or tools are needed to study complex, multi-level interactions within populations that impact obesity?

- Can standardized methods be developed for assessing predisposing behaviors and outcomes in human obesity trials?

- How well do self-reported and observational measurements correlate with biological markers?

- What are the best research designs to study causality in sociological systems?

- Can new instruments be developed to measure health promotion outcomes across communities and populations?

- How can more efficient communication be encouraged between people with diabetes and health care providers?

Future Directions:

➤ Develop and make available advanced technologies for discovering diabetes genes in humans.

- Develop analytical methods for epigenetic processes and other resources to study the relationships among genotypes and phenotypes in humans.

- Establish banks of monoclonal antibodies specific for diabetes-associated proteins.

- Create novel cell lines and related resources for diabetes and obesity research.

- Encourage new approaches to diabetes research and treatment based on stem cell technology.

- Make new technologies available as they arise, including stem cell resources.

- Apply proteomic and metabolomic methodologies to research on diabetes and obesity.

- Develop advanced, noninvasive imaging techniques that can be used in living humans.

- Develop statistical and bioinformatical methods and resources for integrating and analyzing large datasets generated by state-of-the-art technologies.

- Design innovative tools for studying energy balance under real-world conditions.

- Develop new methods for studying the impact of the environment on obesity.

- Improve and standardize measurements for translational research.

- Develop new methodologies for comparative effectiveness research.

- Develop advanced web-based and mobile technologies for capturing clinical data, enhancing education, and facilitating data management.

Animal Models for the Study of Diabetes and Obesity

Key Questions:

- What new small and large animal models are needed to accelerate research on type 1 and type 2 diabetes?

- Can animal models be developed that mimic human obesity etiology and treatment outcomes?

- Can animal models be developed that better simulate complications of human diabetes? Can new biomarkers be defined for complications in both animal models and humans?

- How can functional brain imaging techniques be improved for use in animal models?

- What new resources are needed to improve the phenotyping of animal models for diabetes and obesity?

Future Directions:

- Develop new small and large animal models that better represent the pathology and treatment of human diabetes and obesity.

- Develop *in silico* models of disease pathogenesis in type 1 and type 2 diabetes.

- Standardize research protocols involving diabetes-related mouse models.

- Develop standard definitions of abnormalities in mouse models of diabetes and obesity.

- Develop improved methods and technologies for phenotyping of mouse models.

Distribution and Sharing of Human Data and Biosamples

Key Questions:

- How can communication be fostered between basic scientists and clinical investigators conducting clinical studies and trials?

- How can awareness of and access to human biosamples and data from clinical trials be enhanced in order to facilitate biomarker discovery?

- How can awareness and use of new diabetes and obesity intervention programs and research tools be enhanced?

- What mechanisms or resources are needed to make datasets of de-identified medical records available to researchers?

- How can universal electronic medical records be made accessible for research while safeguarding patient and provider privacy?

Future Directions:

- ➤ Communicate the availability of datasets and biosample repositories and improve access to these resources by qualified diabetes researchers.

- ➤ Improve technology capabilities for dissemination of intervention programs.

- ➤ Develop policies that facilitate research using electronic medical records while protecting individuals' right to privacy.

Public-Private and International Partnerships

Key Questions:

- How can NIH collaborate with clinical care providers and payers to conduct clinical research in real-world settings and to conduct comparative effectiveness research more efficiently?

- How can policies for protecting the privacy of research participants be updated to foster multi-center clinical trials, associated biomarker studies, and the sharing of genetic materials between the public and private research sectors and internationally?

- What new NIH policies are needed to facilitate international collaborations?

- How can regulatory and financial issues be resolved in order to support the development of glucose management technologies, new therapeutics for microvascular complications, agents for glycemic control with adequate information on cardiovascular and other risks, and combination therapies for diabetes and obesity?

- How can NIH support and encourage partnerships between researchers and their local communities?

Future Directions:

- ➤ Build or strengthen partnerships between NIH and other government agencies, the pharmaceutical industry, the health insurance industry, and private foundations with an interest in diabetes and obesity research.

- ➤ Foster practice-based and community-based participatory research to promote the prevention and control of diabetes in vulnerable populations.

APPENDIX G

ACRONYMS AND ABBREVIATIONS

ORGANIZATIONS

ADA	American Diabetes Association	NHLBI	National Heart, Lung, and Blood Institute
CDC	Centers for Disease Control and Prevention	NIA	National Institute on Aging
CIHR	Canadian Institutes of Health Research	NIAID	National Institute of Allergy and Infectious Diseases
CMS	Centers for Medicare & Medicaid Services	NIAMS	National Institute of Arthritis and Musculoskeletal and Skin Diseases
DMICC	Diabetes Mellitus Interagency Coordinating Committee	NIBIB	National Institute of Biomedical Imaging and Bioengineering
EFSD	European Foundation for the Study of Diabetes	NICHD	*Eunice Kennedy Shriver* National Institute of Child Health and Human Development
EU	European Union	NIDCR	National Institute of Dental and Craniofacial Research
FDA	Food and Drug Administration	NIDDK	National Institute of Diabetes and Digestive and Kidney Diseases
HHS	Department of Health and Human Services	NIEHS	National Institute of Environmental Health Sciences
HRSA	Health Resources and Services Administration	NIH	National Institutes of Health
IDS	Immunology of Diabetes Society	NIMH	National Institute of Mental Health
IFCC	International Federation of Clinical Chemistry and Laboratory Medicine	NIMHD	National Institute on Minority Health and Health Disparities
IHS	Indian Health Service	NINDS	National Institute of Neurological Disorders and Stroke
JDRF	Juvenile Diabetes Research Foundation International	NINR	National Institute of Nursing Research
NCCAM	National Center for Complementary and Alternative Medicine	NLM	National Library of Medicine
NCI	National Cancer Institute	ORWH	NIH Office of Research on Women's Health
NCRR	National Center for Research Resources	UNOS	United Network for Organ Sharing
NDF	Netherlands Diabetes Foundation	USPTO	U.S. Patent and Trademark Office
NEI	National Eye Institute	VHA	Veterans Health Administration
NHGRI	National Human Genome Research Institute		

Research Programs and URLs

AMDCC
: Animal Models of Diabetic Complications Consortium
www.amdcc.org

BCBC
: Beta Cell Biology Consortium
www.betacell.org

CIT Consortium
: Clinical Islet Transplantation Consortium
www.citisletstudy.org

CITR
: Clinical Islet Transplant Registry
www.citregistry.org/

DASP
: Diabetes Autoantibody Standardization Program

dbGAP
: Database of Genotypes and Phenotypes
www.ncbi.nlm.nih.gov/sites/entrez?db=gap

DCCT
: Diabetes Control and Complications Trial
http://www2.bsc.gwu.edu/bsc/oneproj.php?pkey=5

DirecNet
: Diabetes Research in Children Network
http://public.direc.net

DPT-1
: Diabetes Prevention Trial-Type 1

DRCR.net
: Diabetic Retinopathy Clinical Research Network
www.drcr.net

EDIC
: Epidemiology of Diabetes Interventions and Complications
http://www2.bsc.gwu.edu/bsc/oneproj.php?pkey=10

FIND
: Family Investigation of Nephropathy and Diabetes

GoKinD
: Genetics of Kidneys in Diabetes Study
www.jdrf.org/gokind

ICR
: Islet Cell Resource Centers
http://icr.coh.org

IIDP
: Integrated Islet Distribution Program
http://iidp.coh.org

ITN
: Immune Tolerance Network
www.immunetolerance.org

MMPC	Mouse Metabolic Phenotyping Centers www.mmpc.org
MMRRC	Mutant Mouse Regional Resource Centers www.mmrrc.org
NDEP	National Diabetes Education Program http://ndep.nih.gov
NGSP	National Glycohemoglobin Standardization Program www.ngsp.org
NHPCSG	Non-Human Primate Transplantation Tolerance Cooperative Study Group
NIDDK Central Repositories	www.niddkrepository.org
Prevention Centers	Cooperative Study Group for Autoimmune Disease Prevention www.niaid.nih.gov/about/organization/dait/Pages/CSGADP.aspx
SEARCH	SEARCH for Diabetes in Youth www.searchfordiabetes.org
T1DGC	Type 1 Diabetes Genetics Consortium www.t1dgc.org
T1DR	Type 1 Diabetes Mouse Resource http://type1diabetes.jax.org
T1D-RAID	Type 1 Diabetes–Rapid Access to Intervention Development www.t1diabetes.nih.gov/T1D-RAID/index.shtml
T1D-PTP	Type 1 Diabetes Preclinical Testing Program www.t1diabetes.nih.gov/T1D-PTP/
TEDDY	The Environmental Determinants of Diabetes in the Young www.teddystudy.org
TODAY	Treatment Options for Type 2 Diabetes in Adolescents and Youth http://todaystudy.org/index.cgi
TrialNet	Type 1 Diabetes TrialNet www.diabetestrialnet.org
TRIGR	Trial to Reduce IDDM in the Genetically At-Risk www.trigr.org

Other Acronyms and Abbreviations

AAT	alpha-1 antitrypsin
ABCC	Administrative and Bioinformatics Coordinating Center
ACE	angiotensin-converting enzyme
CBP	Collaborative Bridging Project
CGM	continuous glucose monitors
CL	cytotoxic lymphocyte
CNS	central nervous system
CVD	cardiovascular disease
DA	diabetes autoantibodies
DKA	diabetic ketoacidosis
DNA	deoxyribonucleic acid
DNPA	Diabetes National Plan for Action
DRWG	Diabetes Research Working Group
DSMB	Data and Safety Monitoring Board
DSMC	Data and Safety Monitoring Committee
EAB	External Advisory Board
EC	Executive Committee
EEC	External Evaluation Committee
eNOS	endothelial nitric-oxide synthase
EPC	endothelial progenitor cell
ES cell	embryonic stem cell
ESEC	External Scientific Evaluation Committee
ESRD	end-stage renal disease
e-SPA	electronic Scientific Portfolio Assessment
FY	fiscal year
GAD	glutamic acid decarboxylase
GLP	glucagon-like protein
GMP	good manufacturing practice
GST	Glucagon Stimulation Test
GWAS	genome-wide association study
HbA1c	Hemoglobin A1c
HIF-1 alpha	hypoxia-inducible factor-1 alpha
HIPAA	Health Insurance Portability and Accountability Act
HLA	human leukocyte antigen
ICU	intensive care unit
IDDM	insulin-dependent diabetes mellitus
IL-2	interleukin-2

IMPAC II	Information for Management, Planning, Analysis, and Coordination
IMT	intimal-medial thickness
iPS cell	induced pluripotent stem cell
IRB	institutional review board
LIPS	Luminescent Immunoprecipitation System
MHC	major histocompatibility complex
miRNA	microRNA
MMTT	Mixed Meal Tolerance Test
MRI	magnetic resonance imaging
NDEP	National Diabetes Education Program
NHS	Natural History Study
NHP	non-human primate
NIP	Nutritional Intervention to Prevent Type 1 Diabetes Study
NOD	non-obese diabetic
NSC	Network Steering Committee
P&F	pilot and feasibility
PA	program announcement
PDA	personal digital assistant
PDR	proliferative diabetic retinopathy
PET	positron emission tomography
PI	Principal Investigator
PL	Public Law
RePORTER	NIH Research Portfolio Online Reporting Tools Expenditures and Results
RFA	Request for Applications
RFP	Request for Proposals
RNA	ribonucleic acid
SAC	Scientific Advisory Committee
SBIR	Small Business Innovation Research
SC	Steering Committee
SCRBCB	Seeding Collaborative Research in Beta Cell Biology
siRNA	small interfering RNA
STTR	Small Business Technology Transfer
T1D	type 1 diabetes
UPR	unfolded protein response
VEGF	vascular endothelial growth factor
VMAT2	vesicular monoamine transporter 2
ZNT8	zinc transporter 8

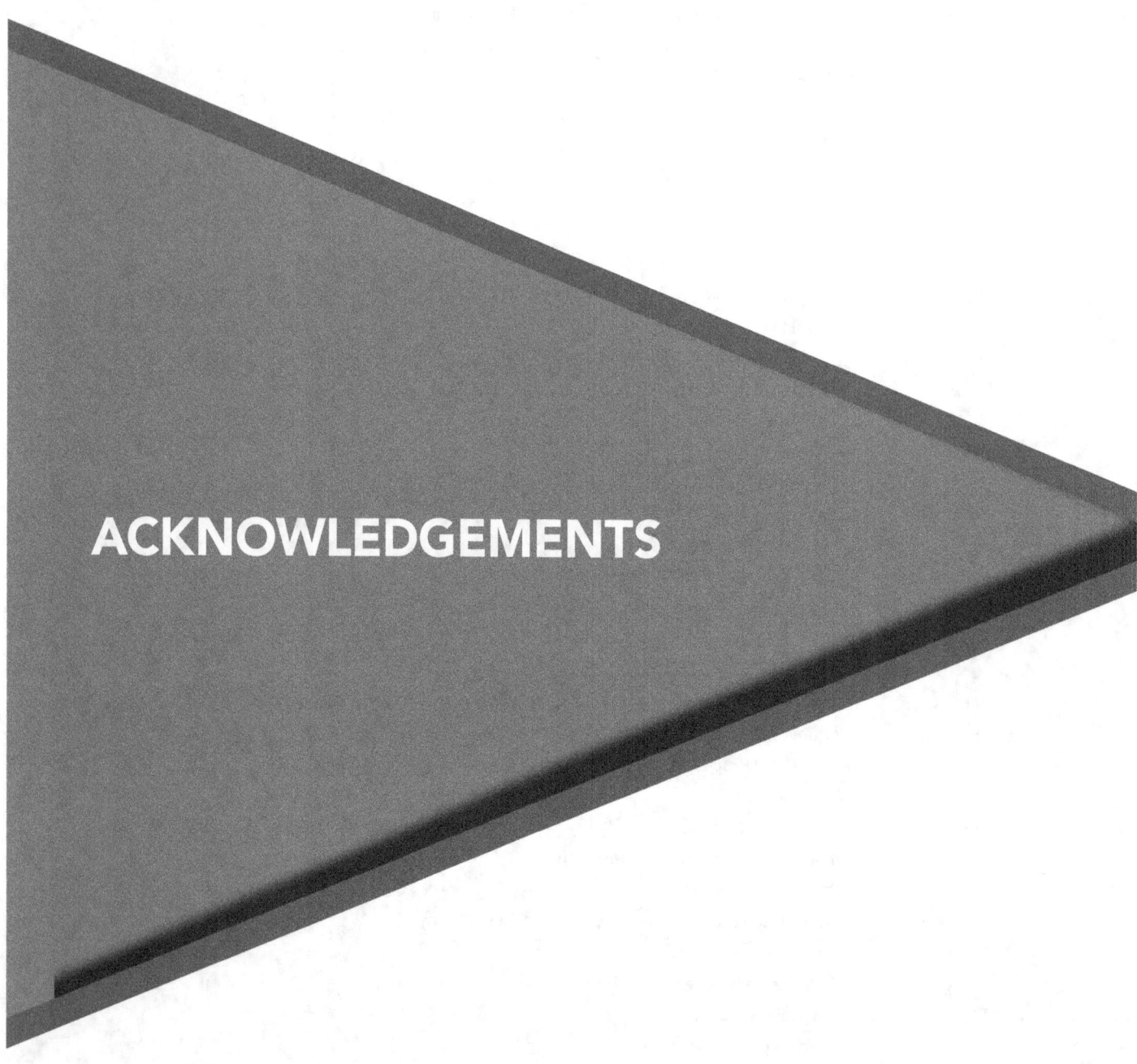

ACKNOWLEDGEMENTS

Acknowledgements

This listing provides names of individuals who contributed to the development, planning, management, implementation, and/or evaluation of the *Special Statutory Funding Program for Type 1 Diabetes Research* since 2006. For a list of prior contributors, please see the "Acknowledgments" section of the 2007 "*Evaluation Report*" on the *Special Statutory Funding Program for Type 1 Diabetes Research* (www.T1Diabetes.nih.gov/evaluation).

Principal Extramural Contributors

Note: In addition to *ad hoc* planning and evaluation meeting participants listed here, many extramural scientists who participated in scientific conferences and workshops contributed to the program planning efforts.

Emmanuel Baetge, PhD[a]
ViaCyte

Elizabeth Barrett-Connor, MD[b]
University of California San Diego

Joseph E. Craft, MD[a]
Yale University School of Medicine

Terry L. Delovitch, PhD[a]
University of Western Ontario

Mark A. Espeland, PhD[b]
Wake Forest University School of Medicine

Paul Fernyhough, PhD[a]
University of Manitoba

Saul M. Genuth, MD[b]
Case Western Reserve University

Ronald G. Gill, PhD[a]
University of Colorado

John B. Harley, MD, PhD[b]
Oklahoma Medical Research Foundation

Peter S. Heeger, MD[b]
Mt. Sinai School of Medicine

Irl B. Hirsch, MD[b]
University of Washington

Diane Mathis, PhD[a]
Harvard University/Joslin Diabetes Institute

Marcia J. McDuffie, MD[a]
University of Virginia

Stephen D. Miller, PhD[a]
Northwestern University Medical School

David M. Nathan, MD[b]
Harvard University/Massachusetts General Hospital

James Neaton, PhD[b]
University of Minnesota

Trevor J. Orchard, MBBCh., MMedSci., FAHA[b]
University of Pittsburgh

Margery Perry[a]
Former Member, NIDDK Advisory Council

Jeffrey L. Platt, MD[a]
University of Michigan

Jane E. Salmon, MD[b]
Hospital for Special Surgery

Ignacio Sanz, MD[b]
University of Rochester Medical Center

Ann Marie Schmidt, MD[a]
New York University Langone Medical Center

Steven E. Shoelson, MD, PhD[a]
Harvard University/Joslin Diabetes Center

Stanislaw Stepkowski, DVM, PhD, DSc[a]
The University of Toledo Medical College

Manikkam Suthanthiran, MD[b]
Weill Cornell Medical College

Megan Sykes, MD[b]
Columbia University

Linda S. Wicker, PhD[a]
University of Cambridge

[a] *Participated in the June 2009 ad hoc planning and evaluation meeting on pre-clinical research.*
[b] *Participated in the April 2008 ad hoc planning and evaluation meeting on clinical research.*

CONTRIBUTORS FROM FEDERAL AGENCIES[39]

Members of the Diabetes Mellitus Interagency Coordinating Committee (DMICC)

The *Special Statutory Funding Program for Type 1 Diabetes Research* is coordinated by the DMICC, which is a statutory Committee that facilitates cooperation, communication, and collaboration on diabetes activities among numerous government components (www.diabetescommittee.gov). This listing provides names of DMICC members as of September 2010.

Chair:
Judith E. Fradkin, MD
National Institute of Diabetes and Digestive and Kidney Diseases

Executive Secretary:
Sanford A. Garfield, PhD
National Institute of Diabetes and Digestive and Kidney Diseases

Members:
Kelly Acton, MD, MPH
Indian Health Service

Ann Albright, PhD, RD
Centers for Disease Control and Prevention

Jane C. Atkinson, DDS
National Institute of Dental and Craniofacial Research

Larissa Avilés-Santa, MD, MPH, FACP, FACE
National Heart, Lung and Blood Institute

---

[39] This listing provides the institutional affiliations of contributors at the time of participation in the evaluation process.

Barbara Bartman, MD, MPH
Agency for Healthcare Research and Quality

Mark Chavez, PhD
National Institute of Mental Health

Irene Dankwa-Mullan, MD, MPH
National Center on Minority Health and Health Disparities

Linda C. Duffy, PhD
National Center for Complementary and
Alternative Medicine

Chhanda Dutta, PhD
National Institute on Aging

Mark Eberhardt, PhD
Centers for Disease Control and Prevention

Zhigang (Peter) Gao, MD
National Institute on Alcohol Abuse and Alcoholism

Garth Graham, MD, MPH
U.S. Department of Health and Human Services

Gilman D. Grave, MD
Eunice Kennedy Shriver National Institute of
Child Health and Human Development

Rachel Hayes, MPH, RD
U.S. Department of Health and Human Services

Jerrold Heindel, PhD
National Institute of Environmental Health Sciences

Jag H. Khalsa, PhD
National Institute on Drug Abuse

Donna Krasnewich, MD, PhD
National Institute of General Medical Sciences

John P. Kugler, MD, MPH
U.S. Department of Defense

Rongling Li, MD, PhD, MPH
National Human Genome Research Institute

Alan McLaughlin, PhD
National Institute of Biomedical Imaging and
Bioengineering

Mary Parks, MD
U.S. Food and Drug Administration

Audrey S. Penn, MD
National Institute of Neurological Disorders and Stroke

John Peyman, PhD
National Institute of Allergy and Infectious Diseases

Leonard M. Pogach, MD, MBA
Veterans Health Administration

Robert C. Post, PhD, MEd, MSc
U.S. Department of Agriculture

Sheila H. Roman, MD, MPH
Centers for Medicare and Medicaid Services

Daniel Rosenblum, MD
National Center for Research Resources

Grace L. Shen, PhD
National Eye Institute

Elliot R. Siegel, PhD
National Library of Medicine

Joan Wasserman, Dr.PH, RN
National Institute of Nursing Research

Baldwin Wong
National Institute on Deafness and
Other Communication Disorders

Samuel Wu, PharmD
Health Resources and Services Administration

Other Federal Contributors

Kristin Abraham, PhD
National Institute of Diabetes and
Digestive and Kidney Diseases

Beena Akolkar, PhD
National Institute of Diabetes and
Digestive and Kidney Diseases

Michael Appel, PhD
National Institute of Diabetes and
Digestive and Kidney Diseases

Guillermo Arreaza-Rubin, MD
National Institute of Diabetes and
Digestive and Kidney Diseases

Olivier Blondel, PhD
National Institute of Diabetes and
Digestive and Kidney Diseases

Aesha Brandy
National Institute of Diabetes and
Digestive and Kidney Diseases

Nancy Bridges, MD
National Institute of Allergy and Infectious Diseases

Catherine Cowie, PhD
National Institute of Diabetes and
Digestive and Kidney Diseases

Thomas Eggerman, MD, PhD
National Institute of Diabetes and
Digestive and Kidney Diseases

Richard Farishian, PhD
National Institute of Diabetes and
Digestive and Kidney Diseases

Gregory Germino, MD
National Institute of Diabetes and
Digestive and Kidney Diseases

Shefa Gordon, PhD
National Eye Institute

Michael Grey, PhD
National Institute of Diabetes and
Digestive and Kidney Diseases

Carol Haft, PhD
National Institute of Diabetes and
Digestive and Kidney Diseases

Mary Hanlon, PhD
National Institute of Diabetes and
Digestive and Kidney Diseases

Mary Horlick, MD
National Institute of Diabetes and
Digestive and Kidney Diseases

Christine Hunter, PhD
National Institute of Diabetes and
Digestive and Kidney Diseases

James Hyde, PhD
National Institute of Diabetes and
Digestive and Kidney Diseases

Giuseppina Imperatore, MD, PhD
Centers for Disease Control and Prevention

Teresa Jones, MD
National Institute of Diabetes and
Digestive and Kidney Diseases

Christian Ketchum, PhD
National Institute of Diabetes and
Digestive and Kidney Diseases

Thomas Klausing
National Institute of Diabetes and
Digestive and Kidney Diseases

Maren Laughlin, PhD
National Institute of Diabetes and
Digestive and Kidney Diseases

Ellen Leschek, MD
National Institute of Diabetes and
Digestive and Kidney Diseases

Barbara Linder, MD
National Institute of Diabetes and
Digestive and Kidney Diseases

Karl Malik, PhD
National Institute of Diabetes and
Digestive and Kidney Diseases

Saul Malozowski, MD, PhD, MBA
National Institute of Diabetes and
Digestive and Kidney Diseases

Merrill Mitler, PhD
National Institute of Neurological Disorders and Stroke

Patricia Mueller, PhD
Centers for Disease Control and Prevention

Beth Paterson
National Institute of Diabetes and
Digestive and Kidney Diseases

Rebekah Rasooly, PhD
National Institute of Diabetes and
Digestive and Kidney Diseases

B. Tibor Roberts, PhD
National Institute of Diabetes and
Digestive and Kidney Diseases

Griffin Rodgers, MD, MACP
National Institute of Diabetes and
Digestive and Kidney Diseases

Daniel Rotrosen, MD
National Institute of Allergy and Infectious Diseases

Karen Salomon
National Institute of Diabetes and
Digestive and Kidney Diseases

Sheryl Sato, PhD
National Institute of Diabetes and
Digestive and Kidney Diseases

Peter Savage, MD
National Institute of Diabetes and
Digestive and Kidney Diseases

Eleanor Schron, PhD
National Eye Institute

Salvatore Sechi, PhD
National Institute of Diabetes and
Digestive and Kidney Diseases

Philip Smith, PhD
National Institute of Diabetes and
Digestive and Kidney Diseases

Lisa Spain, PhD
National Institute of Diabetes and
Digestive and Kidney Diseases

Robert Star, MD
National Institute of Diabetes and
Digestive and Kidney Diseases

Myrlene Staten, MD
National Institute of Diabetes and
Digestive and Kidney Diseases

Julie Wallace, PhD
National Institute of Diabetes and
Digestive and Kidney Diseases

Karen Winer, MD
Eunice Kennedy Shriver National Institute of
Child Health and Human Development

Kevin Wright, MPA
National Institute of Allergy and Infectious Diseases

Hubert Vesper, PhD
Centers for Disease Control and Prevention

Charles Zellers
National Institute of Diabetes and
Digestive and Kidney Diseases

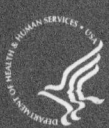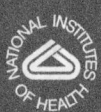NIDDK | NATIONAL INSTITUTE OF DIABETES AND DIGESTIVE AND KIDNEY DISEASES

NIH Publication No. 10-7535
January 2011

www.ingramcontent.com/pod-product-compliance
Lightning Source LLC
Chambersburg PA
CBHW080406290526
45791CB00008BA/2172